NEONATAL SURGERY
A NURSING PERSPECTIVE

NEONATAL SURGERY
A NURSING PERSPECTIVE

Edited by

Carole Kenner, R.N.C., M.S.N.
Assistant Professor, Pediatrics
University of Cincinnati College of Nursing
  and Health
Cincinnati, Ohio

Jeanne Harjo, R.N.
Team Leader Surgical Section, Newborn
  Intensive Care Unit
Children's Hospital Medical Center
Cincinnati, Ohio

Ann Brueggemeyer, R.N., M.B.A., B.S.N.
Instructor, Pediatrics
Good Samaritan Hospital School of Nursing
Cincinnati, Ohio

Grune & Stratton, Inc.
Harcourt Brace Jovanovich, Publishers
Orlando   New York   San Diego   London
San Francisco   Tokyo   Sydney   Toronto

Library of Congress Cataloging-in-Publication Data

Neonatal surgery: a nursing perspective / edited by Carole Kenner,
Jeanne Harjo, Anne Brueggemeyer.
  p. cm.
  Includes index.
  ISBN 0-8089-1893-1
    1. Infants (Newborn)—Surgery.   2. Pediatric nursing.   I. Kenner,
  Carole.   II. Harjo, Jeanne.   III. Brueggemeyer, Ann.
    [DNLM: 1. Critical Care—in infancy & childhood.   2. Neonatology-
  -nurses' instruction.   3. Surgical Nursing—in infancy & childhood.
  WY 161 N438]
  RD137.5.N48 1988
  617'. 98—dc19   87-31410
                                                 CIP

Grune & Stratton, Inc.
Orlando, Florida 32887

Distributed in the United Kingdom by
Grune & Stratton, Ltd.
24/28 Oval Road, London NW 1

Library of Congress Catalog Number   87-31410
International Standard Book Number   0-8089-1893-1
Printed in the United States of America
87   88   89   90   10   9   8   7   6   5   4   3   2   1

CONTENTS

PREFACE

Many authorities have developed guidelines for neonatal patient care but virtually none exist for neonatal nursing care. This book hopes to fill the gap between neonatal medical care and nursing care. Although regional variations in neonatal care occur, the authors have contacted resources across the country to provide the reader with a broad range of practices currently used. This book will offer protocols to help the nurse recognize the newborn with medical and surgical problems, to prevent complications, and to care for these babies and their families. It will help the nurses proceed confidently in the nursing care of the critically ill neonate.

Neonatal nurses often find it difficult to cross the line from neonatal nursing to neonatal surgical nursing. A fear exists among nurses of how to care for the newborn requiring surgery. The principles of neonatalogy remain relevant but a new list of problems is encountered with the "surgery baby". Today, surgery babies are often found in the Newborn Intensive Care Unit along with the premature baby. They are cared for by then same nurses caring for the "premies". This book would be a readily available resource to augment current nursing care. The ready access format facilitates problem solving for the busy N.I.C.U. nurse.

This book would also be used as a ready resource for those who are not involved with the care of the critically ill neonate on a regular basis. This reference would provide them with background information, immediate nursing needs, potential problems to assess for, and parent and family needs.

ACKNOWLEDGEMENTS

We would like to thank the following people for their assistance in the preparation of this book: Lester and Betty Kenner, Edward and Elizabeth Brueggemeyer, and Jim Harjo, without whose support we could not have accomplished this task.

We would also like to thank Dr. Julia George for reviewing the manuscript. Appreciation is extended to Becky Katz, Karen Pattison, Dr. Frances Strodtbeck, and Linda Lefrack who assisted in identifying regional care differences. Special thanks must go to Mr. Thomas Eoyang for editorial assistance and perseverance for seeing this project to its completion.

While many people assisted with the ideas in this text, the authors accept responsiblity for the material presented.

CONTRIBUTORS

Ann Brueggemeyer, R.N., M.B.A., B.S.N.
Instructor, Pediatrics
Good Samaritan Hospital School of Nursing
Cincinnati, Ohio

Pat Gorgone, R.N., B.S.N.
Nutritional Support Team
Children's Hospital Medical Center
Cincinnati, Ohio

Laurie Porter Gunderson, R.N., M.S.N.
Doctoral Student, The Ohio State University
Columbus, Ohio

Jeanne Harjo, R.N.
Team Leader Surgical Section, Newborn intensive Care Unit
Children's Hospital Medical Center
Cincinnati, Ohio

Carole Kenner, R.N.C., M.S.N.
Assistant Professor, Pediatrics
University of Cincinnati College of Nursing and Health
Cincinnati, Ohio

Susan Bondi Schilling, R.N., B.S.N.
Nutritional Support Team
Children's Hospital Medical Center

Chapter 1

Introduction

Carole Kenner   *Jeanne Harjo*
                        Ann Brueggemeyer

Surgical neonatal nursing begins in the delivery room. It is here that nurses first encounter the newborn with a real or potential neonatal problem. Delivery room nurses make the initial assessment of the cardiopulmonary status of the infant by thorough observation and assignment of Apgar scores. It is their role to ease the transition of the infant from intrauterine to extrauterine life and identify many gross anomalies as well as subtle clues—such as skin tags, polydactylia, sluggish response time—that may be suggestive of congenital or chromosomal defects. Nurses must be aware of intrapartal difficulties that may put the infant at risk. These nurses also play a vital role in parent-child interaction and must be honest with the parents if there is a problem and keep them informed of what is being done to the infant. Delivery room nurses provide critical care to the depressed infant in the form of resuscitation or active neonatal support; the wealth of information they can provide to the nursery nurse is often overlooked.

Nurseries are divided into Levels 1, 2, and 3. As the development of regional referral centers (Level 3) attached to university or teaching hospitals has grown, so has the complexity of perinatal health care. If a problem such as meningomyelocele or hydrocephalus is identified in utero by ultrasound or a maternal illness is suggestive of a high-risk delivery, it is conceivable that the mother may be transported, usually prior to the onset of labor, to a regional referral center with a delivery room and Level 3 nursery. The mother and infant can then remain in the same hospital.

If the infant's condition is believed to be uncomplicated or labor has progressed to a point that it is unsafe to move the mother, the birth may take place where a Level 1 or 2 nursery is present. In a Level 1 nursery the facility is primarily geared towards uncomplicated births. Neonates with problems can be supported until a transfer to a center for high-risk neonates can be arranged. Nurses in these

Neonatal Surgery: A Nursing Perspective
ISBN 0-8089-1893-1

1

facilities must develop good assessment and observational skills to identify the poor feeder, the shrill crier, or the baby who just does not act right. Nurses who spend 24 hours each day with the infant are often able to pinpoint problems that need a physician's attention.

Level 2 nurseries can support newborns with greater complications. These nurseries have 24-hour laboratory and x-ray facilities and can support small infants in isolettes or provide oxygen with a head hood. These nurseries can monitor the cardiopulmonary status, but they are not as equipped as an intensive care unit. Nurses in this environment must always be alert to the newborn and be prepared to deal with an emergency code. Knowledge of risk factors is essential if nurses are to care effectively for the potentially ill neonate.

Delivery room, Level-1 and Level-2 nursery nurses have responsibilities in their pivotal position. They must work as a team with obstetricians, pediatricians, neonatologists, respiratory therapists, lab technicians, and transport teams from regional referral centers. They are the keepers of the information—they know if a baby has not passed meconium, is having projectile vomiting, or looks dusky during the feeding—and can provide vital information to physicians and Level 3 nurseries. These nurses are the liaison between their facility, the parents, and the regional center.

Neonatal nursing has come a long way since the 1960s when it began; however, the need to share knowledge remains. Unfortunately, regionalization has at times left a chasm between the small, rural facility and the technologically elite hospital; but this must not continue.

This book is designed to bridge the gap between the delivery room; Levels-1, -2, and -3 nursery personnel; and the parents. Its format provides a quick reference to—not an in depth discussion of—each topic. It serves as a guide to assist perinatal and neonatal nurses in identifying more quickly and more accurately the neonate with surgical problems.

BIBLIOGRAPHY

Stephenson, K. (1983). Neonatal and maternal transport, in K. Vestal & C. A. McKenzie (Eds.) *High risk perinatal nursing.* (pp 22-61). Philadelphia: W. B. Saunders.

Vestal, K. (1983). Regionalization of high risk perinatal care, in K. Vestal & C. A. Mckenzie (Eds.) *High risk perinatal nursing.* (pp 22-61). Philadelphia: W. B. Saunders.

Chapter 2

Assessment of the Critically Ill Neonate

Carole Kenner   *Ann Brueggemeyer*

The assessment of the critically ill neonate is the first step in the care of surgically delivered newborns. It begins with a good understanding of the maternal, paternal, and neonatal risk factors that clues a nurse in on a potential problem. Next comes the physical and gestational exams that help to identify any actual problems and anticipate future problems too. An assessment of the physical status of the infant must also be performed. The physical exam must be thorough and include a head-to-toe assessment and the cardiopulmonary status. Thermoregulation must be a consideration during any examination of the newborn: it is critical to the well-being of the neonate. The gestational exam gives an estimate of the maturity of the newborn in contrast to the age calculated according to the mother's last menstrual cycle. This exam can point out discrepancies and determine whether the newborn is small, large, or average for gestational age; premature; or postmature. Again, this information can be essential for the anticipation, treatment, and possibly even prevention of neonatal difficulties.

Identification of Maternal, Paternal, and Neonatal Risk Factors
Carole Kenner

DESCRIPTION

Assessment of the critically ill or potentially ill neonate must include a detailed maternal, paternal, and neonatal history. Many maternal and paternal factors put the newborn in danger of abnormal fetal development, congenital or chromosomal abnormalities, or postnatal problems. Knowledge of familial and neonatal risk factors allows the nurse to identify high-risk infants and their potential problems more quickly and accurately.

A high-risk infant may be defined as one in danger of developing a neonatal problem because of maternal, paternal, fetal, or neonatal history or one born with a known congenital or newborn condition requiring acute medical care.

ETIOLOGY

Maternal and Reproductive Risk Factors

1. Aged > 35 or < 19 years
2. Weight < 100 pounds or 20 percent over ideal body weight
3. Height < 5 feet
4. Smoker
5. Alcohol consumption
6. Drug usage
7. Exposure to hazardous environmental conditions, such as toxic gases or chemicals, radiation
8. Chronic illness
   a. Heart disease
   b. Anemia
   c. Diabetes (mellitus or insipidus)
   d. Hypertension
   e. Thyroid disease
   f. Psychiatric or emotional illness
   g. Any other long-standing illness
9. Hereditary disease
   a. Sickle cell anemia
   b. Any other inherited disorder
10. Exposure to infection during pregnancy
    a. Toxoplasmosis
    b. Cytomegalovirus
    c. Rubella
    d. Chickenpox
    e. Any other infection contracted or exposed to during pregnancy
11. Positive family history of a genetic disorder
    a. Cystic fibrosis
    b. Down's syndrome
    c. Any other genetic disorder
12. Blood type (may lead to Rh- or ABO-incompatibility problems)
13. Unplanned pregnancy
14. Lack of social support systems (i.e., no spouse, close friends, or extended family)
15. Closely spaced pregnancies: 3 months or less between pregnancies
16. Financial status: unemployed or low income
17. No prenatal care
18. Grand multipariety: over seven pregnancies
19. Previous fetal or neonatal death
20. Previous children with neonatal illness
    a. Respiratory distress
    b. Jaundice
    c. Prematurity
    d. Congenital anomaly
    e. Congenital syndrome
21. Previous cesarean section
22. Infertility
23. Previous multiple births
24. Problems during pregnancy
    a. Bleeding: early (first trimester)
    b. Placenta previa
    c. Abruptio placentae
    d. Toxemia
    e. Pregnancy-induced hypertension
    f. Hydramnios
    g. Inappropriate fetal growth for gestational age
    h. Premature rupture of membranes

Intrapartal Risk Factors

1. Precipitous delivery
2. Prolonged labor
3. Abnormal fetal presentation:
   a. Breech
   b. Footling
   c. Shoulder
   d. Brow or face
4. Prolapsed umbilical cord
5. Intrapartal drugs
6. Multiple birth

Paternal Risk Factors

1. Aged > 40 or < 19 years
2. Blood type (may lead to Rh- or ABO-incompatibility problems)
3. Positive family history of genetic disorder or chronic illness
4. Street drug usage (e.g., cocaine, heroin, marijuana)
5. Alcohol consumption
6. Exposure to hazardous environmental conditions, such as toxic gases or chemicals, radiation

Neonatal Risk Factors

1. History of fetal depression (e.g., bradycardia, acidosis)
2. Multiple birth
3. Low Apgar scores (Charts 2-A and 2-B)
4. Respiratory depression
5. Cardiac depression
6. Small (< 10th percentile) or large (> 90th percentile) for gestational age
7. Bleeding
8. Meconium staining of the newborn or amniotic fluid
9. Foul-smelling amniotic fluid
10. Abnormal appearance or weight of placenta
11. Abnormal number of umbilical vessels
12. Prematurity (< 37 weeks)
13. Postmaturity (≥ 42 weeks)
14. Hydrocephalus or microcephalus
15. Infant of a diabetic mother
16. Obvious congenital anomaly

Reproductive maternal, paternal, and neonatal risk factors can readily be gathered by use of a checklist system (Charts 2-C and 2-D). This checklist system will save time while still achieving a complete history.

Physical and Gestational Exams
Carole Kenner

DESCRIPTION

The performance of thorough physical and gestational exams allows the nurse to assess accurately the current status of the neonate. These exams are essential if potential and actual problems are to be identified rapidly.

Chart 2-A
APGAR Scoring System

Physical Parameters	APGAR Scores		
	0	1	2
Pulse	0	1-99	≥ 100
Respiratory effort	None	Weak cry, slow rate, irregular rhythm	Strong cry, regular rhythm
Muscle tone	Flaccid	Weak flexion of extremities	Strong flexion
Reflex irritability	None	Some response	Strong, active response to stimuli
Color	Pale and/or cyanotic	Cyanotic limited to extremities	Pink without visible cyanosis

Chart 2-B
Implications of Apgar Scores

Score	Implication	Action
0-3	Severe depression	Resuscitation; usually full
4-6	Intermediate depression	Partial resuscitation
7-10	Responding well to transition	Assist or support newborn's own effort

Chart 2-C
Maternal and Reproductive History Assessment Sheet

Place a check mark or fill in the information in the appropriate column.

	YES	NO

1. Age _____

2. Height _____

3. Weight (prepregnant/pregnant) _____

4. Number of previous pregnancies _____

5. Date of last pregnancy outcome _____

For questions 6-11, check whether you have ever had any of the following:

6. Multiple births   _____   _____

7. Abortions   _____   _____

8. Miscarriages   _____   _____

9. Stillbirths   _____   _____

10. Neonatal deaths   _____   _____

11. Previous children with neonatal or genetic problems   _____   _____

If you answered yes to any of the previous questions, please explain in detail.

_____

_____

_____

_____

12. Infertility   _____   _____

If so, what kind of treatment did you receive? _____

_____

13. Gynecological surgery   _____   _____

If so, what kind? _____

14. Blood type _____

	YES	NO

15. Prenatal testing _____ _____

 If so, what kind? _____

16. Diabetes, gestational or other _____ _____

 If so, what kind of treatment do you receive? _____

17. Any chronic illness? _____ _____

 If so, what illnesses? _____

18. Anemia? _____ _____

 If so, during pregnancy only? _____ _____

 Any treatment for the anemia? _____ _____

19. Any exposure to communicable or infectious
 diseases during pregnancy? _____ _____

 If so, what diseases? _____

20. Surgery _____ _____

 If so, what kind(s)? _____

21. Positive family history of chronic/hereditary/
 life-threatening diseases? _____ _____

22. Any medications or drugs currently being used? _____ _____

 If so, what drugs? _____

23. Do you smoke? _____ _____

 If so, how much? _____

24. Do you consume any alcohol? _____ _____

 If so, how much? _____

	YES	NO

25. Any emotional or psychiatric illnesses? _____ _____

    If so, what illnesses? _____

26. Race and cultural background _____

27. Educational level _____

28. Occupation _____

29. Marital status _____

30. Support systems (e.g., spouse, close friends, extended family) _____

    _____

31. Financial status _____

32. Type of living accommodations _____

33. During this pregnancy did you have prenatal care? _____ _____

    Complications? _____ _____

    If so, what kind? _____

Bleeding? _____ _____

    If bleeding, when? _____

Cesarean section? _____ _____

Premature rupture of membranes? _____ _____

Labor (either premature, precipitous, or prolonged)? _____ _____

Fetal presentation? _____ _____

Drugs administered during labor and delivery? _____ _____

    If so, what kind? _____

34. Estimated date of confinement? _____ _____

Chart 2-D
Paternal History Assessment Sheet

Place a check mark or fill in the information in the appropriate column.

	YES	NO

1. Age _____

2. Positive family history of chronic/hereditary/or
   life-threatening disease?   _____   _____

   If so what diseases? _____

3. Blood type _____

4. Any emotional or psychiatric illnesses?   _____   _____

   If so what illnesses? _____

5. Any genetic or chronic illnesses?   _____   _____

   If so what illnesses? _____

6. Do you take any medications?   _____   _____

   If so what medications? _____

7. Have you ever taken any street drugs?   _____   _____

   If so what drugs? _____

8. Do you consume any alcohol?   _____   _____

   If so how often, how much, and what type of alcohol? _____

9. Have you ever had any environmental exposures to
   toxic chemicals?   _____   _____

   If so what toxic chemicals? _____

10. Race and cultural background _____

11. Educational level _____

12. Occupation _____

13. Marital status _____

14. Support systems _____

15. Financial status _____

16. Type of living accommodations _____

The neonatal history information is included in the sections describing physical and gestational exams.
For the implications of the Apgar scoring system please see Chart 2-B.

Physical Exam

The physical exam should begin with observation, followed by the least invasive procedures first. The baby will be much easier to assess in this sequence. Remember to keep the baby warm, preferably under a warming device such as a radiant warmer.

If the infant is not under a radiant warmer or in an isolette, the inspection, auscultation, palpation, and percussion must be done systematically: during the head-to-toe examination, uncovering one portion of the body at a time will generally guard against cold stress. If the baby is in a warmed environment, however, to gain the cooperation of the infant, as much inspection from head to toe should be done before touching the infant. This inspection gives much information rapidly. Then auscultation, palpation, and percussion can be performed. Physical assessment from head to toe should be accomplished first with the exception of any invasive procedures. It may be necessary to do palpal and intrusive procedures such as otoscopic, ophthalmic, and oral exams last. The gestational exam should be conducted concurrently with the physical exam to decrease the chance of cold stress and conserve the neonate's energy. The exam should take place as soon as possible after delivery and the baby's contact with the parents. Examining the newborn when most alert should increase the accuracy of the results.

Gestational Exam

The gestational exam may be conducted using any of the available scales such as the Dubowitz or Ballard scale. This exam indicates the maturity of the infant in comparison to the infant's age by maternal dates (the estimated date of delivery based on the maternal menstrual cycle). Discrepancies in the latter may indicate that the infant is small or large for the gestational age. Also, the nurse can identify the premature infant (36 weeks or less), full-term infant (37-41 or 42 weeks), and the postmature infant (42 weeks or greater). The gestational exam should be performed along with the initial assessment. This strategy conserves the newborn's energy, an important consideration for the infant making the transition from intrauterine to extrauterine life. The initial assessment should take no more than 10 minutes but is critical for identifying potential problems. If difficulties or abnormalities can be identified or potential problems anticipated at this first examination, precious treatment time can be gained.

Neurologic Exam

A neurologic exam may not be accurate during the first 24 hours of life, as the baby is still adjusting to extrauterine life, and this system is the least well developed in the neonate. Further, a complete neurologic exam may not be warranted if there is no indication of other physical problems or no known risk factors. Do only as much of the exam as is absolutely necessary in the critically ill infant—be guided by the infant's response to the exam: if stressed or too irritable, stop the assessment and give the infant a rest.

EQUIPMENT FOR EXAMS

1. Infant stethoscope
2. Infant indirect oscillometric BP measuring devices, doppler for BP with premie or newborn disposable blood pressure cuff
3. Thermometer
4. Radiant warmer, isolette, or warming device
5. Tape measure for head and chest circumference, and length of body
6. Infant scale (in grams)
7. Penlight or flashlight
8. Light source above infant for examination
9. Formula nipple or pacifier
10. Extra diapers
11. Alcohol-soaked sponges
12. Sterile tongue depressors or blades
13. Ophthalmoscope
14. Otoscope with ear piece for newborn
15. Gestational scoring sheet

The following table lists the systems of the neonate, the parts of the physical exam (inspection, auscultation, percussion, and palpation) along with the normal and abnormal manifestations of each system, and the significance of the indices. These normal and abnormal manifestations are not a complete list of all the possibilities but give the examiner guidelines for identifying what the problem might be. See the Bibliography at the end of this chapter for more details about the results of physical and gestational exams.

PHYSICAL EXAMINATION

System	Normal	Significance	Abnormal	Significance
Color: Good indicator of overall status of infant, especially cardiopulmonary system				
Inspection	Pink; in dark-skinned infants, mucous membranes should be pink	No cardiopulmonary compromise	Duskiness or cyanosis (other than acrocyanosis)	Poor circulation or respiratory difficulty or distress
	Acrocyanosis of hands and feet during first 24 hours of life	Sluggish peripheral circulation caused by transition to the cool extrauterine life	Acrocyanosis lasting longer than first 24 hours	Poor peripheral circulation, may have cardiac compromise

System	Normal	Significance	Abnormal	Significance
	Reddish hue (especially noted immediately after birth)	Adjustment in oxygen levels in extrauterine environment	Plethora	Elevated hematocrit or hemaglobin levels, polycythemia levels, or hyperviscosity of blood
			Pale	Cardiopulmonary compromise or failure
	Ecchymosis over presenting part (to differentiate between cyanosis and ecchymosis, apply pressure to darkened area; cyanotic area will blanch while ecchymotic area remains dark)	Pressure over presenting part, causing bruising and trapping of blood in external tissue layers		
	Mongolian spots over buttocks, may extend to sacral region (usually in dark-skinned infants)	Hyperpigmentation		
	Jaundice after first 48 hours of age, receding by days 4-5 (peak will occur later in premie, may be after day 4)	Physiologic jaundice: transition of blood supply to liver, increased RBC count with decreased lifesepan of cells, decreased plasma protein level, and decreased glucuronyl transferase that aids in bilirubin conjugation	Jaundice on day 1 or after day 4	Isoimmunity such as Rh or ABO incompatibility, polycythemia, enzyme deficiencies, excessive bruising or bleeding, Hirschsprung's disease, pyloric stenosis, other intestinal obstructions that increase blood supply or shunt blood to the liver; maternal diabetes, small for gestational age

System	Normal	Significance	Abnormal	Significance
General appearance: indicative of nutritional status, infant maturity, and general well-being				
Inspection	Well-formed and rounded, with presence of subcutaneous tissue; no obvious anomalies	Good nutritional status; generally healthy	Little or no subcutaneous tissue, wasting muscle, loose skin, thin extremities, anomalies	Malnourished or with a variety of congenital defects, such as cleft lip and/or palate, omphalocele, gastroschisis, meningomyelocele; infant stressed in utero
	Vernix	Increases with gestational age		
	Lanugo	Decreases with gestational age		
Posture				
Inspection	Fetal position: fists clenched, arms adducted, flexed, hip abducted, knees flexed (extension of extremities may be normal in premie but abnormal at full term, as extension of legs and then flexion occurs, as development progresses); flexions move upward to arms; spinal column straight	Full term	Opisthotonos, (neck in extension)	Brain damage, birth asphyxia; neurological abnormality
			"Frog position" of legs	Prematurity
			Bulge or curvature of the spinal column	Spina bifida or meningomyelocele
	Spontaneous, symmetrical movement, may be slightly tremulous (flexion and extension should be equal bilaterally)	Full-term newborn activity	No movement; or asymmetrical, irregular, tremulous (jerky motions, unequal movement)	Birth asphyxia; neurological dysfunction; prematurity; drug-induced birth injury

System	Normal	Significance	Abnormal	Significance
Muscle strength and tone				
	Strength and tone strong	May be full term	Strength and tone weak, hypotonia, or flaccid	Birth asphyxia or prematurity
	Palmar grasp strong	Good overall strength; may be full term	Palmar grasp weak	Prematurity
Alertness and cry				
Inspection	Mood ranges from quiet to alert; consolable when upset	Normal newborn activity	Not easily aroused, not very alert	Prematurity; stressed; septic; states of wakefulness from neurologic problem
	Cry: strong	Strong; no increased intracranial pressure	Weak, high-pitched, or absent cry	Brain damage or increased intracranial pressure
			Raspy	Upper airway problem
			Expiratory grunt	Respiratory distress
			Unilateral drooping of mouth when crying	Nerve damage
Cardiopulmonary				
Inspection	Respiratory effort: easy, unlabored rhythm; may be irregular, but periods of apnea > 15 seconds are abnormal; abdominal breathing	No respiratory distress or difficulty	Dyspnea: Accessory muscle retractions, (substernal, supracostal, intercostal, supraclavicular); flared nostrils, stridor, or grunting	Respiratory distress or difficulty

System	Normal	Significance	Abnormal	Significance
	Respiratory rate: 40-60 breaths per minute	Normal rate	Apnea lasting longer than 15 seconds and accompanied by duskiness, cyanosis, or respiratory rate > 60 breaths per minute	Prematurity; respiratory difficulty; sepsis; tachypnea in cesarean section or in full-term infants may be transient (from retention of lung fluid)
	Symmetrical excursion of thorax	Normal respiratory pattern	Asymmetry or unequal chest excursion	Diaphragmatic hernia; pneumothorax; phrenic nerve damage
	AP diameter normal	Normal respiratory pattern	Exaggerated AP diameter: ratio greater than 1:1, barrel chest; hyperinflation equal without exaggeration	Respiratory distress
Auscultation	Clear breath sounds, equal bilaterally, anteriorly, and posteriorly; a few rales may be present the first few hours after birth because of residual fetal lung fluid: no color changes or cyanosis should accompany this finding	Clear lung fields	Rales after first day; rhonchi; expiratory grunting; wheezing	Lung congestion; respiratory distress; pulmonary edema; pneumonia
			Unequal breath sounds	Pneumothorax or diaphragmatic hernia

System	Normal	Significance	Abnormal	Significance
	Heart rate: 100-160 beats per minute; regular, without murmurs (initially may hear slight murmur until ductus arteriosus closes)	Normal cardiac rhythm without significant abnormalities	Bradycardia < 100 beats per minute or tachycardia > 160 beats per minute; murmur (usually heard at left sternal border or above apical pulse)	May be secondary to respiratory difficulty; increased workload of the heart; prematurity; sepsis; congenital heart defect with or without cyanosis
	No bruit in cranium or abdomen	No arteriovenous malformation	Bruit either in abdomen or cranium	Arteriovenous malformation
Palpation	Apical pulse at fourth or fifth intercostal space, midclavicular line, left anterior chest (point of maximum impulse at fourth intercostal space just right of midclavicular line, may be shifted to the right during the first few hours of life)	Normal position of cardiac pulse; no shifting without cardiomegaly	Displaced apical pulse	May have cardiac defect or cardiomegaly
	No thrill	No increased cardiac activity	Thrill after first few hours of life	Increased cardiac activity
	BP: average systolic rate (in beats per minute) 28-32 weeks, 52; 32-36 weeks, 56; full-term, 63; BP equal in all four extremities	Normal cardiac output; good circulation; possibly no cardiac defect	Decreased BP Unequal BP in the extremities, especially between the upper and lower extremities	Shock or hypovolemia Cardiac defect: coarctation of the aorta

System	Normal	Significance	Abnormal	Significance
Percussion	No increased tympany over lung fields	Normal lung field borders	Increased tympany over lung fields	Hyperinflation of the lungs
Skin				
Inspection	Moist, warm to touch, without peeling	Normal, well-hydrated	Dry, peeling, cracked	Postmature infant
			Wrinkled	Intrauterine growth retardation
			Gelatinous with visible veins (transparent skin and visible veins disappear with increasing gestational age)	Prematurity
	Vernix (thick, white cheesy material)	Increases with gestational age	No vernix	Prematurity
	Scant lanugo (fine hair over body)	Full term; decreases with gestational age	Abundant lanugo	Prematurity
	Milia	Blocked sebaceous glands (common in newborns)		
	Erythema toxicum	Newborn rash over body, usually on days 1-3	Nevus-flameus	Hyperpigmentation
			Meconium staining	Fetal distress
			Petechiae	Hematopoetic disorder
			Edematous, shiny, taut skin	Kidney dysfunction; cardiac failure; and/or renal failure

System	Normal	Significance	Abnormal	Significance
			Skin tags	Extra folds of skin, over-growth of tissue; some-times associated with congenital anomalies
	Mottling	May be normal reaction to immaturity	Mottling	May be ab-normal if associated with cold stress, color changes, bradycardia, or apnea
Palpation	Warm (axillary temperature 35.5°-36.5° C)		Cool (< 35.5° C)	Poor peri-pheral per-fusion; prematurity
			Warm (> 37° C)	Hyperthermia or fever
Head				
Inspection	Normocephalic in proportion to body (head circumference for average full-term newborn is 32-38 cm)		Microcephalic	Congenital syndromes or decreased brain growth
			Hydrocephalic	Blockage of the passage of CSF such as in meningomye-locele; or excessive production of CSF
			Anencephaly	Absent cerebral tissue and/ or scant or absent skull
			Encephalocele	Brain and spinal cord that have herniated

Carole Kenner and Ann Brueggemeyer

System	Normal	Significance	Abnormal	Significance
			Bradycephalic	Premature closure of coronal suture line; AP diameter shortened and lateral growth increased
			Craniosynostosis	Premature closure of suture lines
			Molding: cranial distortion lasting 5 to 7 days	Excessive pressure on cranium during vaginal delivery
			Overriding sutures	Excessive pressure on cranium during vaginal delivery
			Caput succedaneum	Edematous region of scalp extending over suture lines, resulting from pressure on presenting part during vaginal delivery
			Cephalhematoma	Trapping of blood in tissues not crossing the suture lines and lasting up to 8 weeks
			Forcep marks; edematous or reddened area	Forcep delivery

System	Normal	Significance	Abnormal	Significance
	Head lag: not greater then 10° in full term (pull newborn up supporting the arms, from supine to sitting position; grade degree of head lag by position of head in relationship to trunk—part of gestational exam)	Head lag: decreases with maturity	Head lag: greater than 10°; little or no support of head	Hypotonia or prematurity
	Hair distribution: over top of head, with single strands identifiable	Full term	Hair distribution: fine fuzzy, may be over entire head	Prematurity
Palpation	Without masses or soft areas over skull bones	Normal	Masses or soft areas such as craniotobes over parietal bones	May be normal variation if no other abnormality present
Auscultation	No bruit	Normal	Bruit	Cerebral arteriovenous malformation
Fontanelles				
Inspection and palpation	Anterior fontanelle (open until 12-18 months of age): diamond-shaped, 5 x 4 cm, along the coronal and sagittal sutures	Normal	Craniosynostosis	Premature closure of suture lines may result from brain-growth retardation
	Posterior fontanelle: triangle-shaped, very small, 1 x 1 cm along sagital and lambdoidal suture lines; or closed at birth	Normal	Bulging fontanelle, usually anterior fontanelle	Increased intracranial pressure
			Sunken fontanelle	Dehydration

System	Normal	Significance	Abnormal	Significance
Facies				
Inspection	Eyes on line with ears; nose midline	Normal	Low-set ears; asymmetry of features	Congenital syndromes such as Down's syndrome, or genetic defect
			Wide-eyed, worried	Postmature; small for gestational age; or intra-uterine growth retardation
			Hypertel-orism > 2.5 cm	Congenital syndrome; genetic disorders
			Hypotelorism < 2.5 cm	Trisomy 13
Oral Cavity				
Inspection (After inspec-tion, gently insert tongue depressor into infant's mouth; then with pen-light examine the oral cavity; this should be one of the last procedures done, as it is upsetting to infant)	Mouth: midline of face, symmetrical	Normal	Mouth: drooping or slanting unilaterally with crying; movement of mouth	Seventh cranial nerve damage; facial nerve damage
	Mouth: shape and size in proportion with face	Normal	Birdlike mouth: shortened ver-million border	Fetal alcohol syndrome
			Wide mouth (macro-stomia)	Metabolic disorder
			Small mouth (microstomia)	Down's syndrome
	Mucous membranes: moist, pink	Well-hydrated and oxygen-ated	Mucous membranes: dry, dusky	Dehydrated or poorly oxygenated
	Chin shape and size in proportion with face	Normal	Micrognathia	Pierre Robin syndrome

System	Normal	Significance	Abnormal	Significance
	Lips completely formed, pink, moist	Normal	Cleft lip	Congenital anomaly: failure of midline fusion during first trimester
	Palate: without arching; intact (determine by palpating	Normal	High-arched palate	Turner's syndrome
			Cleft palate	Failure of midline fusion during first trimester
	Tongue: size in proportion with mouth	Normal	Macroglossia	Hypothyroidism
			Microglossia	Congenital syndrome
	Tongue: midline	Normal; no neurologic dysfunction	Tongue: deviation from midline	Cranial nerve damage
	Uvula: midline rises with crying	Normal function of glossopharyngeal and vagus nerves	Uvula: not midline or does not rise with crying	Neurologic dysfunction
	Gag reflex: present (reflexes generally develop from head to toe during gestation)	Normal neurologic function of glossopharyngeal and vagus nerves	Gag reflex: absent	Neurologic dysfunction
	Sucking reflex present and strong when nipple or finger offered	Normal maturity and intact hypoglossal nerve	Sucking reflex absent	Prematurity or brain dysfunction
	Rooting reflex: present when cheek is stroked: infant turns towards stroking	Normal maturity and intact trigeminal nerve	Rooting reflex: absent	Prematurity or brain dysfunction

System	Normal	Significance	Abnormal	Significance
	Salivation without excess	Normal	Excessive salivation	Tracheo-esophageal fistula; esophageal atresia

Nose

System	Normal	Significance	Abnormal	Significance
Inspection	Position: midline	Normal	Position: off midline	Congenital malformation or syndrome
			Flattened nasal bridge	Congenital syndromes
			Beaked	Treacher Collins syndrome
			Enlarged or bulbous	Trisomy 13
	Nares: bilaterally present	Intact	Nares: not present bilaterally	Congenital malformation or syndrome
	Nares: patent (occlude neonate's nostrils one at a time while holding mouth closed; infant should be able to breathe through one side at a time; passing a catheter into newborn's nares, one at a time, also demonstates patency)	Normal	Nares: not patent	Nasal obstruction; choanal atresia
	Grimace or cry in response to strong odors passed under nose	Intact olfactory nerve	No response to strong odors passed under nose	Olfactory nerve damage

System	Normal	Significance	Abnormal	Significance
Auscultation	Nares: (with a stethoscope auscultate for breathing, one side at a time): breathing detected bilaterally	Patent	Nares: Breathing not detected bilaterally	Not patent; nasal obstruction

Eyes (indicate many systemic problems)

System	Normal	Significance	Abnormal	Significance
Inspection (if newborn's eyes are closed at this point in the exam, save inspection for later during ophthalmic exam; the remainder of the ophthalmic exam is included here, but, other than external inspection, this exam should be saved until last as it is upsetting to the infant)	Sclera clear	Normal	Sclera: Yellow Hemorrhages Blue	Jaundice Birth trauma Osteogenesis imperfecta
	Conjunctiva: clear	Normal	Conjunctiva: Hemorrhage Pink	Birth trauma Conjunctivitis, may be chemical, caused by silver nitrate
	Iris: colored evenly, bilaterally	Normal	Iris: Brushfield's spots (these gold flecks may be normal if not found with other anomalies)	Down's syndrome or congenital syndrome
			Coloboma (opening of pupil which extends into iris on one side)	May be associated with congenital malformation (internal)
	Pupils: equal bilaterally and reactive to light (exam done in darkened room with penlight or flashlight; if done with	Normal; intact oculomotor nerve	Pupils: unequal bilaterally; nonreactive	Brain damage or increased intracranial pressure

System	Normal	Significance	Abnormal	Significance
	newborn in isolette or in nursery, shield baby's eyes as much as possible)			
	Cornea: clear	Intact	Cornea: Hazy Milky	Prematurity Congenital cataracts possibly due to congenital rubella
	Retina: transparent	Intact	Retina: Areas of pigmentation Blood vessels without clear demarcation, or tortuous	Damaged retina Retinal hemorrhage
	Lacrimal duct: patent	Normal	Lacrimal duct: blocked or absent	Congenital obstruction
	Blink reflex: reactive (responds to bright light)	Intact optic nerve	Blink reflex: nonreactive	Facial-nerve paralysis or optic-nerve damage
	Red reflex: present	Lens intact	Red reflex: absent	Congenital cataracts
	Eye lids: without ptosis or edema	Normal; intact oculomotor nerve	Eye lids: Edema Ptosis	Birth trauma Oculomotor-nerve damage
			Epicanthal folds	Down's Syndrome or cri du chat syndrome
	Doll-eye response: present (with infant in supine position turn head from one side to the other side: eyes move to opposite side the head is turned	Normal; intact trochlear, abducens, and oculomotor nerves	Doll-eye response: absent	Damage to trochlear, abducens, and oculomotor nerves

System	Normal	Significance	Abnormal	Significance
	Eye position: without slant	Normal	Eye position: Slant upward Slant down-ward	Down's Syndrome Treacher Collins syndrome
			Sunset eyes (downward slope of pupils below lid)	Hydrocephalus
Ears				
Inspection	Position: ears in straight line with eyes; vertical angle that is greater than straight vertical line; without slant	Normal	Position: set below eyes; ears slant, internally or externally rotated	Down's syndrome
	Skin tags: absent	Normal	Skin tags: present	Congenital renal anomaly
	Cartilage formation: well-curved pinna, sturdy, stiff cartilage, instant recoil	Maturity	Cartilage formation: flattened or folded, slow recoil	Prematurity
	Neonate startles or cries in reaction to loud noise or snapping fingers	Hearing intact; auditory nerve intact	Startles or cries in reaction to loud noise or snapping fingers: absent or little response (further testing can be done with hearing tests done in the crib or other hearing tests)	Deaf or decreased hearing

System	Normal	Significance	Abnormal	Significance
	Otoscopic exam (this exam is often omitted since it is difficult to perform and may be potentially harmful if the examiner is not skilled; ear should be pulled down and back for exam): umbo (cone) of light present, pearl-gray tympanic membrane may have vernix; membrane is moveable without bulging	Normal intact ear without infection	Otoscopic exam: umbo of light: dull or absent; dull or immobile tympanic membrane, may be Red Blue Bulging	Congenital malformation or infection Infection Hemmorhage Infected otitis media
Neck				
Inspection	Shape symmetrical	Normal	Shape asymmetrical	Fetal position
	Head turns from side to side equally, full range of joint motion	Normal	Head lacks full range of joint motion or tilts to one side (torticollis)	Birth injury; muscle spasm resulting in contraction of neck muscles, thus tilting head
	Short without excessive skin	Normal	Short and webbed	Down's syndrome
	Tonic neck reflex: asymmetrical and present but decreases (place infant in supine position; turn head to one side with body restrained; extremities toward side that head is turned are extended, but other extremities are flexed: attemptby newborn to right head when turned to side in position tests Accessory nerve)	Normal	Tonic neck reflex: asymmetrical and strongly present Tonic neck reflex: symmetrical	Prematurity Neurologic dysfunction

System	Normal	Significance	Abnormal	Significance
Palpation:				
	Thyroid: midline	Normal	Thyroid: enlarged	Goiter (rare)
	Lymph nodes: not palpable	Normal	Lymph nodes: palpable	Congenital infection
	No masses	Normal	Mass in neck	Cystic hygroma
			Sternocleido-mastoid enlarged	Torticollis: birth or in-utero injury resulting in hematoma of sternomastoid muscle
	Carotid: pulse rate strong and regular (do not massage carotid artery or neck: can result in reflex bradycardia)	Normal cardiac and circulatory function	Carotid: pulse rate weak or irregular	Cardiac defect or circulatory problem
	Clavicles: even and without "lumps" along bones; symmetrical	No fractures	Clavicles: fracture or lump felt; uneven; asymmetrical	Birth injury
Abdomen and thorax				
Inspection	Chest cir-cumference 30-36 cm	Average for full-term neonate	Chest circum-ference < 30 cm	Prematurity; or small for gestational age
			Chest circum-ference > 36 cm large for gestational age	Barrel chest: respiratory difficulty for gestational age
	Equal excursion of diaphragm	Normal	Unequal excursion of diaphragm	Phrenic nerve damage

System	Normal	Significance	Abnormal	Significance
	Ribs: symmetrical	Normal	Ribs: asymmetrical	Birth injury or congenital syndrome
	Breast: Nipple spacing on line without extra nipples	Normal	Breast: Nipple spacing not on line, or extra nipples	
	Areola: raised and without discharge	Full-term infant	Areola: flat and/ or discharge	Prematurity or discharge from hormonal influence
			Hypertrophy	Maternal hormonal influence
	Abdomen: rounded, contoured, symmetrical	Normal	Abdomen: scaphoid	
			Distended (if suspected, measure the abdominal girth every 4 hours to detect change)	Intestinal obstruction, renal problem; ascites: edema caused by a variety of problems including congenital kidney or cardiac defects, prematurity, fetal hydrops)
			Distension in left upper quadrant	Pyloric stenosis or duodenal or jejunal obstruction
			Asymmetrical	Abdominal mass
	Umbilical cord:		Umbilical cord:	
	3 vessels (2 arteries, 1 vein)	Normal	2 vessels (1 artery, 1 vein)	Internal congenital anomalies possible
	Bluish-white	Normal	Meconium-stained	Distress in utero
			Reddened with discharge	Infection
			Thick cord	Large for gestational age
			Small cord	Small for gestational age or malnourished

System	Normal	Significance	Abnormal	Significance
			Mass Hernia of the cord through which abdominal viscera, intestines, and sometimes other organs enter	Hernia Omphalocele
			Hernia (lateral to the cord of abdominal contents)	Gastroschisis
	Abdominal musculature: strong	Normal	Abdominal musculature: weak	Prune-belly syndrome, may have associated renal problems including hypo-plastic kidneys
			Visible abdominal-wall defect over bladder area	Exstrophy of the bladder
	No visible peristaltic waves	Normal bowel activity	Visible peristaltic waves	Intestinal obstruction, usually not present immediately after birth
Auscultation	Bowel sounds: present	Normal	Bowel sounds: Absent	Obstruction
			Hyperactive (unless just after feeding)	Obstruction or hypermotility
	Abdomen: no bruit	Normal	Abdomen: bruit	Arteriovenous malformation
	Renal: no bruit	Normal	Renal: bruit	Renal-artery stenosis
Palpation:	Xiphoid process: present	Normal; intact	Xiphoid process absent or depressed	Fracture (sometimes due to resuscitation)

System	Normal	Significance	Abnormal	Significance
	Ribs: without masses or crepitous	Intact, without defects or "air leaks"	Ribs: masses or crepitous	Fractures, or mass; subcutaneous air due to air leaks from pulmonary dysfunction
	Breast tissue: 1 cm	Normal; full term	Breast tissue: < 1 cm, may be ≤ 5 mm	Prematurity
	Abdomen Soft and not tender	Normal	Abdomen Tense, rigid, tender	Intestinal deformity or obstruction
	Without masses	Normal	Masses	Renal or urinary tract deformity
			Separation of abdomino-rectus muscles (diastasis recti)	Common in newborns, especially premature
	Kidneys: 4-5 cm in length; right kidney lower than left, found in abdomen and posteriorly in lumbar or flank area (palpate with newborn's legs flexed in fetal position to relax infant)	Normal	Kidneys: Enlarged	Polycystic
			Absent	Potter's syndrome
	Liver: sharp edge just above right costal margin; firm	Normal size	Liver Below right costal margin Hard Liver damage or cardio-pulmonary problems	Respiratory distress or congestive heart failure
	Spleen: 1 cm below left costal margin	Normal spleen size	Spleen: absent or not palpable	Congenital heart defects

System	Normal	Significance	Abnormal	Significance
	Bladder: not distended (unless just prior to void)	Normal kidney and urinary tract system	Bladder: distended; may be visible above pubic bone	Urinary tract obstruction
	Groin: Femoral pulse rate strong and regular bilaterally	Normal	Groin: Femoral pulse rate weak or absent bilaterally	Coarctation of the aorta
	No hernias or groin masses	Normal	Bounding femoral pulses Groin masses	Patent ductus arteriosus Inguinal hernia
Percussion	Gastric bubble: just below the left costal margin and toward midline; tympanic	Normal	No tympany	Esophageal atresia or gastric de-formity
	Abdomen: tympanic except dull over liver, spleen, and bladder	Normal liver, spleen bladder, no masses (indi-cated by dullness)	Abdomen: Increased tympany Increased areas of dullness (if liver or spleen is en-larged, the dull-ness extends below the costal margins; if bladder is en-larged, dullness extends towards umbilicus: be sure to reexamine after void)	Increased presence of fluid or air Masses or enlarged abdominal organs, located where the dullness is increased

Genitourinary (GU) tract

Inspection, of female newborn	Labia majora: present and extend beyond labia minora	Full-term	Labia majora: smaller than labia minora	Prematurity

System	Normal	Significance	Abnormal	Significance
	Labia minora: present and well formed	Full-term	Labia minora: larger than labia majora	Prematurity
	Clitoris: present, may be enlarged	Full-term or prematurity		
	Urethral meatus: present in front of vaginal orifice	Normal	Urethral meatus: displaced	Urinary malformation
	Vagina: patent with or without white discharge	Normal	Vagina: not patent, with or without slight bleeding	Hormonal influence
	Genitalia: distinguishable as female or male	Normal	Genitalia: not clearly distinguishable as to sex, may have organs of both sexes	Ambiguous
	Perineum: smooth	Normal	Perineum: dimpling or extra opening	Urinary or genital malformation, or urinary fistula
	Anus: Midline, patent (test by inserting small finger)	Normal	Anus: Shifted anteriorly or posteriorly	Anal defect
			Nonpatent or dimpling	Imperforate anus
	Anal wink: present (lightly stroking of anal area produces constriction of sphincter)	Normal sphincter	Anal wink: absent	Poor muscle strength of sphincter
Inspection of male newborn	Penis: straight; proportionate to body (length 2.8-4.3 cm)	Normal	Penis: Curved Enlarged	Chordee Renal problem

System	Normal	Significance	Abnormal	Significance
	Urinary meatus: midline and at tip of glans (if neonate is uncircumcised, gently retract foreskin; if circumcised, also check for edema or bleeding)	Normal	Urinary meatus: displaced To ventral surface To dorsal surface	Hypospadias Epispadias
	Urinary stream: straight from penis (first void should occur no later than 24 hours postnatal)	Normal urinary pattern	Urinary stream: Not straight or from opening in abdomen or perineum Failure to void within first 24 hours of life	Urinary fistula Renal or urinary obstruction or malformation
	Testes and scrotum: Full, numerous rugae	Full term	Testes and scrotum: Flaccid, smooth or few rugae	Prematurity
	Darkly pigmented	Normal	Bluish testes or scrotal sac Enlarged or edematous Dimpling	Torsion of the testicles Hydrocele; Breech delivery Torsion of the testicles
	Perineum: smooth	Normal	Perineum: dimpling or extra opening	Urinary or genital malformation, or urinary fistula
	Anus: Midline, patent (test by inserting small finger)	Normal	Anus: Shifted anteriorly or posteriorly Nonpatent or dimpling	Anal defect Imperforate anus
	Anal wink: present (lightly stroking of anal area produces constriction of sphincter)	Normal sphincter	Anal wink: absent	Poor muscle strength or sphincter

System	Normal	Significance	Abnormal	Significance
Palpation of male newborn	Testes descended on at least one side	Full term	Testes not palpable (may be found high in the inguinal canal)	Prematurity or unde- scended

Upper extremities:

System	Normal	Significance	Abnormal	Significance
Inspection:	Length: in proportion to each other; lower extrem- ities and body symmetrical	Normal	Length: shortened extremities or asymmetrical	Diabetic mother; congenital syndrome; maternal drug use
	Full range of joint motion: (includes abduc- tion, adduction, internal and exter- nal rotation, flexion, and extension as applicable to resoec- tive joint; (full flexion of upper extremities comes with maturity)	Normal	Limited range of joint motion:	Birth injury or trauma
			Limited range of flexion	Prematurity
	Full range of joint motion of: Shoulder	Normal	Limited range of motion or flexion of shoulder	Dystocia; brachialplexus damage
	Clavicles	Normal	Clavicles	Clavicle injury; osteogenesis imperfecta
	Elbow	Normal	Elbow	Birth injury or fetal position
	Wrist (test for square window by flex- ing infant's wrist on forearm, then measure angle according to gestational exam chart, i.e., 0° angle for term)	Normal	Wrist	Birth injury or fetal position
			Square window: angle greater than 0°	Prematurity

System	Normal	Significance	Abnormal	Significance
	Hand	Normal	Hand	Hand injury or fetal position
	Grasp reflex: present, strong, and equal bilaterally	Maturity	Grasp reflex: weak or absent, or unequal bilaterally	Prematurity or birth injury
	Scarf sign: elbow short of midline (grasp infant's hand and gently pull hand around neck towards the opposite shoulder; observe position of elbow to chest; grade position according to gestational chart)	Maturity	Scarf sign: elbow beyond midline	Prematurity
	Arm recoil: (quick flex neonate's fore-arms for 5 seconds, next pull them to full extension, then release; recoil time is graded)	Maturity	Arm recoil: slow	Prematurity
	Palm: no simian creases	Normal	Palm: simian creases	Down's syndrome
	Fingers: 10 digits and without webbing; equal spacing	Normal	Fingers: More than 10 digits (polydactylia) Webbed, digital tags (syndactylia), or unequal spacing	May be part of syndrome Congenital syndrome
	Carpals and metacarpals: present and equal bilaterally	No fractures; bone formation normal	Carpals and metacarpals: absent or unequal bilaterally	Fractures or absence of bone, may be associated congenital syndromes

System	Normal	Significance	Abnormal	Significance
	Nails: extend beyond nailbeds	Normal; full term	Nails: Short spoon shaped	Congenital syndromes, fetal alcohol syndrome
			Absent	May have absent radius
			Meconium stained	Fetal distress
	Nailbeds: pink, brisk capillary refill (3 seconds), equal bilaterally	Normal peripheral perfusion, normal oxygenation	Nailbeds: dusky, or slow capillary refill (> 3 seconds), bilaterally	Poor peripheral perfusion or oxygenation
Palpation (Palpation in the presence of a fracture may produce crying or a facial grimace; observe infant's response)	Clavicles: without fractures or pain; symmetrical	Normal	Clavicles: asymmetrical or pain on palpation	Fractures, Shoulder dystocia, brachialplexus damage or palsy
	Humerus, radius and ulna present; symmetrical and without fractures	Normal bone formation	Humerus, radius, and ulna absent, or asymmetrical; Painful fractures	Absence of any of these bones may be associated syndromes Birth injury
	Pulses: brachial and radial strong and equal bilaterally and in comparison to femoral pulses	Good peripheral perfusion, without obvious cardiac defects	Pulses: Brachial and radial weak, absent, or unequal bilaterally	Poor peripheral perfusion, possible cardiac defects

Lower extremities

Inspection	Length in proportion to body and equal bilaterally; limbs straight	Normal extremity length	Length not in proportion to body: short or unequal; limbs not straight, leg internally rotated or bowed	Congenital syndrome; diabetic mother

System	Normal	Significance	Abnormal	Significance
	Ten toes and without webbing; equal spacing	Normal	More than ten digits or with webbing or unequal spacing	May be associated with congenital syndromes
	Feet: straight	Normal	Feet Turned valgus	Absent fibula or fetal position
			Turned varus	Absent tibia or fetal position
	Ankle dorsiflexion: 0° angle (foot is flexed back on ankle, then angle between foot and ankle is measured)	Maturity	Ankle dorsiflexion: angle > 0,° may be up to 90° in very premature	Prematurity
	Popliteal angle: ≤ 90° (flex newborn's leg then flex thigh; next release and extend leg; measure angle of knee)	Maturity	Popliteal angle: > 90° and ≤ 180° in very immature infant	Prematurity
	Heel-to-ear maneuver: (gently pull leg to ear without forcing; heel will not reach ear but only near shoulder area in full-term infant)	Maturity	Heel-to-ear maneuver: heel reaches ear, or just short of the ear	Prematurity
	Nails: extend to end of nailbed	Normal maturity	Nails: do not extend to end of nailbed	Prematurity
	Nailbeds: pink; brisk capillary refill (> 3 seconds)	Good peripheral perfusion	Nailbeds: dusky, or slow capillary refill (< 3 seconds)	Poor peripheral perfusion

System	Normal	Significance	Abnormal	Significance
			Pedal edema	Pressure due to fetal position, also can be associated with poor peripheral perfusion, syndromes, such as Turner's syndrome
	Plantar creases: cover the sole	Maturity	Plantar creases: few or only anterior third of sole	Prematurity
	Buttocks: creases symmetrical	Normal hips	Buttocks: creases asymmetrical	Congenital hip dysplasia
Palpation	palpation in the presence of a fracture may produce crying or a facial grimace; observe infant's response			
	Fibula, tibia, trochanter, and femur: present and equal bilaterally	No fractures; bone formation normal	Fibula, tibia, trochanter, and femur: absent or unequal bilaterally	Fractures or absence of bone, may be associated with congenital syndrome
	Tarsals and metatarsals present and equal bilaterally	No fractures; bone formation normal	Tarsals and metatarsals absent or unequal bilaterally	Fractures or absence of bone, may be associated with congenital syndromes
	Full range of joint motion (includes abduction, adduction, internal and external rotation, flexion and extension as applicable to respective joint of legs, knees, ankles, feet, toes)	Normal; maturity	Limited range of joint motion	Birth injury or trauma
			Flexion of legs knees, ankles, feet, toes	Prematurity

System	Normal	Significance	Abnormal	Significance
	Hips: without clicks, and full range of joint motion (Ortholoni's maneuver: flex newborn's hips and knees then adduct and adduct hip to detect a slipping of the hip out of the acetabulum or an uneven motion unilaterally; Barlow's maneuver: flex newborn's hips and knees, then place finger on the femur and trochanter, put hip through full range of joint motion and listen for audible click)	Normal range of joint motion and no clicks	Hips: limited range of motion or positive result of Ortholoni or Barlow maneuvers	Congenital hip dysplasia
	Knee jerk or patellar reflex: present, symmetrical	Normal; mature	Knee jerk or patellar reflex: absent, weak, or asymmetrical	Neurologic deficit or prematurity
	Plantar reflex: present and symmetrical	Normal; mature	Plantar reflex: absent, weak or asymmetrical	Neurologic deficit or prematurity
Back				
Inspection	Spinal column: Straight	Normal alignment	Spinal column: Curved	Altered alignment that should gradually resolve if resulting from the fetal position

System	Normal	Significance	Abnormal	Significance
	No visible deviations or defects	Intact	Visible defects: mass, dimple, or bulge with or without a tuft of hair	Spina bifida
			Open spinal defect or may be covered with tissues, involving the meninges and spinal cord or just spinal cord	Meningo-myelocele
			Sinus tracts present	Pilonidal cysts
Palpation	Vertebrae present, without enlargement or pain	Normal spinal column	Vertebrae with bulge, enlarged area, or pain	Mass, bulge, or cyst; fracture of a vertebrae; spina bifida; occult meningomyelocele or pilonidal cyst

Anus: see Genitourinary tracts

Buttocks: see Lower extremities

Cardiopulmonary Status
Carole Kenner

DESCRIPTION

Transition to extrauterine life means a lot of rapid changes for the neonate. Suddenly, the infant is thrust into a cool, bright environment. The placenta that has been nourishing and oxygenating the fetus is rendered useless with the clamping of the cord. Thus, the ductus venosus, a fetal shunt that diverts about half of the fetal blood around the portal circulatory path is also rendered nonfunctional. As the cord is clamped, all the blood begins to flow into the liver. The loss of the placenta also results in increased systemic resistance. After the first breath is taken the pulmonary vascular resistance is decreased and blood begins to flow into the pulmonary system in a right-to-left direction, the opposite of fetal circulation.

Pressure on the right side of the heart decreases and left atrial pressure increases, putting pressure on the foramen ovale and closing this fetal shunt between the atria. Exposure to a cool extrauterine environment also facilitates the foramen's closure. As the arterial oxygen levels increase and blood continues to travel in the new right-to-left direction, the ductus arteriosus begins to close. Complete closure may not occur, however, for the first 24-48 hours even in the full-term infant. A premature infant may continue to have a patent ductus arteriosus because hypoxemia, hypotension, or cold stress can delay closure or even result in an intermittently patent ductus arteriosus. It is not uncommon for premies to have their patent ductus arteriosus either surgically ligated (see Chapter 8) or closed with indomethacin.

These dramatic changes in the cardiovascular system can be stressful for a healthy newborn, but to the sick infant the changes can be life-threatening. That is why it is essential that a thorough cardiopulmonary assessment be performed and resuscitation equipment readily available in the delivery room, nursery, or newborn intensive care unit (NICU).

RISK FACTORS

Prenatal

1. Maternal disease, such as diabetes mellitus; chronic illness; accident; or surgery.
2. Maternal age: adolescent or elderly primipara.
3. Grand multipara.
4. Multiple pregnancy (including twins).
5. No prenatal care.
6. Substance abuse (such as alcohol, smoking, drug usage).
7. Pregnancy-induced hypertension.
8. Premature or prolonged rupture of membranes.

9. Rh factor.
10. ABO incompatibility.
11. Poor maternal nutritional status.
12. Preeclampsia or eclampsia.
13. See Assessment of Maternal, Paternal, and Neonatal Risk Factors in this chapter (p. 3) for more specific details.

Intrapartal

1. Maternal hemorrhage or hypotension.
2. Abruptio placentae.
3. Placenta previa.
4. Placenta accreta.
5. Precipitous delivery.
6. Extended labor.
7. Fetal distress: late decelerations or decreased variability.
8. Fetal positioning: especially breech and footling breech.
9. Cephalopelvic disproportion.
10. Cesarean section.
11. Maternal intrapartal drugs (Chart 2-E).
12. Infant of a diabetic mother.
13. Premature infant.
14. Large infant.
15. Meconium-stained infant or amniotic fluid.
16. Prolapsed or compressed umbilical cord.
17. See Assessment of Maternal, Paternal, and Neonatal Risk Factors in this chapter (p. 3) for more specific details.

Neonatal

1. Surgical or medical neonatal problems such as diaphragmatic hernia, meconium aspiration, prematurity.
2. Neonatal hypotension.
3. Cold stress.
4. Low Apgar scores.
5. Traumatic birth.
6. See Assessment of Maternal, Paternal, and Neonatal Risk Factors in this chapter (p. 3) for more specific details.

EQUIPMENT FOR ASSESSMENT

1. Stethoscope.
2. Indirect automatic oscillometric BP measuring device for infants.
3. Warming device such as radiant warmer.
4. Resuscitation and intubation equipment (see the following list).

Chart 2-E
Maternal Intrapartal Drugs and Their Effects on the Neonate

Drug	Type	Neonatal Effects
Meperidine hydrochloride	Narcotic	Neonatal depression
Morphine	Narcotic	Neonatal depression
Diazepam	Tranquilizer	Unstable thermoregulation CNS depression
Sodium thiopental	Anesthetic barbiturate	Hypotension; respiratory depression
Nitrous oxide	Inhalation anesthetic	Neonatal depression
Oxytocin	Oxytocic	Neonatal jaundice; asphyxia; anoxia
Lidocaine	Local anesthetic	Neonatal depression

Note: This list is not comprehensive.

EQUIPMENT FOR RESUSCITATION

1. Radiant warmer with good light source.
2. Oxygen source capable of delivering 100 percent oxygen with humdification and mixbox or blender box.
3. Vacuum source for suction.
4. Premie and infant masks.
5. Inflatable oxygen bag, T-piece, and manometer.
6. Clock.
7. Laryngoscope with sizes 0 and 1 blades and extra light bulbs.
8. Endotracheal tubes sizes 2.5, 3.0, 3.5, and 4.0 mm.
9. Oral airway tubes sizes 000, 00, and 0.
10. Suction catheters sizes 5, 5/6, 8, and 10 French.
11. Sterile gloves.
12. Bulb syringes.
13. Forceps.
14. Stylets.
15. De Lee suctions sizes 8 and 10 French.
16. Umbilical venous cutdown tray with 3.0 or 4.0 silk sutures, sterile 4 x 4 pads, scalpel with handle, tissue forceps, straight scissors, stopcock for venous or arterial line, umbilical catheters 3.5 and 5.0 French, medicine cup, povidone-iodine solution, and isotonic saline solution (0.9 percent) for flushing the line.
17. Syringes: 1, 3, 6, 12, and 35 cc.

18. Monitors for neonatal respiratory and cardiac functions.
19. Tape: paper and plastic.
20. Armboards: infant and premie sizes.
21. IV access equipment: 5 percent and 10 percent dextrose; 22 and 25 gauge IV butterfly needles or angiocaths, IV setup including tubing.
22. Emergency medications (Chart 2-F).

Chart 2-F
Neonatal Resuscitation Drugs

Drug	Action	Dosage
Atropine	Corrects brady-cardia	0.01 mg/kg IV
Calcium gluconate (10%)	Corrects brady-cardia and strengthens cardiac contraction to increase output	1-2 mL/kg IV given slowly
Calcium chloride (10%)	Corrects brady-cardia	0.10-0.15 mL/kg IV given slowly
Epinephrine hydrochloride (1:10,000 dilution)	Corrects brady-cardia	0.1- 0.3 mL/kg IV
Dopamine hydrochloride	Increases cardiac output	5-10 mg/kg/min IV
Plasma protein traction (5%)	Expands volume	10 mL/kg IV
Albumin (5%)*	Expands volume	10-15 mL/kg IV
Sodium bicarbonate†	Corrects metabolic acidosis	1-3 mEq/kg IV given slowly
Naloxone	Reverses narcotic depression§	0.01 mg/kg IV or IM
Glucose (10% or 25%)	Reverses hypo-glycemia	2 mL/kg IV

*If only 25% is available, dilute in a ratio of 1 part albumin (25% solution) to 4 parts normal saline solution.
†Dilute in a ratio of 1:1 with sterile water (less hypertonic than with dextrose, *may* decrease incidence of intracranial bleeding).
§Use with caution in narcotic-addicted mothers as may precipitate acute neonatal withdrawal.

Neonatal depression resulting from narcotics may be treated with naloxone hydrochloride. It should be used with caution. If this drug is given to a neonate following maternal use of heroin or methadone, acute infant withdrawal symptoms may occur. Maternal anesthesia that has been inhaled or local anesthesia that has been absorbed by the neonate and has resulted in neonatal depression may require cardiopulmonary resuscitation. The chart on page 46 lists the most common neonatal resuscitation drugs with suggested dosages. Consult individual hospital protocols for variations in these dosages.

Cardioversion may also be required during resuscitation to reverse ventricular fibrillation or paroxysmal atrial tachycardia: 1 W/sec/kg-10 W/sec is suggested (Epstein, Frantz, & Ostheimer, 1985). If cardiopulmonary resuscitation is necessary, then use the ratio of 1 breath for every 5 cardiac compressions, at a rate of approximately 20-40 breaths per minute and 100-160 heartbeats per minute. An umbilical artery catheter should be placed if the infant is in need of resuscitation or is a potential candidate for neonatal depression or distress.

The following are guidelines for determining when to intervene and how to assist an infant whose heart rate, respiratory rate, or color is diminished.

RESUSCITATION IN THE DELIVERY ROOM

1. Place the newborn in radiant warmer in Trendelenburg position (head down), facilitating postural drainage.
2. Quickly dry infant and assess respiratory and cardiac function.
3. Clear upper airway by suctioning nose and mouth with bulb syringe.
4. If Apgar score is from 8 to 10, then support the infant's own respiratory effort and continue to observe.
5. If Apgar score is from 5 to 7, heart rate is less than 100 beats per minute, or respiratory effort is weak, then attempt to stimulate neonate by stroking or flicking the feet or hands. If heart rate or respiratory effort remain decreased after 25-30 seconds of stimulation, then give the infant continuous positive airway pressure (CPAP), by facial mask, at approximately 8 cm of pressure. If infant is cyanotic prior to stimulation, blowing oxygen to the face may correct cyanosis and increase heart and respiratory rates; this may be attempted prior to CPAP in some instances. If CPAP or bag-breathing is needed, the infant's head should be tilted back only slightly to open the airway; otherwise, the trachea may be compressed and the airway blocked.
6. If CPAP is effective, closely observe the infant.
7. If CPAP is ineffective after 30-60 seconds and infant remains dusky or heart rate or respiratory effort remain decreased, then begin bag-breathing with 100 percent oxygen at a rate of 20-40 breaths per minute. Begin with peak pressures of 20 cm of water and increase until chest excursion is achieved. (Peak pressures that are too high or low may inhibit gas exchange. A pressure that is unable to move the chest will not ventilate the infant; however, pressure

that exceeds the amount necessary to move the chest may contribute to a collapsed lung or pneumothorax.) The pediatrician or neonatologist should be notified, if not already present, as soon as the baby is noted to be in distress.

8. Intubation is necessary if heart rate is less than 100 beats per minute and/or respiratory effort is weak, after approximately 30-60 seconds of bag-breathing. Intubation should only be attempted by those who have been trained in endotracheal intubation.

9. If Apgar score is from 3 to 4, heart rate is from 50 to 90 beats per minute, respiratory effort is weak, or if infant is cyanotic, then bag-breathe with 100 percent oxygen per facial mask at a rate of approximately 20-40 breaths per minute and at a pressure of 20 cm; increase the pressure and/or rate if no response is noted after a few seconds. Be sure the baby's chest is moving with the bag-breathing; otherwise the lungs are not being expanded.

10. If respiratory effort or heart rate remains decreased, then intubation will be necessary.

11. If Apgar score is from 0 to 2, respiratory effort is absent, or heart rate is from 0 to 50 beats per minute, then begin bag-breathing with 100 percent oxygen, pressure of 20 cm (or more only if no chest excursion is noted), at a rate of 20 to 40 breaths per minute. If experienced personnel are present, an intubation may be attempted; however, in many centers bag-breathing is the preferred method of ventilation at this point. Adequate ventilation can be provided by mask and bag-breathing with 100 percent oxygen if chest excursion is observed. No attempt should be made to intubate the infant at this stage if there is any question about the procedure's success. Once ventilation is established, cardiac massage should be started if bag-breathing does not increase heart rate to 100 beats per minute or greater after 30 seconds of bag-breathing. Cardiac massage should be at a rate of 120-160 beats per minute.

12. If bag-breathing is ineffective in correcting cyanosis, heart rate, or respiratory effort, then intubation must be performed.

13. Cardiac massage should be done anywhere along the resuscitation route listed here when the heart rate is less than 100. Cardiopulmonary resuscitation (CPR) is continued until respiratory effort is reestablished, cardiac rate is 100 or greater, cyanosis is lessened or corrected, or emergency measures are deemed ineffective and resuscitation is stopped.

The physician should begin administering emergency drugs to the infant when cardiopulmonary resuscitation has begun (the infant may or may not be intubated) and resuscitative efforts remain ineffective. A rule of thumb is that no longer than 3 minutes should elapse after cardiopulmonary resuscitation has begun and efforts remain ineffective before emergency drugs are administered (Schreiner, Keener, & Gresham 1982) . Check hospital protocol for time when resuscitation medications are to be given.

Remember: the first step in any resuscitation effort is a clear airway. This airway must be free of secretions, opened by a slight tilting of the head. Often the opening of the airway is all the resuscitation that is necessary. Remember too that cold stress increases the likelihood of acidosis and can trigger apnea and/or bradycardia, so it is essential that the newly delivered infant be dried immediately and placed in a radiant warmer.

If resuscitation efforts are ineffective or only a gradual response is noted, consultation with or transfer to a tertiary center may be necessary. If so consult with the pediatrician and call the Level-3 center. Provide all essential information to them: maternal history, Apgar scores, resuscitation efforts, and response. A call to a regional referral center, if only to alert them to a potential transfer, may save precious minutes if such a move is necessary.

NEONATAL DEPRESSION

A brief synopsis of the transition from fetal to neonatal circulation is given in Figure 2-1. Figure 2-2 depicts apnea leading to neonatal collapse.

After Resuscitation

1. Check blood glucose level using Dextrostix, every 2-4 hours after resuscitation; glycogen and glucose stores may have been used to provide energy, thus resulting in hypoglycemia.
2. Intravenous fluids of 10 percent dextrose should be given at 5 mL/kg/h (Phibbs, 1987). Caution: While this amount of dextrose is acceptable in some institutions, this is considered high for fluid volume, delivering 120 mL/kg/d. Recommended fluid maintenance is at least 60-80 mL/kg/for the first 24 hours of life and 120-160 mL/kg/d after that. A small infant has increased insensible water losses and may need as much as 180-200 mL/kg/d. An asphyxiated infant may already have cerebral edema that can be increased by such an amount of fluid; 50-60 mL/kg/d is recommended by some experts. Any fluid restriction should be based on urine output, at least 1 mL/kg/h and urine-specific gravity, 1.005-1.012.
3. Prevent hypothermia by placing the infant under a radiant warmer, with a skin-temperature probe for monitoring and regulating the warmer's temperature, or in an isolette. Skin temperature should be maintained at 35.5-36.5°C. It is essential that the infant be closely observed for the next few hours. These infant warmers provide good visualization as well as warmth.
4. Place a transcutaneous oxygen monitor (TCM) or oximeter, if one is available, on the infant; either may be used to follow trends or to correlate with measurements of arterial blood gases. Neither monitor reading should be done without periodically checking arterial blood gases.
   a. Watch for changes in transcutaneous oxygen levels.
   b. Keep TCM readings at 50 and preferably 70. Remember these readings are close to the partial pressure of oxygen in arterial blood; the oximeter measures oxygen saturation, which should be kept at no less than 90 percent.
   c. If levels are below 50, notify the physician; the amount of oxygen, if being given, may need to be adjusted; if newborn is on ventilator, the pressure or rate may need to be changed.

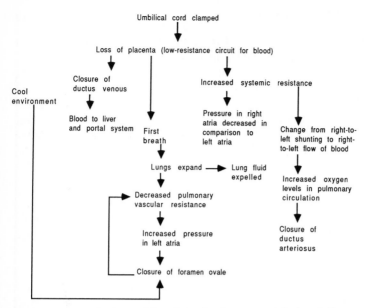

Fig. 2-1. Physical transition from fetal to neonatal circulation.

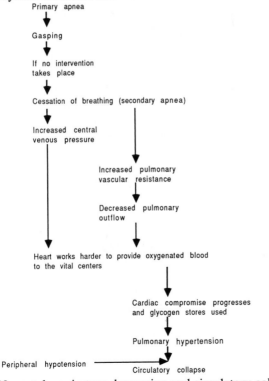

Fig. 2-2. Neonatal respiratory depression and circulatory collapse.

50

    d. If a medical procedure has precipitated a decrease in the oxygen level, note exactly what activity lowered the oxygen level on the monitor, and stop the procedure, allowing infant to rest. Make a notation in the chart and report the incident to other attendants.

    e. If the TCM begins to register 100 or above or if the oximeter reading is in the high 90s, notify the physician. First make sure that the monitor probe is in place. If the monitor probe is in correct position and if the infant is receiving oxygen, the percent of oxygen may need to be decreased gradually. Too sudden a change in oxygen may result in a boomerang effect in which the baby's oxygen levels rise and plummet, thus opening fetal shunts and sometimes resulting in persistent fetal circulation. Remember that wide fluctuations or a rise in arterial tension may contribute to the development of neonatal retrolental fibroplasia.

5. If no TCM or oximeter is available, the arterial blood gases must be closely followed at least every 1-2 hours, and every 15 minutes after every oxygen or ventilator change has occurred. Even if a TCM or oximeter is in use, blood gases should be evaluated every 3-4 hours. (Capillary blood gases are usually not reflective of the oxygen status of a critically ill infant, as peripheral circulation is even poorer than usual in these infants. Capillary blood gas may be useful for pH and $PaCO_2$ determinations but is not the sample of choice for an unstable infant. If such a gas must be drawn, the site for sampling must be well warmed to increase peripheral circulation. Blood should be free flowing with no excessive squeezing of sampling site, as this may cause an inaccurate reading.)

6. Closely observe the infant for any changes in vital signs, thermal status, color, or respiratory effort.

7. Check serum electrolyte levels 2-4 hours after resuscitation, even if no medications were given. Fluctuations in electrolyte levels are not uncommon in a stressed infant.

Thermoregulation

Ann Brueggemeyer

DESCRIPTION

Thermoregulation in the newborn is very important. Dramatic metabolic changes occur during periods of cold stress and hyperpyrexia. The newborn is at special risk for cold stress from the time of delivery until the infant has developed its own ability to maintain body heat. Methods that prevent heat loss can be utilized by health care professionals in all aspects of newborn care.

HEAT PRODUCTION

Heat production in the newborn is related to the amount of cooling of the infant's body and its metabolic response to this cooling. The adult response to cold stress is shivering, but the neonate's ability to produce heat by shivering is limited. Shivering is further inhibited in those neonates exposed to anesthestic agents, receiving certain drugs (e.g., pancuronium bromide), or suffering from brain damage (Graven, 1976).

Brown-fat metabolism in the newborn is the mechanism for heat production. Brown fat is located mainly in the middle to upper thorax. When the infant is suffering from cold stress, the metabolism of brown fat begins in order to maintain normal body temperature. As brown-fat metabolism increases, oxygen consumption also increases, placing a further stress on the infant. Since brown-fat stores are minimal, protection against heat loss is rapidly depleted. Acidosis occurs as glucose is metabolized and a buildup of lactic acid occurs. The production of surfactant declines during cold stress, leading to an increase in respiratory distress.

Physiologic responses of infants to cold stress include peripheral vasoconstriction, diminished cerebral blood flow, alteration in acid-base balance, decrease in renal function, diminished ability for normal metabolism, gastrointestinal disturbances, and decreased nerve conduction (Holdcroft, 1980).

HEAT LOSS

Infants are at risk for heat loss because of their large body surface area in contrast to that of an adult. Heat is lost by (1) conduction, (2) convection, (3) evaporation, and (4) radiation.

Conduction losses occur from body tissues to objects in contact with the infant's skin. Linens and bed surfaces should be prewarmed to prevent heat losses to these objects. Infants placed on cold examination tables and x-ray plates can lose a great deal of heat, especially if they are unclothed for any period of time.

Convection loss occurs as air currents pass over exposed skin surfaces. Air currents are most noticeable near air vents and air conditioners. Infants in open cribs should not be placed near them. Administration of oxygen can also be a source of heat loss to the infant: cool air currents passing over the head can cause a great deal of heat loss, even with head coverings in place. Oxygen should be warmed to a few degrees less than environmental temperature.

Evaporative losses occur when wet skin surfaces are exposed to dry air. At the time of delivery, infants should be dried and wrapped to prevent this.

The heat loss due to radiation is the most difficult to prevent. Heat losses can occur from the infant's skin to surfaces not in contact with the infant. Losses occur when incubators are placed near cool windows or air vents.

WARMING THE NEONATE

Rapid rewarming of a cold infant is not without risks. Apnea has been associated with too rapid rewarming and dramatic environmental temperature swings (Perlstein, Edwards, & Sutherland, 1970). The exact mechanism for this effect is not well defined. The infant being warmed continues to accept the flow of heat from the environment until death ensues: the infant has no ability to store heat. Optimum body temperature is defined as between 36°-37.8° C (Swyer, 1978). If the infant continues to gain heat beyond this level, fever, dehydration, and cardiorespiratory failure ensue.

The infant may safely be rewarmed 1° C every hour (Holdcroft, 1980). Temperature readings may be taken axillary or rectally. Electronic thermistors may be secured to the abdomen or toe to monitor temperature changes. Metallic thermistors should not be in contact with any surface other than the infant's skin. Fluid spilled on the thermistor may also yield inaccurate results as its own evaporation causes heat changes.

PROTECTING AND MAINTAINING THE NEONATE'S BODY TEMPERATURE

The first goal of the delivery room nurse is to protect the newborn from heat loss; second, to maintain a neutral thermal environment to prevent the complications secondary to cold stress. In the delivery room, the normal infant's core temperature declines to approximately 35° C. External cooling can take place even before the core temperature has begun to decrease. This immediate cold stress can delay restoring normal thermoregulation for several hours.

Wrapping the dry infant in a cotton blanket is probably the least effective method of maintaining body heat (Besch, Perlstein, Edwards, Keenan, & Sutherland, 1971). Even prewarmed incubators are less effective than using an insulation swaddler (Besch et al., 1971). Infants can be wrapped in plastic sheeting, plastic bags, silver swaddlers, and "bubble" insulator bags.

After delivery, the infant is placed foot first into the bag. The clear plastic bag permits the nurse to visualize the infant while still wrapped. In the silver swaddler, a thin layer of reflective liner helps reflect heat back to the infant, but prevents visualization. In the clear plastic varieties, a small rip can be made in the bag to apply name bracelets, take foot prints, and provide care; later, the bag can be repaired with tape. If the head is also covered, the bag provides a major shield against heat loss. The infant must also be placed under a radiant warmer to maintain normal temperature.

Once in the nursery the infant should remain in the plastic shield in a warming bed until the newborn's temperature stabilizes. Routine care can be provided through small holes in the plastic. Warm-water baths should not be attempted until several hours after delivery.

After the temperature has stabilized, the mature infant can be dressed in a cotton shirt and diaper. Cotton blankets are then used to provide sufficient wrapping to maintain normal temperature. The small or premature infant is unable to maintain a healthy body temperature. The infant must be placed under a radiant warmer or in an incubator. Size and gestational age both play a part in the infant's ability to maintain body heat. The infant weighing less than 1800 g is expected to need external heat sources to maintain proper temperature (Swyer, 1978).

If an infant requires transport to another health facility, special considerations must be taken to ensure the arrival of a warm baby. Every effort must be taken to provide a neutral thermal environment for the infant prior to transport. This is sometimes difficult because many health care workers place an infant in a position that is readily accessible to them and not what is best for the infant; close observation of the infant may mean keeping the infant unwrapped. The simple procedure of starting an IV infusion may provide an extended period of exposure for the infant. Despite these interruptions in maintaining a neutral thermal environment, every effort should be made to protect the infant from heat loss.

The process of transport is a major source of potential cold stress to the infant. Despite sophisticated modern equipment, the standard transport incubator is not completely capable of heat retention. A great deal of heat can be lost by radiation within the transport vehicle itself, whether ambulance or air carrier. If the team must move the equipment through unheated entry accesses, the incubator again may lose a great deal of heat. At times, it may be impractical to wait the full length of time to reheat the incubator at the transferring institution.

Since the incubator must be opened to place the infant inside, a great deal of heat is lost as the door or hood is opened. This can be further compounded by the time spent straightening out lines and tubes and making sure the infant is situated in the incubator before closing the hood or entry port. If possible, the infant should be wrapped or clothed prior to transfer into the transport incubator. In some cases, it may be necessary to use portable warming mattresses to improve the heating capability of the transport incubator (Nielsen, Jung, & Atherton, 1976). The use of additional heating sources must also be followed by carefully observing the delicate newborn's skin for burns.

REFERENCES

Cardiopulmonary Status

Epstein, M. F., Frantz III, I. D., & Ostheimer, G. W. (1985). Resuscitation in the delivery room. In J. P. Cloherty & A. R. Stark (Eds.), *Manual of neonatal care* (pp. 73-89). Boston: Little, Brown.

Phibbs, R. H. (1987). Delivery room management of the newborn. In G. B. Avery (Ed.), *Neonatology: Pathophysiology and management of the newborn* (3rd ed.) (pp. 212-231). Philadelphia: J. B. Lippincott.

Schreiner, R. L., Keener, P. A., & Gresham, E. L. (1982). Resuscitation. In R. L. Schreiner (Ed.), *Care of the newborn* (pp. 59-68). New York: Raven.

Thermoregulation

Besch, N., Perlstein, P., Edwards, N., Keenan, W., Sutherland, J. (1971). The transparent baby bag. *The New England Journal of Medicine, 284*(3), 121-124.

Graven, S. (1976). Heat and body temperature. In N. Dahl & S. Frazier (Eds.), *Neonatal thermoregulation: Module I* (pp. 17-22). White Plains, NY: The National Foundation/March of Dimes.

Holdcroft, A. (1980). *Body temperature control in anaesthesia, surgery and intensive care* (pp. 17-18.) London: Bailliére Tindall.

Nielsen, H., Jung, A., & Atherton, S. (1976). Evaluation of the Porta-warm mattress as a source of heat for neonatal transport. *Pediatrics, 58*, 500-504.

Perlstein, P., Edwards, N., & Sutherland, J. (1970). Apnea in premature infants and incubator-air-temperature changes. *The New England Journal of Medicine, 282*(9), 461-466.

Swyer, P. (1978). Heat loss after birth. In J. Sinclair (Ed.), *Temperature regulation and energy metabolism in the newborn.* New York: Grune & Stratton.

BIBLIOGRAPHY

Apgar, V. (1953). A proposal for a new method of evaluation of the newborn infant. *Current researches in anesthesia and analgesia, 32*, 260-267.

Hodson, W. A., & Truog, W. E. (1983). *Critical care of the newborn* (pp. 8-14). Philadelphia: W. B. Saunders.

Moyer-Mileur, L. J. (1986). Nutrition. In N.S. Streeter (Ed.), *High-risk neonatal care* (pp. 263-296). Rockville, Maryland: Aspen.

Reid, R. J. (1986). Transport of the high-risk neonate. In N. S. Streeter (Ed.), *High-risk neonatal care* (pp. 477-511). Rockville, Maryland: Aspen.

Spitzer, A. R., & Fox, W. W. (1986). Infant apnea. *Pediatric Clinics of North America, 33*, 561-581.

Chapter 3

Parent Care: Anticipatory Guidance for the Neonate and Family

Carole Kenner   *Laurie Porter Gunderson*

When a baby is born with a physical deformity or is acutely ill, the parents' expectations are shattered. The family may well perceive this event as a crisis and experience an anticipatory-grief reaction. If there are siblings, they may feel forgotten and confused and experience a crisis as well. The nurse is the pivitol person to assist the family to cope with the unexpected neonatal problem.

Anticipatory guidance, as an intervention strategy, is used to examine the topics Anticipatory Grief, Bonding in the NICU, The Forgotten Siblings, Psychosocial Needs of the Family in Crisis, and Transition from NICU to Home. Anticipatory guidance as a strategy provides a means whereby the family and nurse can work together to anticipate parental concerns before they become overwhelming. Parents are encouraged to share their concerns with the nursing staff. Mutual goals are set between parents and nurses to promote the parents' progress and comfort with their infant. The parents are viewed as a vital part of the health care team. Their input and concerns are highly valued as issues to be addressed before they impinge on parent-child interaction. Anticipatory guidance makes parents active participants in a team effort to meet the challenge of parenting in a high-risk situation. This parental participation helps combat the feelings of helplessness they often feel. It may even help the parents to better cope with the unexpected "imperfect child." Their active participation, even to a limited degree, in a teaching-learning situation leads to a more productive outcome.

Obviously, each family should be treated as an individual unit, with unique responses. Not every family will be able to or want to verbalize feelings or participate in an anticipatory effort. Cultural differences and values play an important role in how a family reacts in a crisis. This individualized outlook must be taken into consideration if effective nursing care is to be provided to the family.

Neonatal Surgery: A Nursing Perspective
ISBN 0-8089-1893-1

Anticipatory Grief
Carole Kenner

DESCRIPTION

Anticipatory grief or bereavement is a response to a perceived potential loss—the parents' anticipation of their baby's death before the clinical circumstances warrant such a conclusion. It may be precipitated by the birth of a newborn with physical deformities or illness that may or may not be life-threatening. This grief reaction may be experienced by both parents, as the perfect child has not been born. Even the older siblings may feel cheated when the baby that they expected does not come home right away. Adults often forget that children often pick up on the parent's grief and yet are afraid to ask their already-upset parents about the baby.

This parental grief response may be seen by the nursing staff as unwarranted if they feel the baby is in no real danger of death. The parents, having less experience with sick infants, do not care that to the nurse it is just a little cleft lip that can easily be repaired. They do not care that Baby A is a 28-week premie struggling for its life in the next isolette. They do care that their child has a problem and they do not know what to expect for this infant. The loss of their expected, perfect child is very real (Johnson, 1986).

The anticipatory grief response may act as a defense mechanism to shield the parents from the reality of their imperfect child. It may also may be considered part of the same bereavement process that takes place any time there is an actual or predicted impending death of a person. The stages of the grief process, whether precipitated by fear of impending death or the death itself, must be worked through if successful parental adaptation is to take place (Johnson, 1986). Otherwise, bonding and attachment can be severely affected.

STAGES OF THE GRIEF PROCESS

1. Denial: "This problem could not be true!" is a typical response at this stage. Parents may refuse to see the baby in the hospital, thus avoiding confirmation of the problem.

2. Anger: "Why did this happen to us? How dare we have a deformed baby?" are two common responses of parents in this stage, which may be manifested by any of these scenarios:
   a. Anger at the obstetrician or delivery room nurses
   b. Anger at the transport team for taking the baby away
   c. Anger at the NICU staff for causing the problem or making it worse
   d. Anger at the partner for the failure in producing a perfect child
   e. Anger at God for allowing this horrible problem to happen

3. Bargaining: "We'll do anything you want if only the baby can be OK" is a common plea by parents at this stage. Bargaining with God (e.g., to go to church more often) is common too. They make a pact with God to gain time for the baby.

4. Acceptance: "OK, we hear what you are telling us, now what do we do about the baby's problem?" is often heard from parents entering this phase.

Note that parents vacillate between these stages. This process is not always orderly and sequential.

SYMPTOMS

Identification of the presence of these symptoms is necessary to determine what, if any, intervention is necessary. The need for nursing intervention may be based upon the degree of concern expressed by the parents or how severely the parent-child interaction is being affected. Even if no signs of anticipatory grief are currently present, their development must be expected. Early intervention can prevent future parent-child interaction problems. Symptoms of anticipatory grief include the following:

1. Inability to accept the infant's condition

2. Refusal to see the infant

3. Distancing techniques to avoid attachment or to avoid a potentially painful confrontation with reality:
   a. Physical withdrawal: avoiding the baby; or psychological withdrawal: seeing the baby but avoiding making eye contact with or touching the baby
   b. Excessive or uncontrollable crying
   c. Flat affect
   d. Depression

4. Fear of impending death of their newborn

5. Calling the clergy to see the infant even if the infant's life is not in danger

6. Mobilizing family resources to face death (even when death is not probable), for example:
   a. Gathering family members to come to the hospital
   b. Refusing to leave the baby's bedside to take care of themselves

ASSESSMENT

Before any interventions can take place a detailed assessment of the family must be conducted. The following is a list of questions that provide the nurse with the necessary information upon which to develop a plan of care.

1. Assess the family:
   a. Was this a planned child? If not, the parents may feel doomed to lose the baby because the baby was initially unwanted.

b. What was their fantasy child like? The further removed the newborn actually is from this child, the more the family may feel a loss.
c. What does the family know about the child's condition? If there was a suspicion of a problem during the pregnancy, they may be better prepared to deal realistically with the situation; however, the parents may have denied the problem during the pregnancy and now cannot escape the actual occurrence.
d. Have the parents seen the baby? Early visual contact with the infant is important. Seeing the baby may alleviate exaggerated fears of gross physical abnormalities or concerns that the infant will appear less than human.
e. Has the family experienced a fetal or neonatal loss before? If so, this will influence how they react to the new baby. Do not assume that their past experience will lessen anticipatory grief this time around. In fact, the response may be greater, since their other child actually died.
f. How do they usually cope with a difficult situation: with anger? rage? withdrawal? Do they blame others? Seek emotional support? Their past coping mechanisms will be called into action by this anticipatory grief. If the nurse knows what is the norm for this family, then an appropriate response can be formulated and the family's reaction better anticipated. Nurses then may not take the parents' anger and rage personally, which often happens and only leads to a vicious cycle of the parents and nurse fighting for control of the baby's care (Sammons & Lewis, 1985).
g. What role is this baby to play in the family? Cultural values and expectations dictate certain roles for children, even an infant. It is this loss of the child's role in the family that may set anticipatory grief into action. The nurse can use this information to strengthen psychosocial support for the family to include their cultural beliefs and values. Thus a more holistic and realistic approach is given to the care; the chances for successful care are greater too.

2. Anticipate an anxiety response from the family:
   a. Assess the parents' understanding of the baby's condition. If the parents were together in the delivery room, they may already know or suspect there is a problem.
   b. Assess the delivery room environment for potential stressors. There is a tendency for the staff to become task-oriented and to forget the parents in the delivery room when a baby is in trouble. Swift movements in an emergency situation may convey anxiety to the parents.
   c. Assess any inconsistencies in the parents' verbal and nonverbal behavior.
   d. Assess their current expectations of the infant now.

INTERVENTION STRATEGIES

The first strategy is anticipating the parents feelings and actions. Anticipatory guidance allows the nurse to plan for each family according to their grief reaction. Once parents have begun to display grief, the nurse must work even harder to identify and alter the response to prevent problems in long-term parent-child interaction.

Early Visual Contact

1. This contact between parent and neonate must be supported by the nurse staying with the family to answer questions and provide positive comments.

2. If the baby is to be transferred to a special care nursery or regional referral center, the nurse should make certain the parents see and touch the infant prior to the separation.

3. If the baby's condition prevents physical contact, a photograph may help the parents adjust to a more realistic picture of their baby's condition at the time of transport and throughout the early stages of the infant hospitalization. This photograph is something the parents can hold when they may not be able to touch their infant. It is also helpful to the mother who is still in the postpartum unit and may be asked by others where her baby is.

Facilitating Communication

1. Give factual information as this may help to decrease the parents' guilt feelings and ultimately reduce their blaming each other for the child's problem or defect.

2. Inform parents of the problem in an open and honest manner. Keep them informed of the infant's progress whether they are in the delivery room, nursery, or separated from the infant in the recovery room or postpartum unit.

3. Gradually tell them what the problem is and what treatment is necessary; this may help to prevent informational overload.

4. Repeat this information often. Shock precludes taking in and grasping information; so the parents may not even hear, much less remember what was initially said.

5. If a transfer is to be made:
   a. Prepare parents for this. Tell them what equipment to expect, what it will look like and why it is necessary to have this amount of equipment that is carried for any infant to be transferred.
   b. Show a picture of the transport isolette and equipment; if none is available, consider having a picture on hand.
   c. Explain in lay terms the functions of the members of the transport team; very few people know what a respiratory therapist, transport nurse, neonatal nurse practitioner or a neonatal resident or fellow is. Anticipating the parents' fears of the equipment and team may decrease the anxiety and alleviate some stress for the family.

d. Provide the transport team with complete information on how the parents are reacting to the transfer and what preliminary work has been done with the parents. This information usually takes more space than the one line that is often given on transfer sheets.

e. Keep lines of communication open to the transferring hospital if the mother is still confined there. Remember, it is difficult for nurses to help a mother if they do not know what is happening with the infant.

6. Keep lines of communication open between the parents themselves:

a. Encourage them to talk about their concerns for the baby, their relationship with each other, and their concerns about their other children.

b. Help them understand that friends and family members need to know how to help since they want to be useful yet often feel very uncomfortable and in the way. (Unfortunately, it is often up to the parents to relieve this discomfort at a time when they themselves are emotionally exhausted.)

Assisting the Grief Response

1. Accentuate the positive—not false hopes. All babies do have positive characteristics (e.g., good color, strong cry).

2. Do not force the parents through the grief process; rather, evaluate where they are in the process and what might help them at that stage and in the days ahead. Let them set the pace.

a. Allow privacy for the parents.

b. Encourage them to verbalize their fears.

c. Help them to feel better by explaining that the grief reaction is necessary and normal. Assist the process, do not arrest it.

d. Conduct care conferences with other disciplines to keep them informed of the parents' stage in the grief process.

e. Be an advocate for the baby and the parents, yet allow the parents to assume their rightful role in caring for the baby. They should not be seen as inconveniences but rather as central figures in the outcome, especially the psychological outcome, of this infant. Work with the parents, not against them.

3. Discuss the progress of the infant with the parents:

a. Develop progress charts that parents can fill in at the infant's bedside, or keep the chart with the mother in her hospital room. These charts demonstrate to the parents the passing of developmental milestones—the first bottle, the first pound gained, the discontinuation of an IV infusion.

b. Coordinate meetings between parents and other disciplines (e.g., social workers, chaplains, physicians) so that a coordinated approach is made in keeping the parents informed of their infant's condition;

4. Anticipate parental reactions, such as being angry with friends who have "normal" babies or other parents who can take their infants home from the hospital:

   a. Encourage ventilation of what they consider negative feelings.
   b. Acknowledge their right to be angry.
   c. Touch the parents (e.g., put your arm around them) to reassure them.
   d. Let the parents know it is OK to cry.

5. Encourage them to become involved in parent support groups.

Bonding in the NICU
Carole Kenner

DESCRIPTION

Bonding is the first phase of the attachment process between parent and child. Nurses have an important role in helping families in this phase but must be careful not to impose their own sense of the proper progress that the parents should make. Sometimes nurses have made parents feel obligated to bond or unite with a baby whom they do not even recognize as their own. For some parents the baby may be a complete stranger from the one they created in their dreams during the prenatal period.

Literature abounds with information on neonatal attachment and bonding. For a while it was believed that if a parent and infant did not bond in the first few minutes of life they were doomed for psychological discomfort the rest of their lives. Parents of a sick infant are thus likely to feel intense guilt because their child is whisked away, and they cannot touch or hold the baby during the so-called critical moments. Other ways of inducing guilt in parents relate to the high technological environment of the neonatal intensive care unit (NICU) where it is not difficult to make parents feel inadequate. After all, expert care is required. Many parents, however, are experts at parenting. They just need support in their attempts to build a relationship with their infant. Nurses can make a significant difference in the development of this new parent-child relationship.

Bonding is a process that begins during the gestational period and is only embellished in the neonatal period (Greenspan, 1985). The latter bonding is a critical component in the parent-child relationship; however, when the contact must take place in the NICU much consideration needs to be given to the environmental influences on the parents and their infant. Chances for successful bonding are high if nurses attune themselves to the parents' and newborn's needs. In the NICU, nurses must be creative to lessen the overstimulation that the NICU environment gives to parents and their infant. Intervention strategies should be aimed at providing a quiet, private, and yet supportive atmosphere for the bonding.

SYMPTOMS

Signs of healthy bonding as well as danger signals must be identified:

Assessment	Healthy Bonding Behaviors	Danger Signals
How do the parents hold and touch the infant?	Parents touch and explore the infant usually by first touching the baby with the fingertips in a circular manner over the extremities and the head; this progresses to whole-hand exploration with the palm open, moving over the rest of the baby's body	Parents do not engage in close cuddling and hold baby at a distance from their bodies
How do the parents look at the infant?	Parents use en face position in looking at infant and lower own body to baby's level if unable to hold infant.	Parents hold baby away from en face position
How do the parents vocalize with the infant?	Parents talk and sings to the baby; baby responds reciprocally when able	Parents do not direct any vocal expressions to the baby; infant does not respond positively to parental talking
Are the parents able to identify the infants' cues?	Parents do not disturb infant during sleep; the infant moves and looks toward the parents when they speak.	Parents attempt to talk to or wake infant during sleep
Are parents able to soothe infant?	Parents provide comfort when infant is irritable; parents use pacifier to calm infant; infant quiets to parents' touch; parents stroke the child and talk in a soft voice	Parents do not attempt to soothe infant when fussy; negative comments are made by the parents about the infant; parents do not become involved in the infant's care; infant does not calm to parents' voice or touch.

INTERVENTION STRATEGIES

Goal	Intervention
Facilitate parent-child interaction before, during, and after transfer	1. Allow parents to see and touch infant as soon as possible after delivery; if there is a congenital anomaly, prepare the parents for what to expect but accentuate the newborn's positive charcterisitics 2. Remain with the parents for the first few minutes with their baby to answer questions and give support 3. Then, provide privacy to the parents 4. If possible, allow the parents to see the baby before the transport team arrives 5. Give the parents time to really look at and touch their newborn; in some cases, this may be the only time they see their baby alive; let them view their baby, however sick, in a supportive environment

6. Offer to take a picture of the infant as soon as possible so that the parents can have something tangible to hold on to after the transfer has occurred

7. Encourage the parents to visit the baby and let them know they are welcome; supply parents with rules and regulations for visiting: these should be in writing, as little of what is verbally told them will be retained; put these "rules" in a positive way so that parents feel encouraged to visit and feel more like they belong in the unit and have a place with their baby

8. Keep the referring hospital informed of the baby's progress if the infant is separated from the parents; if nurses in the referring hospital know what is happening with the baby, they can provide emotional support and more holistic care to the parents

9. If the mother is hospitalized, encourage the father to take pictures of the baby to keep her updated on the infant's progress

Encourage positive feelings toward the infant

1. Once in the NICU, parents need support in confronting their real child as they still may be clinging to their "fantasy" baby; encourage expressions of feelings regarding the discrepancy between the two children; the reconciling of the actual child versus the expected one facilitates bonding and eventually allows the attachment process to occur (Mercer, 1981)

2. Encourage the parents to express negative as well as positive feelings regarding the appearance of their child; some babies, especially very premature ones are not very attractive; parents need to know that these feelings are normal

3. Parental views of infants are often intimately tied to cultural values; these values must be considered if appropriate family-centered care is to be given

4. Call the baby by name; this encourages parents to see their infant as a unique individual, and it also gives the parents a sense of warmth and caring on the part of the nurse, which will be the foundation for a trusting relationship

5. Give positive reinforcement to the parents and baby when a reciprocal rhythm or response pattern occurs; show the parent what is soothing to an irritable baby, or what makes a quiet baby come to an alert state; parents may feel that they are failures if the baby does not respond to their attempts

Encourage parental contact with the infant

1. Encourage them to talk and stroke their baby; very few babies, however sick, will be harmed by such behavior

2. Explain to the parents what the baby can do and not what he cannot do; encourage them to assist in the infant's care in relation to diaper changes, mouth care, turning, etc.

3. Teach parents the responsiveness of their newborn; if premature, tell them that the baby may not respond to their touch at first, but that it is still important

4. Demonstrate to the parents how the baby responds to their voice or their touch; praise them for their attempts to soothe their child

5. Encourage parents to make tapes of their voices to be kept in the bed and played to the newborn

6. Allow parents time with their infant before the routine care is initiated; usually 5-10 minutes will not cause a critical delay in an infant's care but it may be critical to the bonding process

7. Call the parents if they have stopped visiting or calling the unit; the overture of just calling them may let them know that nurses are concerned about the parent's welfare as well as that of their baby

8. Encourage parents to bring in clothes for the baby; the clothes make the baby more real to the parents and give the parents something that they can contribute to their baby; allow the parents to dress the infant or place a bow in the baby's hair

9. Have the baby "write" a note to the parents; notes that they can keep make the baby more a part of them (Jenkins & Tock, 1986)

Manipulate the environment to facilitate parenting	1. Acknowledge the overstimulation of the environment: the noise, the bright lights, the movement of the staff, and its effect on both the parents and the baby 2. If possible, provide a private area 3. Encourage open visiting hours; parents sometimes have a great need to see their baby at any time of the day or night; this should be encouraged; if hospital policy will not allow open visiting, encourage them to telephone the unit at any time 4. Assess the nursery environment: Do parents visit often? Are parental visits extremely short? Are the walls decorated with cheery animals or bright colors? If a nursery is depressing, or the environment is viewed as negative, bonding and subsequent attachment will be difficult
Promote as nearly normal growth and development as possible	Educate the parents in the use of infant stimulation principles; the use of stuffed animals, mobiles, and pacifiers supplied by the parents not only serves to meet the needs of the infant but makes helpless parents feel worthwhile
Build the confidence of the parents in relation to their ability to parent the infant	1. Allow the parents to practice care in a supervised and supportive environment to decrease their feelings of role failure 2. Help the parents to understand the effect that an intensive care unit may have on their interaction with the child 3. Teach the parents that sick newborns may not always be the sociable baby that we have all come to expect; it will take time for the baby to get to know the parents 4. Help the parents to recognize a baby's attempts to respond, such as the grasp of a hand and the quiet behavior that infants exhibit while held securely against the parent's body 5. Teach the parent's about normal newborn responses such as the sucking reflex, rooting reflex, and about the sleep-wake patterns of newborns in an intensive care unit 6. Help the parents to understand that building a relationship with a child takes time and is a learning experience (Greenspan, 1985), in which each participant tests the other one in getting to know each other
Promote the expression of individual needs	1. Encourage the parents to take time for themselves; having an infant in an NICU can be a draining experience; parents may need permission to have personal needs away from the baby; often, parents feel they will be labeled as bad parents if they are not present every day 2. Encourage the parents to talk about their other children; parents may resent the other children for making demands on their time

Bonding is a reciprocal relationship between people. Attachment is the end product of successful bonding. Like any other relationship a parent-child relationship must be nurtured to become positive. Nurses are the patient advocates who must anticipate the needs of the parents and their child. It is the nurses who must provide a calm, reassuring, positive environment in the midst of a noisy, bright, stressful NICU. Too easily can we make parents feel guilty by discouraging visitation, indicating they are interrupting our work, referring to our baby instead of theirs, discounting their importance to the infant, and failing to acknowledge their feelings of inadequacy and anxiety. Nurses can either make parents feel guilty or foster a positive, non-judgmental atmosphere in which the parent-child relationship can grow and blossom.

While only parental bonding has been addressed here, grandparent and sibling bonding and attachment must be encouraged in the same manner.

The Forgotten Siblings
Carole Kenner

DESCRIPTION

Siblings of a sick newborn are often forgotten in the turmoil of the family crisis. Their routines are disrupted. They may be shunted to relatives or friends, separated from their parents. Depending on the children's developmental stages, they may not understand why they are being sent away or why their parents are so upset. Children often feel that they are being punished for something they do not remember doing. Suddenly, a happily anticipated arrival of a new baby brother or sister is fraught with discomfort and sadness.

Helplessness, powerlessness, guilt, and anger are all felt by the siblings of a critically ill newborn. Resentment towards the new baby may build as parents spend less and less time with them and more time at the hospital. When the baby does not come home, the children are disillusioned about the reality of the new baby. They may equate the baby's not coming home with their own potential departure from home (i.e., they fear leaving or being sent away since the baby doesn't come home).

The feelings of these children must be acknowledged and expressed. They must be encouraged to visit their new sibling. Parents must understand their children's need to see the baby, after all, they have fantasized too about the baby. Their fears must be allayed by directly confronting them. Attention must be paid to the siblings' developmental stages if holistic, family-centered care is to be provided. A sound knowledge of growth and development must be used to help meet the siblings' needs and assist parents to care for the older children as well as the new baby. It is nurses that can be instrumental in this process.

SYMPTOMS

1. Regression or acting out behavior of siblings

2. Increased sibling rivalry in the home

3. Withdrawal from parents

4. Multiple guardians, resulting in mood swings in the children

5. Anger expressed openly or covertly to parents

6. School problems

7. Nightmares or fears of being sent away

8. Anger at the baby, once brought home

INTERVENTION STRATEGIES

1. Determine the developmental stages of the siblings to determine appropriate intervention strategies.

2. Assess the family composition and their understanding of the developmental process.

3. Help parents identify the needs of their other children and how they can best realistically meet the needs.

4. Encourage the parents to talk with the children, according to their developmental stages, about the baby and why the infant has not come home.

5. Encourage the parents to bring the children to the hospital to see the baby:
   a. Children, too, need to see the baby to reconcile fantasy and reality.
   b. If the children are in the preoperational phase, the baby may not be real to them unless they see the infant.
   c. Help the parents prepare the children for a visit to the NICU. Many units across the country now have sibling visitation programs. The only requirements for visitation are to check that the children's immunizations are current and that no exposure to communicable diseases has occurred. A brief health assessment of the children should be done prior to entering the unit. This exam is often conducted by the nurse with the help of the parents.
      This strategy allows the children to get to know their baby brother or sister's nurse before they see the baby. Sibling visitation can facilitate a decrease in parental guilt for always having to leave the other children at home. If no sibling visitation program is in place, then bring the children to the NICU where the infant, in an isolette or radiant warmer, may be viewed through a viewing window, door, or enclosed area. Research studies conducted after such sibling visitations demonstrate that children

concentrate on the positive aspects of the baby and not on all the tubes, wires and, equipment that adults focus on. Remember, fear is usually learned. If the children are treated in a positive manner and prepared in simple terms for the visit, such a meeting with the newborn can be very rewarding and positive.

6. Help the parents to realize that small children may think that the parents' crying or sadness is their fault and that their being removed from the home environment and placed with neighbors or relatives may be a form of punishment.

7. Help the parents to realize that it is all right to spend time with family members and away from the hospital.

8. Help parents to feel OK about explaining to their other children how tired they are, and how sorry they are that they have to be away so much. Children will respond to this honesty if they know they are not to blame for the disruption in family life.

9. Encourage parents to attend parent support groups where such issues as sibling problems can be discussed openly and with people experiencing the same difficulties.

10. Encourage parents to have the children, if old enough, draw pictures for the new baby and to draw pictures to express their feelings.

11. Encourage the parents to have the children to talk to their friends about the new baby. This strategy helps the baby become more real to them.

12. Encourage the parents to talk about the tendency to overprotect the new baby once home:
    a. Parents need to realize that children have a need to help with the new baby—this may be done with careful supervision. This strategy will decrease the chances for the parents to become frustrated with the children. Otherwise, parents may give negative reinforcement to the siblings, and the children may feel that they are in the way.
    b. Foster the parents' self-esteem by including them in the infant's care.

13. Encourage the parents to discuss problems they may be having with their children:
    a. Inform parents that their other children may regress developmentally during the hospitalization of the newborn.
    b. Prepare parents for anger or acting out behavior that may occur with their children. It may be helpful for the parents to talk with their children about why they are acting out.
    c. Encourage the parents to plan family activities so that the children feel like they are members of the family.

14. Encourage parents to keep lines of communication open between the parents and their children and the parents and their children's teachers:
   a. Parent-teacher conferences may help prevent school problems.
   b. If parents cannot visit the school, a phone call may be sufficient.

Psychosocial Needs of a Family in Crisis
Carole Kenner

DESCRIPTION

Crisis occurs when previous problem-solving or coping techniques fail to produce an equilibrium (Aguilera & Messick, 1986). What constitutes a crisis for one person may not result in a crisis for another. Often, the situation is defined by the individual's values and beliefs. Crisis is usually a turning point, either in a positive or negative direction. A change in role or role expectations is one precipitating factor that may constitute a crisis. For parents, the act of giving birth and taking on a role of mother or father even for a second time may result in crisis whether the baby is healthy or not. Parenthood is an experience that requires change and adaptation to a new role. This new role may cause disequilibrium as old coping mechanisms may not work in the new situation. The addition of a new child changes how parents relate to their other children. New expectations of their time and energy can be overwhelming. Yet, health care professionals often assume that if parents have other children, they do not need as much support as first-time parents. They are, however, a new family, one that has changed composition overnight, and so need support.

Adjustment to the new role is difficult enough if the baby is healthy, but one who is premature, or who has a surgical problem can make the situation a very stressful event. Nurses need to assess the developmental needs of the mother and her self-concept, as these may affect her approach to motherhood. One of the tasks of a mother is to develop her own identity. This task may severely be affected if her baby is less than perfect. Nurses can make this assessment by observing the mother and talking with her about her feelings. Assessment of the mother's expectations regarding her new role is necessary; if her expectations do not coincide with reality, a crisis may result. Her knowledge of child development will affect her expectations of herself and her child. Nurses further need to assess the mother's readiness to assume her new role. The mother may need time before she is able to participate in her infant's care if she has not worked through the tasks of pregnancy completely. This incompletion of tasks is especially true if the infant is premature and the mother has not yet created an image of the baby as a separate human being with a separate identity. A situational crisis may result if intervention is not started (Aguilera & Messick, 1986).

Fathers also undergo a rapid psychological change once the baby is born. For them the baby may not be real until it is born. Having fathers present at the birth helps with the transition into fatherhood. When the baby experiences a problem, however, and forces a separation between the mother and baby, the father may be caught in the middle, running between two hospitals or two units. The father often feels guilty for spending time away from other responsibilities to be either with the baby or with the mother. Expected to be "superman," he is often the one who must continue to work, take responsibility for the home, the other children, make decisions about treatment for the baby and console his wife about their baby's condition. It is no wonder that parents under these circumstances find themselves in crisis in which prior coping mechanisms fail to work. It is unlikely that most of their experiences up to this point adequately prepare parents to face this kind of upheaval.

Nurses must be cognizant of the psychosocial needs of parents in crisis if holistic, family-centered care is to be given. Nurses must anticipate that a crisis is likely if they do not provide this support. Anticipatory guidance can be an effective strategy to reduce some of the family's stress and in some instances, avert a full-blown crisis.

SYMPTOMS

1. Feelings of helplessness, powerlessness

2. Withdrawal from newborn

3. Excessive crying, anger, unrealistic expectations of themselves or of the baby

4. Denial of a problem with the baby

5. Blaming of the partner for the baby's condition

6. Distrust of the health care professionals

7. Refusal to care for themselves or to leave the newborn's bedside

8. Disheveled appearance

9. Discrepancy between verbal and nonverbal cues

10. Failure to bond with infant

11. Turning away from previously held religious beliefs

12. Withdrawal from friends and family

13. Withdrawal from partner

14. Concealment of feelings

15. Preoccupation with retelling the birth experience

16. Expressions of role failure to produce a perfect child

17. Anticipatory grief

INTERVENTION STRATEGIES

1. Assess and identify the developmental needs of the parents:
   a. Support their self-esteem and self-concept by including them in the focus of the plan of care.
   b. Include parental needs when planning infant care and encourage their participation in care activities as the parents become ready for responsibility.

2. Assess the parents' expectations regarding their new role; if these expectations do not coincide with reality, a crisis may result.

3. Assess the parents' knowledge of child development, as this will affect expectations of the parent-child relationship.

4. Prepare the parents for what to expect from their baby and from the staff in the NICU.

5. Assess the parents' readiness to assume their new role:
   a. Encourage the parents to ask questions about their baby.
   b. Encourage the parents to express their concerns about the newborn's condition.
   c. Allow the parents to express ambivalence about the baby and the neonatal problem.

6. Assess and observe interactions between the mother and father for signs of failure to cope with the stressful situation:
   a. Excessive use of defense mechanisms on the part of one or both parents may threaten their relationship.
   b. Encourage open communication of feelings between the partners.
   c. Make referrals to social services, clergy, or psychologists as appropriate for emotional support. Parents often need reassurance from financial counselors about payment arrangements before they can cope with their baby's problem.
   d. Explore social support systems available to parents; a strong support system is necessary to circumvent a crisis.

7. Explore the parent's dreams and expectations of their child prior to birth to assist the parents in adjusting to the realities of their newborn.

8. Allow the parents to express their feelings openly and honestly without fear of being judged bad parents:
   a. Let them know it is OK to be angry and hurt that their child has a problem.
   b. Let them know that it is perfectly normal to resent other new parents who have "perfect" children.
   c. Let them know it is natural to feel emotionally and physically drained and to have friends or relatives take care of their other children for a time.
   d. Discourage the "super parents" syndrome, in which only they can do all things for the family, the other children, the baby, and each other.

9. Encourage parents to express their own personal needs; let them know it is acceptable to set aside time for themselves and each other.

10. Anticipate the parents' fear of their baby's death or illness once home; help them work through these feelings before time for discharge.

11. Discuss with the parents the role of the siblings with the new baby:
    a. Encourage parents to express problems they may be having with the children while the baby is hospitalized.
    b. See the Forgotten Siblings section (p. 67) for more specific guidelines.

12. Discuss the family's use of coping mechanisms; explore what strategies have worked best in the past and together plan what strategies can work under the present circumstances.

13. Anticipate what knowledge the parents need to care for the infant in the hospital and once home. Knowledge is a good defense against anxiety and may help avert a further crisis situation.

14. Provide psychosocial support for the whole family. A team approach may be necessary to utilize the resources within the institution. Religious organizations, social services, and other ancillary health team members can provide individual, family, or group support. The use of parent and grandparent support groups can serve to facilitate open communication that may alleviate anxiety.

Transition from the NICU to Home

Carole Kenner   Laurie Gunderson

DESCRIPTION

Transition from an NICU to home can be a frightening experience. It can be anticipated that parents will be quite relieved when the infant is ready for discharge, yet quite anxious about their ability to care for the baby. The dependency on high technology supports the idea that parents cannot easily assume responsibility of the care.

Infant care and parent care go hand and hand. The needs of one cannot be met without meeting the needs of the other. Health care professionals have a responsibility to provide family-centered care through assessment, identification and communication of the family's needs to all health care persons involved. Better continuity in care and discharge planning is then provided. The goal of parent care is the promotion of a psychologically comfortable transition to parenthood in the hospital and then home, and a healthy parent-child relationship.

Nurses must begin discharge planning from the day of admission. If they get into the habit of including parents as part of the care-giving team, the parents gradually learn infant care as the baby progresses and in a supervised environment. They may feel confident in their ability to meet their infant's needs and better able to take the infant home. Hurried instructions to the parents at the baby's discharge are rarely remembered or followed. Parents need an adjustment time before they are solely responsible for caring for their baby.

Parents must also be prepared for the transition by understanding that their infant may be different from the baby that has never been in the NICU environment. It is up to nurses to explain the reasons why the baby needs noise or a light left on in the room. After all, the baby may never have been in the dark since birth. Parents need to know that such infants often appear unresponsive in the new home environment since this home atmosphere is so quiet in contrast to the hospital unit. Parental expectations and need for support once at home must be explored prior to discharge if the transition from the NICU to home is to be a positive experience. Nurses can make a difference in the outcome of the homecoming.

SYMPTOMS

1. Anxiety as relates to the planned homecoming: anxiety may be exhibited in the form of decreased visiting, nonverbal facial clues such as frowns or grimaces, inability to retain information, short attention spans during teaching sessions; or making excuses for why the baby should remain in the hospital one more day.

2. Expression of fear that the baby will become ill or die once home.

3. Concern over how the siblings will respond to this vulnerable new family member.

4. Fear of failure as parents.

5. Fear of leaving the infant with sitters, friends, or relatives.

6. Withdrawal from the infant as discharge approaches.

INTERVENTION STRATEGIES

1. Begin to anticipate discharge needs upon admission of the mother to the hospital: assess the parents readiness and need for knowledge. This assessment is an ongoing process throughout the hospital stay.

2. Include parents as members of the care team from the beginning of the hospitalization; allow them to provide as much of the care as they feel comfortable with.

3. Teach parents gradually and with repetition the skills necessary for caring for the baby:
   a. Teach normal newborn care such as baths and umbilical cord care.
   b. Determine what special care needs the child will have at home, and prepare the parents for these care needs (e.g., for gastrostomy tube, tracheostomy, stoma care).
   c. Inform the parents that the infant may need to have a night-light left on in the room for the first few days at home as the baby has not been in the dark since birth. A radio may also help soothe the infant.
   d. Teach the parents about the habituation of noise in the home environment; their baby is used to shutting out noise in the NICU and so at first may be unresponsive to noises at home.

4. Provide parents with positive reinforcement as they attempt to care for the infant.

5. Explain the disease process or surgical problem and the signs and symptoms they must recognize that may signal a problem, once the baby is home.
   a. Help the parents to understand what long-term care needs and/or problems the child might have.
   b. Realistic expectations help the parents mobilize their resources effectively and plan for the future.

6. Encourage the parents to be realistic in their self-expectations:
   a. Exhaustion in new parents is the norm, but when a sick newborn goes home parents become oblivious to taking time for themselves.
   b. Remind them of the importance of their own needs including rest periods.
   c. Explore the support systems—such as church or synagogue, neighbors, friends, and family members—available to the parents and encourage the use of these resources to allow parents to recuperate from the hospital stay, the excitement of the homecoming, as well as the demands of the new baby.
   d. Help the parents to identify individuals who can give the parents "break time" from the infant, at least several hours every week. Parents need to understand this is not selfish but absolutely necessary for their psychological well-being.

7. Inform the parents that they can call the nursing and medical staff of the NICU for advice once the baby is home:
   a. Encourage open communication with the private pediatrician either via the parents or a summary of progress from the NICU directly to the physician.
   b. Give the parents emergency numbers to keep at the telephone, so that they may feel that help is available.
   c. Teach cardiopulmonary resuscitation to the parents if deemed necessary, or to offer them peace of mind. In some institutions it is necessary to obtain physician permission before cardiopulmonary resuscitation training is instituted within the institution.
   d. Encourage questions from the parents. Often parents are embarrassed about

calling physicians with "silly" questions but may feel less anxious if their NICU or nursery nurses are available by telephone to answer questions.

8. Make appropriate community referrals for follow-up care or resource support for medical supplies:
   a. Community agencies, hospital clinics, public health nurses, and surgical pharmacies are all good resources for parents.
   b. If a referral is made to a community agency, a discharge summary should be sent stating the follow-up needs of the family; this strategy increases the continuity of care for the family.
   c. Home follow-up is being done by some discharging hospitals, as infants are being discharged earlier under the constraints of Diagnostic-Related Groups System for determining hospital lengths of stay. If this is the hospital protocol, then have the visiting nurse meet the family prior to departure from the unit. This strategy increases the comfort of the parents.

9. Give parents a follow-up call 1 week after discharge. This call should be made by the primary nurse from the NICU or a nurse known to the parents. This strategy is not only good public relations for the hospital and encouragement for the parents, but may be an avenue of averting a crisis if a problem has arisen.

If these interventions are followed, parents and health care professionals alike can be confident in their ability to successfully make the transition from the high technological environment of the NICU to the supportive surroundings of home.

REFERENCES

Aguilera, D. C., & Messick, J. M. (1986). *Crisis intervention: Theory and methodology* (5th ed.). St. Louis: C.V. Mosby.
Greenspan, S. I. (1985). The ties that bind. *Working Mother*, January, 90-94.
Jenkins, R. L. & Tock, M. K. S. (1986). Helping parents bond to their premature infant. *Maternal Child Nursing, 11*(1), 32-34.

Anticipatory Grief

Johnson, S. H. (1986). *Nursing assessment and strategies for the family at risk: High-risk parenting* (2nd ed.) (pp. 15-60, 129-156). Philadelphia: J. B. Lippincott.
Sammons, W., & Lewis, J. (1985). *Premature babies: A different beginning*. St. Louis: C.V. Mosby.

BIBLIOGRAPHY

Adams, M. (1963). Early concerns of primigravida mothers regarding infant care activities. *Nursing Research, 12*, 42-77.

Barnard, K. W. (1984). The family as a unit of measurement. *Maternal Child Nursing, 9*, 21.

Borg, S., & Lasker, J. (1981). *When pregnancy fails.* Boston: Beacon.

Brown, C. C. (Ed.). (1984). The many facets of touch. Pediatric round table: 10. Somerville, NJ: Johnson & Johnson Baby Products.

Cohen, M. R. (1982). Parents' reactions to neonatal intensive care. In R. E. Marshall, C. Kasman, & L. S. Cape, (Eds.), *Coping with caring for sick newborns* (pp. 15-30). Philadelphia: W. B. Saunders.

DeWet, B., & Cywes, S. (1985). The birth of a child with a congenital anomaly. Part I. Some difficulties experienced by parents in the maternity home. *South African Medical Journal, 67*(8), 292-296.

Gardner, S. L., & Merenstein, G. B. (1986). Perinatal grief and loss: An overview. *Neonatal Network, 15*(2), 7-15.

Gennaro, S. (1985). Maternal anxiety, problem-solving ability, and adaptation to the premature infant. *Pediatric Nursing, 11*, 343-348.

Goodman, R. M., & Gorlin, R. J. (1983). *The malformed infant: An illustrated guide.* New York: Oxford University Press.

Horowitz, J. A., Hughes, C. B., & Perdue, B. J. (1982). *Parenting reassesed: A nursing perspective* (pp. 85-118). Englewood Cliffs, NJ: Prentice-Hall.

Jackson, P. L. (1985). When the baby isn't perfect. *AJN, 85*(4),396-399.

Julian, K. C., & Young, C. M. (1983). Comprehensive health care for the high-risk infant and family: Follow-up of the high risk family. *Neonatal Network, 2*(3), 32-35.

Kayiatos, R., Adams, J., & Gilman, B. (1984). The arrival of a rival: Maternal perceptions of toddlers' regressive behaviors after the birth of a sibling. *Journal of Nurse-Midwifery, 29*(3), 205-213.

Kelting, S. (1986). Supporting parents in the NICU. *Neonatal Network, 4*(6), 14-18.

Klaus, M. H., & Kennell, J. H. (1983). *Bonding: The beginning of parent-infant interaction* (3rd ed.). St. Louis: C. V. Mosby.

Kubler-Ross, E. (1969). *On death and dying.* New York: MacMillian.

Litchfield, M. L. (1983). Family-infant bonding. In K. Vestal & C. A. McKenzie (Eds.), *High risk perinatal nursing: The American association of critical-care nurses.* Philadelphia: W. B. Saunders, 64-79.

Maloney, M. J., Ballard, J. L., Hollister, L., & Shank, M. (1983). A prospective controlled study of scheduled sibling visits to a newborn intensive care unit. *Journal of the American Academy of Child Psychiatry, 22*(6), 565-570.

Mercer, R. T. (1981). The nurse and maternal tasks of early postpartum. *Maternal Child Nursing, 6*(5), 341-345.

Montgomery, L. V. (1983). Crisis periods and developmental tasks of the family of the premature infant. *Neonatal Network, 2*(3),26-31.

Rushton, C. Y. (1986). Promoting normal growth and development in the hospital environment. *Neonatal Network, 4*(6), 21-30.

Shiff, H.S. (1978). *Bereaved parent.* New York: Penguin Books.

Ventura, J. N. (1986). Parent coping: A replication. *Nursing Research, 31*(5), 269-273.

Wallisch, S. (1983). Stress: The infant, family, and nurse. In K. Vestal & C. A. McKenzie (Eds.), *High risk perinatal nursing: The American association of critical-care nurses* (pp. 97-117). Philadelphia: W. B. Saunders.

Chapter 4

Alterations in Effective Breathing Patterns

Jeanne Harjo   *Carole Kenner*
                    Ann Brueggemeyer

Respiratory distress in neonates can be caused by a wide variety of surgical problems. Obstructions or deviations can occur at any point along the respiratory tract. Other organs and tissues may exert pressure on the respiratory system, impeding air flow. It is most important to recognize and treat these problems as soon as possible. Providing a clear airway is essential. Stabilization of the infant must occur before surgical intervention is possible. In non-life-threatening problems surgical intervention may be postponed, but early recognition and treatment may improve outcome.

TRANSPORT

See Appendix A for guidelines.

ADMISSION SETUP

See Appendix B. In addition to the regular admission setup, intubation equipment should be available. Specific diagnostic and lab tests are also necessary for the infant with altered breathing patterns.

1. Intubation equipment:
   a. Laryngoscope with extra batteries
      i. straight blades, sizes 0-1
      ii. extra light bulbs for the laryngoscope

Neonatal Surgery: A Nursing Perspective
ISBN 0-8089-1893-1

   b. Intubation forceps
   c. Stylets
   d. Endotracheal tubes, sizes 2.5 (<1000 g), 3.0 (≤2500 g); 3.5 (≤4000 g)
   e. Lubricating ointment
   f. Stethoscope
   g. Securing devices:
     i. Benzoin, tape and sterile applicators
     ii. Logan bars
     iii. Suture material, size 4.0 black silk with straight needle

2. Diagnostic measurements and lab tests:
   a. Blood gas analysis, preferably arterial sample, for baseline
   b. Complete blood cell count (CBC) with differential
   c. Type and crossmatch
   d. Chest radiograph
   e. Urinalysis
   f. Baseline serum electrolyte levels and other tests as indicated

---

CHOANAL ATRESIA

Jeanne Harjo

DESCRIPTION

In choanal atresia, there is a blockage of the posterior nares. It may be due to a web, membrane, cartilage, or bone structure. The defect can be unilateral or bilateral. Unilateral defects may be undetected in the newborn period unless routine suctioning or passing of a catheter is performed. Bilateral lesions are frequently evident at the time of birth since infants are obligate nose-breathers.

ETIOLOGY

During the sixth to eighth week of gestation the oral-nasal cavity undergoes a separation. This process involves the formation of a partition between the palate and nasal chambers. In addition a wall is formed in the midline of the nasal cavity leaving a passageway, or choana, on either side. Failure to separate these two distinct passages results in an atresia of the choanae (Sadler, 1985).

INCIDENCE

Choanal atresia occurs in 1 of every 5000 live births, with it occurring more commonly in females having a positive link with familial pattern (Schaffer, Avery, & Taeusch, 1984).

SYMPTOMS

1. The inability to pass a nasogastric tube or a suction catheter beyond the posterior nares may be indicative of choanal atresia.

2. Mouth breathing (normal neonates are obligate nose-breathers).

3. The infant may be pink when awake and crying, as the mouth is open.

4. The infant may be cyanotic and retracting chest when asleep, as the mouth is closed.

5. Thick mucus in the nose may be found extending from the external nares to the point of the blockage.

DIAGNOSIS

1. Place a radiopaque orogastric tube to straight drainage to maintain gastric decompression and prevent aspiration.

2. Obtain anteroposterior (AP) and lateral radiographs of the head and neck. These will determine the presence of a nasal obstruction and its degree of severity.

3. To visualize soft-tissue obstructions that may not have been detected on x-ray film, insert methylene blue (3 drops) into nares. The inability to see the blue dye in the posterior pharynx is suggestive of choanal atresia.

4. Attempt direct visualization of the airway of the infant to rule out other forms of airway obstruction.

5. Insertion of an oral airway should result in improvement of the color of the infant.

6. An absence of air exchange on auscultation at the external nares is suggestive of choanal atresia.

7. Observe the newborn for associated defects: CHARGE syndrome (DiGeorge); coloboma, heart anomalies, atretic choanae, mental retardation, genital hypoplasia, and ear anomalies (Goodman & Gorlin, 1983).

TRANSPORT

The goal during transport is to maintain a patent airway and prevent respiratory compromise.

1. Insert an oral airway, size 0 or 00. If an airway tube is not avaliable, a rubber nipple with the end cut off may be used.

2. Maintain patency of the oral airway and nares (especially if the atresia is unilateral) by frequent suction. Avoid trauma to the airway as edema may further obstruct it.

3. Elevate the neonate's head to improve air exchange.

4. Allow for visualization of the head to assess the color of the lips and mucous membranes.

5. Provide respiratory support as dictated by the infant's condition.

6. If intubation is required, place the endotracheal tube orally (size 2.5, 3.0, or 3.5 depending on the size of the infant).

7. If NPO, start an IV site prior to transport. For specific guidelines see Chapter 9.

8. Parent care:
   a. For specific guidelines see Chapter 3.
   b. Explain to the parents the need for an oral airway.

ADMISSION EQUIPMENT

1. See Appendix B.

2. Oral airway tubes, sizes 0 and 00, should be kept available.

3. Use cloth tracheostomy tape to secure the oral airway.

4. Intubation equipment: see pages 79-80.

PREOPERATIVE STABILIZATION

Preoperative stabilization includes the maintenance of a patent airway and prevention of respiratory compromise while providing appropriate nutrition via oral or gavage feedings.

1. Respiratory status:
   a. Assess respiratory status: chest retractions, nose or mouth breathing, color, inability to pass catheter down one or both nares, presence of excess mucus in the nose, inability to auscultate air exchange at the nares. Reassess the neonate's color and respiratory status after insertion of an oral airway.
   b. Provide humidified oxygen or if no oxygen is needed place the infant in an oxygen hood with room-air mist to liquify nasal secretions.

2. Fluids, nutrition, and electrolyte levels:
   a. To maintain adequate hydration, give IV fluids if NPO status is necessary due to intolerance of feedings.
   b. To maintain adequate nutrition, keep infant on gavage feedings if tolerated.
   c. For more specific fluid and electrolyte level guidelines, see Chapter 9.

3. Infection:
   a. The infant is prone to aspirate if nipple feedings by bottle are attempted or if gavage feedings are given too rapidly (infants are obligate nose- breathers and so cannot breath and eat simultaneously).
   b. Respiratory infection may occur if secretions are not liquified or if the infant is not suctioned appropriately, at least every 2 hours.
   c. Mouth care with sterile water and petroleum ointment applied to the lips every 2-4 hours helps keep the mucous membranes moist and intact. This serves as a barrier to infection.
   d. Broad-spectrum antibiotics may be given: ampicillin 100 mg/kg/d IV in divided doses and gentamicin 5 mg/kg/d IV in divided doses, or according to hospital policy. Many institutions do not routinely administer preoperative antibiotics unless an infection is present.

SURGERY

The extensiveness of the surgery depends on the characteristics of the blockage. If the passage is occluded by a thin membrane, then a simple procedure is performed to open the passage. If bone or cartilage block the opening, then extensive surgery may need to be performed to remove the solid obstruction. If extensive surgery is needed, nasal passage areas may become swollen for long periods of time or may reclose. Inflammation may result over a long period of time leading to scar tissue formation physically closing the passage. In some cases, it is necessary to provide the infant with a temporary or permanent airway via a tracheostomy. In most cases, stints are placed in the nasopharynx to provide an open passage until tissue swelling has subsided and a permanent opening in the posterior nares has healed (Fig. 4-1).

POSTOPERATIVE STABILIZATION

Prevention of airway obstruction remains an important aspect of the immediate postoperative care of the infant.

1. Respiratory status:
   a. To maintain a patent airway, suction frequently (every 15-30 minutes) through the stints and around the stints, for the first 8 hours, then every 1-2 hours until secretions decrease. This may be necessary up until the time of the patient's discharge from the hospital.
   b. Stints will need to be manipulated in and out to maintain patency of the nares. Spectific guidelines are usually given by the surgeon.
   c. Vital signs, including the blood pressure, are checked every 15 minutes four times, every 30 minutes four times, every hour four times, and then every 2 hours for the remainder of the first 24 hours after surgery.

2. Fluids, electrolyte levels, and nutrition:
   a. Maintain IV fluids and electrolyte levels while infant is NPO according to the guidelines in Fluid and Electrolyte Status (p. 268) in Chapter 9.
   b. Feedings may be started as early as 24 hours after surgery. Nipple feedings may be given safely if the stints are kept patent. Oral gavage feedings are given if the infant is unable to nipple-feed. See Chapter 9 for specific guidelines on feedings.

3. Infection:
   a. To maintain suture-line integrity do not force nipple feedings. Instead, provide gentle oral gavage feedings and mouth care with sterile water every 2-4 hours.
   b. Antibiotics, as described in Preoperative Stabilization in this section can be given if there are signs of infection; otherwise, they are usually not prescribed.

4. Parent care:
   a. Involve the parents in the care of their infant.
   b. Encourage them to hold the baby.
   c. To promote home management, teach the parents the following:
      i. Suctioning of the stints (Fig. 4-1).
      ii. Signs and symptoms of blocked stints: respiratory difficulty, color changes, or the inability to pass a suction catheter down the stints.
   d. Help the parents obtain equipment necessary for home care, such as suction catheters and a suction machine.
   e. For more specific information about parent care see Chapter 3.

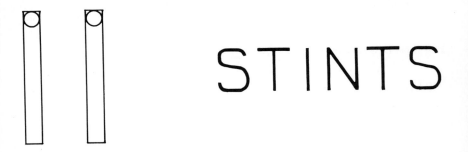

One stint is placed in each nare to provide a patent airway.

Fig. 4-1. One stint is placed in each nare to provide a patent airway.

Pierre Robin Syndrome
Carole Kenner

DESCRIPTION

Pierre Robin syndrome consists of micrognathia (small lower jaw), mandibular hypoplasia with associated shortened mandibular muscle, and cleft palate, which may or may not be present. The underlying problem of this syndrome is the maintenance of an airway. This is due to the tongue falling back into the posterior pharynx and occluding the esophagus, which creates a vacuum.

PATHOPHYSIOLOGY

Congenital mandibular hypoplasia is usually associated with a posterior tongue position. This combination may result in upper airway obstruction. Cleft palate may accompany this defect.

INCIDENCE

Mandibular hypoplasia often accompanies other syndromes, making it difficult to estimate the exact incidence.

SYMPTOMS

1. Receding chin with birdlike facies.

2. Respiratory difficulty in flat or side-lying position.

3. Choking, gasping, and respiratory distress during feedings.

4. Inability to feed due to posteriorly placed tongue.

DIAGNOSIS

1. Physical assesment of the palate for cleft.

2. External inspection of the chin and jaw for receding chin and shortened jaw.

3. Respiratory distress in the flat or side-lying position.

4. AP and lateral head and neck radiographs to rule out other upper respiratory obstructions.

5. Study of the baby sleeping, to determine the presence of obstructive apnea.

6. Transcutaneous oxygen monitor (TCM) study to determine oxygen and carbon dioxide status during sleep, position changes, and feedings.

TRANSPORT

The nurse should maintain a patent airway for the neonate by preventing occlusion by the tongue.

1. Place infant in the head-down position to allow the tongue to fall forward.

2. Place an oral airway or nasopharyngeal tube to stop a vacuum from occurring in the esophagus.

3. Suction nasopharyngeally and orally to maintain a patent airway.

4. See Appendix A for transport setup.

ADMISSION EQUIPMENT

1. Oral airway, sizes 0 and 00.

2. Cloth tape to secure oral airway.

3. Sutures if the tongue is to be sutured and secured.

4. See Appendix B for admission setup.

PREOPERATIVE STABILIZATION

1. Assess respiratory status to maintain a patent airway and facilitate ventilation:
   a. Keep the newborn's head down.
   b. Maintain the patency of the oral airway or nasopharyngeal tube by suctioning every 1-2 hours and as needed.
   c. Check vital signs every 2-4 hours.
   d. Provide oxygen as dictated by the infant's condition.
   e. Take AP and lateral neck x-ray films to identify structural airway anomalies.

2. Fluids, nutrition, and electrolyte levels:
   a. To provide adequate hydration, maintain IV fluids if NPO.
   b. Feed by nasal gavage, if tolerated by the infant, to provide nutritional support.
   c. For specific guidelines see Fluid and Electrolyte Status (pp. 263-290) in Chapter 9.

3. Parent care (See Chapter 3 for specific guidelines):
    a. To encourage parental involvement, keep communications open.
    b. To provide positive reinforcement, encourage the parents to visit and hold their baby.
    c. Offer explanations often. Be prepared to repeat the information frequently as little is retained at such a stressful period of time.
    d. Verify informed consent for surgery.

NONSURGICAL INTERVENTION

Nonsurgical intervention involves the use of either a nasopharyngeal tube or sutures placed in the tongue and then secured in extension to keep the airway patent. If no surgery is to be performed, the preoperative care can still be used with the addition of maintaining the position of the infant to insure extension of the tongue.

SURGERY

A tracheostomy is the usual form of surgical intervention. A gastrostomy tube may be placed if oral feedings are not possible.

POSTOPERATIVE CARE

Nursing care postoperatively focuses on the maintenance of a patent airway.

1. Respiratory status:
    a. If a tracheostomy is performed, maintain the patency of the trachea by sterile suctioning every 30 minutes to 1 hour, until the secretions have decreased.
    b. Mucus may be bloody at first due to the trauma of surgery.
    c. Report frank bleeding around or from the trachea to prevent aspiration pneumonia and maintain patency of airway.
    d. Check for edema around the tracheostomy tube which may apply pressure to the trachea and occlude the airway.
    e. Check for cyanosis or any color changes and respiratory difficulty such as retractions, decreased breath sounds, lung congestion, or nasal flaring.
    f. Do not change the tracheostomy ties while sutures are still in place. Such an action could result in trauma or displacement of the tracheal tube creating a blind canal.
    g. Do not place dressing around the tracheostomy while the sutures are in place. Direct visualization of the ostomy is essential. Attempts to dress the stoma may disrupt the suture line.

h. Check vital signs every 15 minutes four times, every 30 minutes four times, every hour four times, every 2 hours until 24 hours after surgery, and then every 4 hours if stable.

i. Give oxygen and ventilatory support as needed to maintain gas exchange.

2. Infection:

a. To prevent infection, maintain skin integrity by cleansing the stoma with hydrogen peroxide, placing antimicrobial ointment every 2-4 hours around the stoma, and using lubricating ointment around the stoma for a waterproof seal. The use of an ointment may not be recommended in some institutions due to the potential for obstruction of the stoma. Excessive use of ointments may also lead to aspiration pneumonia.

b. Keep the newborn's skin dry and free of mucus buildup to maintain skin integrity.

c. Antibiotics may be given as a precautionary measure. These dosages are suggested: ampicillin 100 mg/kg/d IV in divided doses and gentamicin 5 mg/kg/d IV in divided doses or according to hospital protocol. Many institutions do not use prophylactic antibiotics.

3. Fluids, electrolyte levels, and nutrition:

a. Continue the IV infusion for the first 24 hours after surgery to maintain fluid and electrolyte balance.

b. To provide nutrition, begin gavage feeding slowly.

c. A gastrostomy tube may be placed surgically at a later time if the infant is not tolerating gavage feedings. See Chapter 12 for gastrostomy-care guidelines (pp. 347-349).

d. Nipple feedings may be introduced as tolerated, when the infant no longer requires oxygen and is no longer having respiratory difficulty.

e. For a baseline check on fluid and electrolyte status, check serum electrolyte levels at least once every day. Serum electrolyte levels should be checked at least once a day while the newborn is receiving IV fluid therapy.

f. For specific guidlines see Fluid and Electrolyte Status in Chapter 9 for postoperative considerations (pp. 271-272).

PARENT CARE

1. To prepare for home management, teach the parents hygienic tracheostomy care and suctioning (see Tracheostomy Care in Chapter 12).

2. Help the parents obtain necessary equipment for the home such as suction equipment and gastrostomy equipment (see Gastrostomy Care in Chapter 12, pp. 347-349 for a list of specific supplies).

3. To prevent complications once home and to promote health maintenance, teach the parents the symptoms of respiratory distress or difficulty such as nasal flaring, color changes, and chest retractions.

4. Encourage the parents to call and visit the baby in the hospital.

5. For more specific information see Chapter 3.

Cleft Palate and Lip
Carole Kenner

DESCRIPTION

Cleft palate or lip results from a lack of proper development and fusion of the upper lip and/or palate. This fusion failure occurs during the 5th to 12th week of gestation. They are considered midline defects.

The cleft in the palate can either occur in the soft palate only or in both the hard and soft palate, as fusion occurs in the anterior-to-posterior direction. The cleft palate may be unilateral or bilateral if it is a complete (both palates) cleft. The cleft lip may also occur as unilateral incomplete (not extending into the nasal floor) or unilateral or bilateral complete (extending into the nasal cavity).

The cleft may be expressed as cleft lip, cleft palate, or both, or as a part of a congenital syndrome (Williams, Shprintzen, & Goldberg, 1985)—such as the Pierre Robin syndrome, with the co-existent cleft palate, or other midline defects such as found in Hirschsprung's disease (Goldberg & Shprintzen, 1981). Studies have shown that a greater percentage of children with clefts have other defects than found in the general population (Guzzetta, Randolph, Anderson, Boyajian, Eichelberger, & Avery, 1987).

ETIOLOGY

The etiology is unclear, but an autosomal recessive or a dominant inheritance has been suggested if the defect occurs by itself and not as a part of a syndrome. Besides genetic or familial factors, other factors such as drugs taken or diseases contracted by the mother during the second and third months of pregnancy have been shown to be significant in animal studies. Excessive intake of vitamin A has also been implicated.

INCIDENCE

Cleft palate or lip occurs in 1 of every 1000 to 1 of every 2500 live births. The defect is twice as common in male as in female newborns.

SYMPTOMS

The cleft palate or lip is usually readily visible. Only when the cleft occurs just in the soft palate does the cleft go undetected until an oral exam is made.

DIAGNOSIS

The diagnosis is made by direct observation; however, a cleft in the soft palate may go undetected unless observation is accompanied by a thorough oral exam. If either of these defects is present, a thorough exam should be done for other midline defects (internal and external).

TRANSPORT

1. See Appendix A.
2. Transport to a tertiary center may not be necessary since this is generally not a life-threatening problem. Corrective surgery will generally not be done until a minimum of 2 weeks after birth, and in many institutions not for 2-3 months in the case of cleft lip and later for the cleft palate. The palate repair is delayed to decrease the chance of disruption of tooth-bud formation and disturbance of normal facial growth.
3. If the baby is transported, no special precautions need to be observed unless another defect is present. If another defect is present, consult the appropriate section for transport information.

ADMISSION EQUIPMENT

See Appendix B. No special equipment is necessary.

PREOPERATIVE STABILIZATION

1. The goals preoperatively are to provide adequate nutrition, prevent aspiration or infection, and decrease or minimize speech-pattern disturbances.
2. Feeding difficulty is the primary problem:
   a. A regular or premie nipple may be used if only a cleft lip is present. Some surgeons do not allow infants to be fed with nipples as it is believed that the sucking on a pacifier or nipple increases the spread of the cleft lip.

b. A lamb's nipple (an elongated nipple that fits well into the infant's mouth) or an asepto syringe with a rubber tip may be necessary for palatal infants; sucking may not be achieved if a complete cleft is present. (Lamb's nipples are long and firm and may evoke the gag reflex. Other nipples and feeders for babies with cleft palates are available that allow for oral feeding without gagging the infant. Some parents may find these unacceptable methods of feeding as they set their child up as being different from the "normal" infant.)

c. If a syringe is used, direct the tip to the side of the mouth and give the feeding slowly while holding the infant in an upright position.

d. Burp the newborn frequently, every 5-10 minutes, as a lot of air is swallowed.

e. Feeding a baby with a cleft lip or palate can be long and frustrating, especially for the parents, so praise their efforts.

3. Aspiration is a danger in these children due to the regurgitation of formula that occurs up through the palatal opening and in the nasal passages:

a. To prevent infection, clean mouth with water after each feeding to remove any excess formula.

b. To prevent aspiration, place the baby in an upright position in an infant seat, elevate the head of the bed, or place the baby on the abdomen after feedings.

4. Ear infections are more likely in these infants as the eustachian tube is short and easily accessible to bacteria from the nasal and oral cavities. If the palate, which creates a barrier between the oral and nasal cavities, is not present, the chances for infection are greater.

a. Assess the infant for signs of ear infection, such as excessive crying, fever, or increased irritability.

b. To prevent complications and promote health maintenance, teach the parents about ear infections, their signs and how to keep the oral and nasal cavities clean after feedings.

c. Polyethylene tubes may be necessary.

5. Speech-pattern disturbances are possible in the baby with a cleft palate and should be discussed with the parents in the preoperative period.

6. To prevent long-term orthodontia problems, teach the parents to observe tooth formation and to consult a dentist for follow-up care even in the baby's early months of life.

7. Parental support: The nurse needs to educate the parents about the long-term treatment expectations and the need for multidisciplines to be involved: surgeons, dentists, orthodonists, speech/language therapists, pediatricians, otolaryngologists, social workers, psychologists, nurses, audiologists, and genetic counselors all may eventually treat the child.

SURGERY

Cheilorrhaphy (ki-loráh-fe) or Z-plasty is a staggered Z-shaped suture line that unites the edges of the cleft lip. A splint or Logan bar may be used to maintain the position of the lip for healing. Revisions of the lip may be necessary in adolescence. Surgery for a cleft lip usually takes place at the age of 2-3 months. A rule of 10 is often used: 10 pounds, 10 g/dL hemoglobin and 10,000 mm³ WBC. Some physicians do perform the surgery when the baby is only 2 weeks old (Guzzetta, Randolph, Anderson, Boyajian, Eichelberger, 1987).

Palatal surgery involves uniting the palatal segments. The exact procedure varies with the type of defect. It may be a one- or two-stage procedure. Initial surgery occurs at 18-24 months of age. However, some physicians delay surgery until the fourth year or longer to promote normal facial growth (Jorgenson, Sharpiro, & Odinet, 1984) . This surgery is later than the lip repair, as earlier surgery would interfere with the growth pattern of the palate, maxilla, and tooth bud. Revisions of the surgery usually take place at age 8 years.

POSTOPERATIVE STABILIZATION

The postoperative goals are to maintain adequate nutrition, to prevent infection and trauma of the suture line, to prevent respiratory distress and hemorrhage, and to decrease parental anxiety.

1. Monitor the vital signs closely: Check the temperature, pulse, respiration, and BP every 15 minutes four times, every 30 minutes four times, every hour four times, every 2 hours until stable, and then every 4 hours.

2. Maintain IV access:
   a. Give maintenance fluids to keep the baby hydrated (usually necessary the first 24 hours after surgery).
   b. For specific guidelines see Fluid and Electrolyte Status in Chapter 9 for postoperative considerations (p. 271-272).
   c. Antibiotics may be given prophylactically: penicillin IV days 1-3, then IM for 2-7 days.

3. To prevent disruption of the suture line, restrain the neonate's arms—usually elbow restraints are used:
   a. Pin arm restraints to diaper or clothing to keep infant from rubbing the suture line.
   b. Check neonate's arms and hands for circulation status every 2 hours.

4. Feedings should be done with an asepto syringe or cleft lip or palate feeder for approximately 3 weeks to prevent pressure on suture line:
   a. Feedings should generally be restarted 24 hours after surgery.
   b. Discourage the baby from sucking—no pacifier.

    c. Palate surgery may necessitate a high-calorie liquid diet for approximately 1 month to meet nutritional needs during the healing process.

    d. To prevent suture-line trauma, no metal utensils, plastic cups, straws, or glasses should be used to feed the baby.

5. Cleanse suture line to prevent infection:

    a. Swab with rolled sterile applicator moistened with water and hydrogen peroxide. Antiseptic ointment may be used. Do not rub suture line. Such an action may result in trauma and disruption of the healing process.

    b. To prevent infection, rinse the baby's mouth with water or saline solution after feedings.

    c. Apply antibiotic ointment to the lip to guard against infection.

6. Observe lip and/or palate for bleeding or separation of suture line.

7. Try to keep the baby from crying as it puts a stress on the suture line.

8. To prevent trauma to lip repair, position the baby in an infant seat or on the baby's back but never on the abdomen as the infant will rub the suture line.

9. Increased mucus and edema may occur—suction gently, if absolutely necessary, to avoid traumatizing the suture line.

    a. To promote circulation and decrease tissue swelling provide humidified air.

    b. Elevate the head of the bed to decrease the incidence of aspiration of mucus.

10. Observe for the two major complications of the postoperative period—hemorrhage and respiratory distress.

11. To prevent long-term complications of hearing loss, assess for signs of otitis media, as the eustachian tube may be partially blocked after palatal surgery:

    a. Fever

    b. Increased irritability

    c. Pulling at the ear (if the child is older)

    d. Excessive crying

12. Long-term considerations include psychological support for the older child and family:

    a. The body image for the child may be altered; parents need to understand this.

    b. Multiple hospitalizations may be necessary to complete the repair.

    c. The nurse needs to coordinate the multidisciplines involved in the care (see Preoperative Stabilization for the specific disciplines that may be involved).

    d. The child's speech may be altered, setting the child apart from others; hypernasal speech, especially affecting the p, b, d, t, sh, h, and g sounds, often occurs after palatal surgery.

PARENT CARE

1. See Chapter 3 for specific guidelines.

2. Bonding with the infant may be difficult for parents, as the visible defect is a constant reminder of their child's problem.

3. Grief for the loss of the "perfect child" is natural:
   a. Encourage the parents to verbalize their feelings.
   b. Allow them to express guilt especially if there is a positive familial history of cleft palates or lips.
   c. Allow the parents privacy and time to sort out their feelings.
   d. Involve the parents only when they are ready and praise their efforts. Remember it is not easy to feed a baby with a cleft lip or palate.

4. Examine support systems for the parents:
   a. The cost of the treatment of these children may be in the tens of thousands of dollars.
   b. Agencies such as Crippled Children's and Medical Insurance Companies as well as some welfare monies can assist families financially.

Tracheoesophageal Fistula
Jeanne Harjo

DESCRIPTION

Tracheoesophageal fistula (TEF) is a term commonly used for a variety of defects of the trachea and esophagus. It occurs either as esophageal atresia with tracheal fistula, as esophageal atresia alone, or with fistula alone.

There are five types: (1) esophageal atresia with distal tracheoesophageal fistula; (2) esophageal atresia without tracheoesopheal fistula; (3) tracheo-esophageal fistula without esophageal atresia, H-type; (4) esophageal atresia with proximal and distal fistula; and (5) esophageal atresia with proximal fistula.

ETIOLOGY

Tracheoesophageal fistula occurs during the middle of the first trimester from a failure of the foregut to divide into separate digestive and respiratory segments.

INCIDENCE

The defect occurs in 1 of every 1500 live births, with an equal ratio in male to female newborns (Schreiner, 1982).

RISK FACTORS

1. Maternal history of polyhydramnios.

2. Neonatal cardiac and gastrointestinal (GI) anomalies. Tracheoesophageal Fistula is often found in conjunction with cardiac and GI anomalies.

Esophageal atresia with distal tracheoesophageal fistula is the most common variety of TEF. It is used here as an example for nursing care. Any variations are noted under the subsequent sections Tracheoesophageal Fistula without Esophageal Atresia and Esophageal Atresia without Tracheoesphageal Fistula, as these defects provide the most comprehensive examples of surgical nursing care.

Esophageal Atresia with Distal Tracheoesophageal Fistula
Jeanne Harjo

DESCRIPTION

Esophageal atresia with distal tracheoesophageal fistula is the most common esophageal anomaly found in the newborn. In this defect the upper esophagus ends in a blind pouch (atresia). There is an abnormal connection (fistula) that joins the distal esophagus and stomach to the trachea.

SYMPTOMS

1. Identification can be made before birth by
   a. Ultrasound.
   b. Maternal history, especially polyhydramnios. (The excess amniotic fluid occurs because the fetus is unable to swallow due to the esophageal atresia.)

2. Excess saliva and mucus. After delivery, the newborn's inability to swallow results in a buildup of mucus and saliva being collected in the blind pouch.

3. Inability to insert a nasogastric tube: the pouch will not allow a nasogastric tube to be inserted beyond it because there is no communication between the upper and lower esophagus.

4. Choking and aspiration during feeding: when the infant is fed, formula will collect in the pouch and the baby will choke and may experience respiratory difficulty.

5. Aspiration pneumonia may occur due to: (1) esophageal atresia, which allows fluid to spill over into the lungs, or (2) reflux due to the distal TEF connecting the trachea to the distal esophagus. This allows acidic gastric juices to reflux into the lung, creating pneumonia.

DIAGNOSIS

Early confirmation is extremely important to prevent aspiration pneumonia.

1. Pass a radiopaque tube, size 10 double lumen, into the esophageal pouch. Do not force the tube.

2. Aspirate the tube. The secretions will be cloudy mucus or saliva. Record the amount and characteristics of the aspirate and discard.

3. Inject 5-10 cc of air with a 12-cc syringe and clamp the tube. (If contrast material is to be used for injection in place of air, it should be injected with great caution. This step can be hazardous, with overflow from the esophageal pouch and aspiration into the lungs. Therefore it is rarely recommended.)

4. Obtain an AP radiograph that includes the neck, chest, and abdomen.

5. Keep the head of the newborn's bed elevated during this procedure.

TRANSPORT

Once a TEF is suspected, the infant should be immediately transferred to a tertiary facility for surgical intervention. The quicker the transport is accomplished the more likely it is to prevent respiratory compromise. The nursing goal during transport is to prevent aspiration and promote ventilation.

1. See Appendix A.

2. Place a double-lumen tube, size10, into the esophageal pouch until resistance is met. Aspirate every 15-30 minutes.

3. Position the infant prone or with head elevated to prevent reflux.

ADMISSION EQUIPMENT

1. See Appendix B.

2. Wall suction unit, either continuous or intermittent; double-lumen catheter. This equipment is secondary to regular suction equipment for esophageal decompression.

PREOPERATIVE STABILIZATION

Initially a gastrostomy tube should be inserted to prevent aspiration pneumonia resulting from reflux.

1. Admission workup:
   a. See Appendix B.
   b. To determine the extent of the atretic area and the position and extent of the fistula, obtain AP chest, neck, and abdominal radiographs.

2. To prevent aspiration:
   a. Place a double-lumen esophageal tube to low-intermittent or low-continuous suction. Irrigate the tube with 2 cc of air every 1-2 hours to maintain the patency of the tube.
   b. Increased secretions around the esophageal tube indicate an obstruction. Aspirate and irrigate with air or sterile water to dislodge the blockage of the tube. (Using sterile water for irrigation prior to surgical repair is not acceptable in all institutions as aspiration may occur. Hospital protocol should be consulted.) If tube becomes dislodged or blocked, reinsert catheter with great care to avoid perforation of the esophageal pouch.
   c. Keep the newborn's head elevated at 40°, even when obtaining radiographs, to prevent aspiration.

3. Respiratory support as needed: Use minimal pressure with mask or endotracheal tube to ventilate. Use just enough pressure to move the chest. Minimal pressure helps prevent rupture of the esophageal pouch and overdistention of the stomach with ensuing reflux through the fistula.

4. Fluids and electrolytes:
   a. See Chapter 9 for specific guidelines.
   b. Give supplemental fluids to compensate for the loss of esophageal secretions as well as maintenance fluids for hydration.

5. Antibiotic therapy:
   a. Broad-spectrum antibiotic therapy is necessary for resolution of pneumonia and for prevention of infection prior to surgery.
   b. In general, ampicillin 100 mg/kg/d IV in divided doses is given along with gentamicin 5mg/kg/d IV in divided doses. These are just guidelines and must be adapted to each infant and each hospital protocol.

6. Parent Care: See Chapter 3 for specific care.

SURGERY

Repair of the defect involves the insertion of a gastrostomy tube. A central-line catheter may be placed if gastrostomy feedings cannot be started in a few days. Repair of TEF involves exposure and ligation of the fistula through a right thoracotomy; the fistula will be tied off so there is no longer a connection between the distal esophagus and the trachea. Repairing esophageal atresia involves an end-to-end anastomosis. The two parts of the esophagus are joined to make a complete pathway to the stomach. When the esophageal ends cannot be connected because of too great a distance, other procedures are needed. Before anastomosis, the esophagus should be dilated and stretched daily with a size 10-12 red rubber catheter. To allow for growth, a cervical esophagostomy may be performed before the anastomosis. This procedure is described later in this section (p. 105).

POSTOPERATIVE STABILIZATION

Nursing care in the postoperative period focuses on maintenance of ventilation, prevention of disruption of the suture lines, and maintenance of gastric decompression.

Gastrostomy Tube

1. Prevention of infection.
   a. The resolution of any pneumonia is imperative to prepare the infant for repair of the defect.
      i. Observe for and report any fever.
      ii. Evaluate the character of respirations, noting any chest retractions or nasal flaring.
      iii. Ausculate the lungs and note any diminished breath sounds; any congestion; rhonchi or rales.
      iv. Note any cyanosis of the mucous membranes, nailbeds, or skin.
   b. Close observation of the gastrostomy tube is needed to detect any infection.
      i. Evaluate abdomen for presence of bowel sounds.
      ii. Observe gastrostomy site for any redness or drainage.

2. Maintain fluid and electrolyte balance: see Chapter 9 for specific guidelines.

3. Promote oxygenation and prevent respiratory compromise:
   a. Administer chest physiotherapy, vibration of the chest to loosen mucus, every 2 hours for infants with atelectasis.
   b. Suction to the end of the esophageal pouch. Use a marked catheter—measured against one marked by the surgeon to the depth just short of the end of the esophageal pouch. Use a No. 8 for suctioning every 2 hours and as needed.
   c. Turn the newborn from side to side every 2 hours to promote ventilation.
   d. Provide oxygen as required, using the preoperative precautions as described in Preoperative Stabilization (p. 97) in this chapter.
   e. Obtain arterial or capillary blood gas levels every 2-4 hours and 30 minutes after each oxygen or ventilator change to detect any changes in respiratory status.

4. Maintain gastric decompression: The gastrostomy tube is a No.12-16 malencot or "mushroom" catheter, which serves to decompress the stomach and abdomen:
   a. Irrigate the gastrostomy tube every 2-4 hours with 2 cc of air to keep the tube patent.
   b. Place the gastrostomy tube to straight gravity drainage.
   c. Observe and record the amount, color, and consistency of the drainage; then discard secretions. Never clamp the gastrostomy tube: reflux from the stomach to the lungs through the fistula may occur. Fistula ligation may be performed at the time of the original surgery. In some instances it is deferred until the infant is stabilized.

5. Prevention of aspiration
   a. Maintain patency of the esophageal tube by irrigating with 2 cc of air every 2 hours.
   b. Care remains the same as in the preoperative period.
   c. Continue to position the tube with the baby's head elevated.

6. Parent care: see Chapter 3 for specific care.

Fistula Ligation and Anastomosis

One-to-one nursing care is strongly suggested for the first 24-72 hours to prevent postoperative complications.

1. Nasopharyngeal suction with a marked catheter (No. 8 marked by the surgeon for the depth to suction to prevent breakage of the suture line) may be necessary as frequently as every 15-30 minutes for the first 6-8 hours, then every 1-2 hours as needed for 3-4 days to minimize secretions and to keep the anastomosis open. Suctioning should be tailored to individual needs.

2. Respiratory support may range from heated room-air mist (to liquify secretions) to endotracheal intubation, depending upon the baby's preoperative condition and complications encountered in surgery. If the baby is intubated, suction the endotracheal tube every 1-2 hours without the marked catheter. Use minimal pressure as described in previous sections.

3. If reintubation is necessary, the most qualified person should be called to perform the procedure to protect the suture line. The surgeon, neonatologist, or anesthesiologist should be available for this procedure.

4. Chest tube or tubes for drainage may be inserted during the surgical repair. Thoracic surgery may result in a compromise in the respiratory system such as atelectasis, pneumothorax, or collection of air or fluid in the pleural space. Chest tubes will facilitate the reexpansion of the lung or promote fluid drainage.
   a. Maintain the patency of the chest tube by placing the tube to low, continuous wall suction and stripping the chest tube every 4 hours.
   b. Record and report the amount, color, and consistency of the chest-tube drainage.

5. Intravenous therapy for hydration and electrolyte balance is necessary. If the infant is to remain NPO for a prolonged period, hyperalimentation may be required. See Chapter 9 for specific guidelines.

6. To prevent infection, broad-spectrum antibiotics may be given postoperatively. See Preoperative Stabilization antibiotic therapy (p. 97).

7. Position newborn to promote removal of secretions and prevent aspiration:
   a. Keep newborn supine and with the head of the bed elevated 40°.
   b. Change infant's position every 2 hours. Do not apply pressure on the chest tube or suture line.

8. Gastrostomy care to promote gastric decompression and prevention of electrolyte imbalance:
   a. Place gastrostomy tube to gravity drainage. Irrigate tube every 2 hours with 2 cc of air.
   b. Record and report the amount, color, and consistency of the gastric drainage every 8 hours. Discard and replace fluid loss via IV infusion see Fluid and Electrolyte Status (p. 263-274) in Chapter 9 for a discussion of gastric drainage and fluid losses.

9. Feedings:
   a. Seven to 10 days after surgery, an attempt should be made to give a clear liquid, colored with dye (e.g., Pedialyte®, 15 cc with 2 drops of methylene blue), by mouth. Then observe the gastrostomy and chest-tube drainage. Blue drainage from the chest tube signifies a suture-line leakage. Blue drainage from the gastrostomy tube shows an intact suture line.
   b. Gastrostomy feedings:
      i. Give feedings by IV slow drip for a period of 20 minutes. Feedings must be given slowly to prevent gastric distention, which may lead to vomiting, aspiration, or disruption of suture line.
      ii. Aspirate the gastrostomy tube before feedings; record and report characteristics of drainage, and reinsert the aspirate. Excessive amounts of retained gastric feedings indicate a lack of intestinal absorption. Aspirates are reinserted to maintain the balance of electrolyte levels as stomach acids could be discarded along with feeding.
   c. Nipple feedings:
      i. Before nipple feeding, an upper GI series is done to document an intact suture line.
      ii. Begin nipple feedings gradually with 10 percent of the feeding offered by mouth; the narrowed site of the anastomosis with dilated upper esophagus may make swallowing difficult for the baby. Use the gastric drip for the remainder of the feedings. The sucking reflex may be weak as the infant has not been fed orally and may not have used a pacifier. Much encouragement may be necessary to begin nipple feedings. Oral feedings require a great deal of energy. Infants should not be forced to nipple-feed for an extended period of time, as this increases caloric consumption and may lead to weight loss.

iii. Increase the amount taken by nipple as tolerated by the infant. For specific progression of the feedings see Chapter 9.

Observing for Complications

1. Signs of leakage of the fistula ligation:
   a. Formula drainage from the chest tube with the feedings.
   b. Duskiness or choking with feedings.
2. Signs of narrowed esophageal anastomosis:
   a. Increased oral mucus and saliva.
   b. Difficulty swallowing feedings; choking and spitting with feedings.

PARENT CARE

See Chapter 3 for specific guidelines.

DISCHARGE PLANNING

The nursing goal is to familiarize the parents with the signs of complications and need for follow-up. Parental anxiety may be lessened as common complications for this problem are anticipated.

1. Educate the parents about signs of fistula leakage or the narrowing of the esophageal anastomosis.
2. Demonstrate an upright position for the infant and explain the need for this to prevent reflux.
3. Explain the need for frequent esophageal dilatations if anastomosis is narrow.
4. Explain that there is a characteristic "barking" cough due to narrowing and edema of the esophagus. Explain that this barking is normal and will decrease with age.

Tracheoesophageal Fistula Without Esophageal Atresia
Jeanne Harjo

DESCRIPTION

H-type tracheoesophageal fistula is an intact esophagus with a fistula from the trachea to the esophagus.

SYMPTOMS

1. Repeated pneumonia from aspiration.
2. Coughing and choking with feeding.

DIAGNOSIS

1. Bronchoscopy can pinpoint the fistula.
2. Barium swallow or water-soluble contrast also locates the fistula but the barium or contrast dye may be aspirated into the lungs through the fistula; water-soluble contrast may be preferred.

TRANSPORT

The nursing goal during transport is to prevent aspiration and promote ventilation.

1. See Appendix A.
2. Position infant with the head elevated to prevent reflux.
3. Place a nasogastric tube to suction or gravity drainage to decompress the stomach and thus prevent aspiration.

PREOPERATIVE STABILIZATION

1. Admission setup: see Appendix B.
2. Feedings may be given by gavage with a No. 8 feeding tube, removed after each feeding. Oral feedings are contraindicated because of the potential for aspiration. Nutrition can be maintained easily with intermittent gavage feedings.
3. Keep the baby's head elevated especially during feedings to prevent further pneumonia.
4. Turn the baby from side to side evey 2 hours to improve gastric motility, promote adequate ventilation, and prevent skin breakdown.
5. Broad-spectrum antibiotic therapy is utilized to resolve the pneumonia (these are just guidelines and must be adapted to each infant and each hospital protocol):
   a. Ampicillin 100 mg/kg/d IV in divided doses
   b. Gentamicin 5 mg/kg/d IV in divided doses

6. Administer chest physiotherapy and suction every 2-4 hours to resolve the pneumonia if present.

SURGERY

Surgery involves the transcervical division and suture closure of both sides of the fistula. Usually it does not require a thoracotomy.

POSTOPERATIVE STABILIZATION

The postoperative course is relatively short depending upon the preoperative condition and surgical complications. See the Postoperative Stabilization (p. 99) Esophageal Atresia with Distal Tracheoesophageal Fistula in this chapter.

PARENT CARE

See Chapter 3 for guidelines.

Esophageal Atresia Without Tracheoesophageal Fistula
Jeanne Harjo

DESCRIPTION

In esophageal atresia without tracheoesophageal fistula the upper portion of the esophagus ends in a blind pouch; there is no connection between the upper and lower esophagus. There is no fistula between the trachea and the esophagus.

SYMPTOMS

1. Maternal polyhydramnios.

2. Increased mucus production.

3. Inability to pass a nasogastric tube to stomach.

4. Cyanosis and difficult breathing if baby is fed.

DIAGNOSIS

1. Obtain a radiograph of the chest, neck, and abdomen after insertion of the size 10 double-lumen tube into the esophageal pouch. At the end of the radiopaque

tube is a blind pouch with no connection to the stomach. Occasionally, a small portion of the distal esophagus is visible above the stomach.

TRANSPORT

Nursing-care goals focus on prevention of aspiration and promotion of adequate ventilation:

1. See Appendix A.

2. Place a size 10 double-lumen tube into the esophageal pouch until resistance is met. Aspirate every 15-30 mintues. If suction is available, low-continuous or intermittent suction may be used.

3. Position newborn prone or with head elevated to prevent aspiration.

PREOPERATIVE STABILIZATION

1. Admission workup: see Appendix B.

2. Place the double-lumen esophageal tube to low-intermittent or continuous suction. Irrigate tube with 2 cc of air every 1-2 hours to maintain patency.

3. Increased secretions around the esophageal tube indicate an obstruction. Aspirate and irrigate the tube to clear. If unable to remove obstruction, remove the tube and irrigate to unblock, or change the tube. Reinsertion must be performed with great caution to avoid perforation of the esophageal pouch.

4. Keep neonate's head elevated, even when obtaining radiographs, to prevent aspiration.

SURGERY

A gastrostomy tube is inserted to allow for feedings. An end-to-end anastomosis of the esophageal ends is performed. Cervical esophagostomy may be performed if the esophageal segments cannot be joined. Some institutions may continue to use a double-lumen catheter to aspirate esophageal pouch secretions.

POSTOPERATIVE STABILIZATION FOR ANASTOMOSIS

1. Suctioning with a No. 8 as often as every 15-30 minutes may be necessary for the first 6-8 hours and then every 1-2 hours. This suctioning should be individualized as needed to keep the anastomosis open. This catheter should be marked by the surgeon for the depth of suctioning required.

2. Gastrostomy feedings must be given slowly for a period of 20 minutes. Rapid gastric distention may lead to vomiting, aspiration, or disruption of the suture line.
   a. Check gastric aspirate before each feeding. Large amounts of retained stomach contents may indicate a lack of intestinal absorption.
   b. Record findings and reinsert aspirate. If stomach contents are discarded, important electrolytes may be lost.
3. Nipple feedings are started when an upper GI series has documented an intact anastomosis.

POSTOPERATIVE STABILIZATION FOR ESOPHAGOSTOMY

Cervical esophagostomy is the surgical opening of the upper portion of the esophagus onto the lateral neck via a small stoma. It is performed to allow oral secretions to drain without the use of an indwelling esophageal catheter.

1. To promote skin integrity, provide esophageal care every 4 hours or as needed, including the following steps:
   a. Apply petroleum jelly to skin after cleansing skin with water, to create a barrier to irritating secretions.
   b. Apply absorbent dressing to absorb secretions and to prevent rash caused by the secretions.
   c. Report any decreased esophagostomy secretions as this indicates the need for dilatation of the stoma.
2. Gastrostomy tube feedings:
   a. Begin with slow gastric drip feedings for a period of 20 minutes. Rapid gastric distention leads to dumping into the intestine, causing diarrhea and malabsorption of nutrients.
      i. Check gastric aspirate before each feeding to determine the amount of gastric absorption.
      ii. Record findings and reinsert aspirate to prevent loss of gastric electrolytes and fluids.
   b. Clamp the gastrostomy tube after feedings to promote absorption.
3. Oral feedings for stimulation of sucking and swallowing should be offered to the baby; however, all feedings taken by mouth will drain from the esophagostomy and should not be recorded as intake.

PARENT CARE

See Chapter 3 for specific guidelines.
1. Gastrostomy care: teach the parents the following procedures to prepare them for home management:

   a. Cleanse the skin around the tube and change dressing every day and as needed to promote skin integrity. See Gastrostomy Care (pp. 347-349) in Chapter 12.

   b. If the gastrostomy tube is dislodged, place an absorbent dressing, bib, or washcloth over the opening to absorb any stomach contents. Bring the infant to the emergency room to replace the tube. The tube must be replaced as soon as possible while the tract to the stomach is open. (In some cases, parents are taught how to replace the tube when traveling distance may preclude their return to the hospital.)

2. Gastrostomy feedings:
   a. Give gastrostomy feedings with syringe or meat baster for a period of 20 minutes.
   b. See Gastrostomy Feeding (pp. 350-351) in Chapter 12.

3. Esophagostomy care (to prevent skin breakdown and infection at the site):
   a. Prevent infection and rash by cleansing skin with water every 4 hours or as needed. Use a bib or washcloth to absorb secretions.
   b. Place petroleum jelly around the stoma every 4 hours to create a barrier from irritating secretions.

4. Oral feedings:
   a. Encourage nipple feedings to stimulate the sucking and swallowing reflexes.
   b. Be alert to observe whether formula is draining from the esophagostomy when bottle feeding; otherwise, the stoma may not be patent.

5. Complications:
   a. Decreased secretions from the esophagostomy indicate the stoma's closure. This will require dilatation. If this condition is allowed to continue, infection and aspiration may occur.
   b. A closure of the esophagostomy may also be indicated by a failure of oral feedings to drain or an increase in oral secretions.

6. An end-to-end anastomosis should be done when the newborn grows.

VACTERL SYNDROME

Some infants with tracheoesophageal fistulas have other associated anomalies as well. These associated anomalies are classified as Vacterl Syndrome:

V   Vertebral anomalies
A   Anal anomalies such as imperforate anus
C   Cardiac anomalies
T   Tracheal anomalies as described in this section
E   Esophageal anomalies as described in this section
R   Renal anomalies such as polycystic kidneys
L   Limb deformities such as absent radii

Diaphragmatic Hernia
Jeanne Harjo

DESCRIPTION

Diaphragmatic hernia, or hernia of Bochdalek, is the herniation of the posterolateral aspect of the diaphragm, which causes the presence of abdominal contents in the chest cavity above one or both diaphragms. The stomach and both large and small intestines are most often found in the chest cavity. Spleen, liver, kidney, and other abdominal organs are less frequently found there. This herniation most often occurs through the left diaphragm. It may be the most urgent of all neonatal surgical emergencies. It often progresses rapidly into fatal respiratory distress. At other times, if the lung is not markedly compromised, the symptoms are minimal and may only be detected by a routine radiograph.

ETIOLOGY AND PATHOPHYSIOLOGY

During the second to third month of gestation the diaphragm forms. It serves to separate the thoracic cavity from the abdominopelvic cavity. First a partition forms between the peritoneal and pericardial cavities, called the septum transversum. Next the septum transversum joins together with pleuroperitoneal membranes to complete the separation from the thoracic, abdominal, and peritoneal cavities. When the pleuroperitoneal membranes fail to fuse with the septum transversum, a diaphragmatic hernia results. This weakened area allows abdominal contents to herniate. The lung development on the affected side may be impaired as the abdominal contents are found in the thoracic cavity, thus giving the lung no room to develop. The amount of abdominal contents that freely enter into the thoracic cavity depends upon the size of the area of pleuroperitoneal membranes that remain open. The most common site for the herniation is in the area of the left lung, the posterolateral segment of the diaphragm.

INCIDENCE

Diaphragmetic hernia occurs in approximately 1 of every 2000 births, with male newborns more commonly affected than female newborns.

SYMPTOMS

The onset of symptoms is related to the severity of the defect. Those who develop severe respiratory distress within hours of birth have a much more serious defect than those who are more than 24 hours of age before the problems arise. The following are characteristic of the defect:

1. Usually a normal pregnancy with a full-term infant.

2. Respiratory distress, from moderate to severe:
   a. Cyanosis.
   b. Tachypnea: respiratory rate >60 breaths per minute.
   c. Chest retractions.
   d. Decreased or absent breath sounds on the affected side. The use of oxygen via face mask or oxygen hood will usually not show an improvement if the affected lung is hypoplastic.

3. Increased chest diameter with asymmetry.

4. Abdomen flat or scaphoid.

5. Bowel sounds may be heard in the chest (rare).

6. Heart sounds may be heard from the right side of the chest if the hernia is on the left.

DIAGNOSIS

The only diagnostic procedure required is obtaining an AP chest and abdominal radiograph to identify any of the following:

1. Loops of bowel in the chest

2. Heart displaced to the right if hernia is on the left

3. Only a small spot of the lung is visible on the affected side

4. Abdominal cavity filled with air

5. Mediastinal shift

TRANSPORT

The nursing goal for transporting this infant is to maintain gastric decompression and adequate ventilation. These goals may be difficult to accomplish since the infant can be very unstable and require continuous ventilatory assistance.

1. See Appendix A.

2. Give warm humidified oxygen to keep the baby's skin pink and allow for easy respiration:
   a. Do not ventilate the baby with a face mask. This will force air into the stomach and intestines, increasing their volume in the chest and causing more compression in an already compressed lung.

b. Use endotracheal ventilation if required.

3. Insert a size 10 double-lumen tube for nasogastric decompression to prevent further distention of the stomach.

4. Position the baby with head elevated to prevent aspiration and to allow for easier respiration.

ADMISSION EQUIPMENT

1. See Appendix B.

2. See the beginning of this chapter for special equipment.

3. The baby may need to be admitted immediately to the operating room.

PREOPERATIVE STABILIZATION

The nursing goal during the preoperative period is to support the respiratory system as needed and to continue gastric decompression.

1. Respiratory support: continue as on transport:
   a. If administration of 100 percent oxygen via endotracheal ventilation does not increase PaO_2, the infant probably has a hypoplastic lung, which decreases the survival chances.
   b. To determine the status of gas exchange, arterial blood gases should be closely monitored. The frequency of drawing blood depends upon the status of the gas exchange. This infant may be very acidotic, hypercarbic, and hypoxic.
   c. A rapid rate of ventilation may be required to improve gas exchange.
   d. The minimal ventilation pressure necessary to maintain adequate ventilation should be used even in such an unstable infant. Use the amount of pressure necessary to observe chest excursion. Remember this excursion may be unilateral due to the location of the hernia and contents of the chest cavity.
   e. A sudden worsening of respiratory condition suggests a pneumothorax. This requires prompt diagnosis and insertion of a chest tube.
   f. Regardless of the degree of improvement obtained with a period of intense preoperative care, operative correction should be undertaken promptly.
   g. Position the infant with unaffected side slightly elevated. This position may be accomplished by placing a small roll behind the infant's back, allowing maximum chest excursion and ventilation. The infant should not be placed completely on the affected side as this will compromise ventilation.

2. Continue with nasogastric decompression:
   a. Connect nasogastric tube to continuous-low (40-60 mm Hg) suction.

b. Irrigate the tube every 1-2 hours with 2 cc of air or normal saline solution to maintain patency of the tube.

3. Monitor vital signs closely, every 15-30 minutes, to detect any change in status:
   a. Check the newborn's temperature, pulse, respiration, and BP. Blood pressure should be included as these infants may become shocky.
   b. To fully assess status, include color, breath sounds, and respiratory effort with each measurment of vital signs.

4. Maintain IV access to promote hydration and have a route for emergency administration of medications and fluids.
   a. Give antibiotics, according to institutional policy, to prevent infections. Some institutions may not give these medications prophylactically. Realistically, there may not be time to give medications prior to surgery.
   b. If the BP level is <50 mm Hg systolic, the infant may require a volume expander such as Plasmanate®.
   c. If the arterial pH level is <7.35, sodium bicarbonate may be needed to correct metabolic acidosis. If the acidosis is respiratory, sodium bicarbonate is not used.

5. To prevent delays in getting the infant into surgery, obtain essential preoperative lab work. Blood type and crossmatch are most important. If time allows a CBC and serum electrolyte levels may be done.

6. Parental support:
   a. See Chapter 3 for specific guidelines.
   b. Verify surgical consent.

SURGERY

Transthoracic or transabdominal incisions are made to explore the abdominal thoracic cavities. The abdominal wall is stretched to increase the size of the abdominal cavity, and reduction of the abdominal viscera is performed. The lung on the affected side is inspected. A chest tube is inserted for drainage. No attempt is made to inflate this lung. Ventilatory support is directed at providing adequate oxygenation. Forced ventilation usually does not expand the affected lung and may produce a pneumothorax of the opposite lung, greatly decreasing the chances of survival. Insertion of arterial lines, if not done preoperatively, is performed.

POSTOPERATIVE STABILIZATION

The "honeymoon period" occurs for several hours after surgery when surgery has been well tolerated and the infant appears stable. A rapid deterioration can occur heralded by increased hypoxia and acidosis, right-to-left shunting of blood, and the development of a pneumothorax. Pulmonary artery hypertension is usually present. The major cause of death is respiratory insufficiency, usually associated with hypoplastic lungs. Associated anomalies also contribute to a poor prognosis.

1. Respiratory support to achieve and maintain hyperoxia and alkalosis:
   a. Use manual or mechanical endotracheal-tube ventilation to keep PaO_2 > 100, $PaCo_2$ < 30-40, and pH at 7.45-7.60. This closely controlled ventilation may be required for several days or weeks. Respiratory assistance is aimed at decreasing the right-to-left shunting, thus decreasing pulmonary artery hypertension. In place of manual ventilation, extracorporeal membrane oxygenation (ECMO) may be used if available. This system serves to bypass the shunting mechanism, allowing adequate oxygenation and gas exchange until pulmonary hypertension resolves. See Extracorporeal Membrane Oxgenation (pp. 304-313) in Chapter 10 for more information on this system.
   b. Auscultate breath sounds every 1-2 hours. Be alert to decreased breath sounds as a sign of pneumothorax. Be alert to congestion, which could signify atelectasis.
   c. Provide suction as needed, as evidenced by ausculation.
   d. Administer pancuronium bromide, a smooth-muscle relaxant, to produce paralysis and allow for controlled ventilation, thereby decreasing oxygen consumption and avoiding pneumothorax. Dosage of pancuronium bromide is usually 0.1 mg/kg IV push.
   e. Administer tolazoline hydrochloride as a vasodilator. Test dose is 1-2 mg/kg/h. This drug should be given in an upper extremity or scalp vein. These sites avoid the right-to-left shunting mechanism that is present. Side effects of this drug are multiple. Bleeding is a major concern. This bleeding may be within the GI or pulmonary system. Thrombocytopenia may be present. The platelet count along with a CBC should be closely monitored. Renal compromise is another side effect. Monitoring the serum electrolyte levels, especially blood urea nitrogen (BUN) and creatinine, is essential.
   f. Administer dopamine hydrochloride as a vasopressor; dose is usually 5 μ/kg/min IV.
   g. Insert chest tube to underwater seal for drainage and to prevent pneumothorax.

Note: These drugs and their dosages are only suggestions. Check institution protocol and recommended dosages.

2. Closely monitor vital signs and intake and output to observe for potential side effects of medication and status changes.
   a. Record temperature, pulse, respiration, and BP every 15 minutes four times, every 30 minutes four times, every hour four times, every 2 hours until stable, and then every 4 hours.
   b. Accurately record intake and output. Report to the surgeon any urine output <1 cc/kg/h.

3. Maintain IV lines to:
   a. Promote adequate hydration.
   b. Maintain electrolyte balance.
   c. Provide an administration route for antibiotics. These should be given according to hospital protocol.
   d. Monitor BP and gas exchange, and maintain arterial lines—usually radial arterial line and/or umbilical arterial line.
      i. Provide constant infusion with a heparinized solution unless lines are used for maintenance fluid access.
      ii. Dressings may be placed around the site to maintain sterility of site and prevent infection. Some institutions include antibiotic ointment at the site with each dressing change.
      iii. Observe the extremity distal to the infusion site for perfusion. A blanching or mottled appearance of this extremity may indicate arterial spasm, occlusion, or compromised perfusion. This sign should be reported immediately as the infant could experience resulting tissue hypoxia, necrosis, and eventual loss of digit or limb. The buttocks should also be observed if an umbilical line is in place, as perfusion may be compromised in this area as well. An arterial line should be removed immediately by a physician (according to most hospital protocols) if there is any question as to the integrity of the line or the tissue perfusion.

4. Feedings
   a. Wait to begin feedings until weaned from the ventilator to avoid the risk of aspiration.
   b. Advance slowly, starting with Pedialyte® or clear infant electrolyte solution and change to breast milk or formula as tolerated.
   c. May require periodic gavage due to residual respiratory distress with increased respiratory rate and the possibility of gastroesophageal reflux.
   d. Nipple feed as tolerated. Note respiratory rate and respiratory effort. Gavage feed if respiratory rate >60 breaths per minute.

PARENT CARE

See Chapter 3 for specific guidelines. The nursing goal for planning the infant's discharge from the hospital is to educate the parents about the potential complications so that appropriate follow-up is conducted. Parents may need extra teaching regarding feeding considerations to promote home management, such as:

1. Special feeding needs: you may need to teach the procedure for gavage.

2. Symptoms of complications (the parents should report any of these problems to the physician):
   a. An increased respiratory rate or effort.
   b. Cyanosis: Does it occur during feeding? At rest?
   c. Feeding intolerances—vomiting or refusal to eat.

Cystic Hygroma

Carole Kenner   Jeanne Harjo

DESCRIPTION

Cystic hygroma is a congenital defect of the lymphatic system. One or more fluid-filled cysts form in the area of the neck posterior to the sternocleidomastoid muscle. These cysts in the lymphatic system, however, may be found in the axilla, mediastinum, or groin, areas of high-density lymphatic tissue. The fluid from the hygroma may actually invade the surrounding normal tissue, making it difficult to distinguish normal tissue from abnormal tissue. The cystic hygroma is usually visible at birth. It may be large enough in the lateral neck to impede the airway.

ETIOLOGY AND PATHOPHYSIOLOGY

Cystic hygroma results from failure of the lymphatic channels to develop properly. Fluid-filled cysts result in the lymphatic tissue, causing a visible swelling to appear. The signs and symptoms vary, depending on the location of these cysts, which may be singular or multiple. If the neck region is involved, an obstructed airway is possible. The cystic hygroma is usually visible at birth and continues to grow in the postnatal period. These infants have a predisposition to infection due to the impaired drainage of the lymphatic tissue.

INCIDENCE

No exact incidence has been reported.

SYMPTOMS

1. Depends on the site of the cystic hygroma.
2. Visible swelling in the lateral neck or supraclavicular region.
3. Visible swelling in the groin.
4. Lateral neck radiograph demonstrating a mass pushing on the laryngeal or subglottic airway.
5. Respiratory distress due to the airway obstruction.
6. Discoloration of the mass: hemorrhage.

DIAGNOSIS

The diagnosis can be made both on observation and with confirmation on radiograph. An AP chest radiograph should be obtained to determine if the mass extends or is located in the mediastinal region. A lateral neck radiograph should be obtained to determine if encroachment of the airway is present.

TRANSPORT

The nursing goal during transport is to maintain a patent airway:

1. See Appendix A.
2. Position infant so that the airway is free: this may involve the placement of a small roll under the neck to hyperextend the airway. The infant will usually assume a position that optimizes the patency of the airway. Do not try to change the position if resistance is met.
3. No other special measures are necessary for transport.

ADMISSION EQUIPMENT

See Appendix B.

PREOPERATIVE STABILIZATION

Preoperatively the nursing goal is to maintain patency of the airway and prevent infection:

1. Monitor vital signs closely every 2-4 hours for first 24 hours after admission, as these infants are prone to infection.
2. Assess and observe for signs of infection such as change in the vital signs from baseline, increased irritability, subtle color changes, and unstable temperature.
3. To prevent infection administer antibiotics prior to surgery: see Chapter 9 for specific guidelines. Some institutions only recommend use of antibiotics preoperatively in the presence of an infection.
4. To promote ventilation and gas exchange, assess for signs of respiratory distress:
   a. Grunting
   b. Nasal flaring
   c. Increased chest retractions
   d. Cyanosis

e. Tachypnea

f. Stridor

5. Hyperextend the baby's neck so that the airway remains patent.

6. Assist in taking x-ray films by supporting the airway: position infant so that the airway remains open during the procedure; a small roll under the neck may hyperextend the neck, keeping airway patent.

7. Feedings, if tolerated, may be continued; gavage is the method of choice as pressure may be exerted by the hygroma on the esophagus, making nipple-feeding dangerous.

8. Intravenous fluids may be necessary if feeding by bottle is not feasible, also this is the method of administration of antibiotics prior to surgery.

9. Make the baby NPO 4-6 hours prior to surgery.

10. Observe for signs of discoloration of the cyst as this is indicative of hemorrhage.

11. Parents should be informed about the appearance of the cystic hygroma, how it will continue to grow, and how it may change in color prior to surgical intervention:

    a. Encourage them to hold the infant as they may be afraid they will obstruct or harm the baby's breathing. Demonstrate proper positioning techniques to lessen their fear.

    b. Encourage parents to express their feelings about the baby's visible deformity.

    c. For specific guidelines see Chapter 3.

NONSURGICAL TREATMENT

The cystic hygroma being fluid-filled makes it conducive to aspiration of the fluid and injection of sclerosing agents such as hypertonic glucose or saline solutions. If aspiration is unsuccessful, surgery is indicated.

SURGERY

Excision of the mass is the treatment of choice. Total removal of the hygroma in one operation may not be possible, however, since complete dissection of the mass may involve damage to underlying tissue and nerves. Multiple revisions of the initial excision may be necessary to remove the residual tissue. Penrose drains may be inserted for drainage of the lymphatic fluid. Some institutions prefer a closed drainage system to protect the infant from infection. This drainage could be serous. These drains are usually left in from 5 to 7 days. Prognosis for these infants is good if complete removal of hygroma can be achieved.

POSTOPERATIVE STABILIZATION

Postoperatively the nursing goals are to maintain the patency of airway and to prevent infection:

1. Vital signs must be monitored closely, every 15 minutes four times, every 30 minutes four times, every hour four times, and every 2 hours for the remainder of the first 24 hours.

2. To maintain patent airway, assess for signs of respiratory distress. These infants are prone to edema and obstruction of the airway especially in the immediate postoperative period.
   a. Increasing chest retractions, tachypnea or apnea
   b. Color changes

3. Infant may be intubated for several days postoperatively:
   a. Suction the endotracheal tube every 2 hours or as necessary.
   b. Suction the oral and nasopharyngeal area with care to prevent bleeding.

4. Draw levels of arterial blood gases every 2 hours, more often if newborn is unstable or ventilator changes have been made.

5. Position infant to maintain patent airway and to protect incision line; the exact position will vary with the location of the suture line.

6. To prevent fluid and electrolyte imbalance, obtain serum electrolyte levels. The infant may experience excessive losses from the wound in the postoperative phase.

7. Continue IV antibiotics for 7-10 days: see Antibiotics section in Chapter 9 (pp. 290-293) for specific guidelines.

8. Intravenous fluids should be given to maintain fluid and electrolyte balance:
   a. See Chapter 9 for specific guidelines.
   b. Losses from a Penrose or closed-system drain need to be replaced to maintain fluid and electrolyte balance.

9. Intake and output should be recorded every 4-8 hours:
   a. Specific gravity should be measured every 4-8 hours to determine hydration status.
   b. Urine output should be maintained at 1 cc/kg/h, report immediately if output falls.
   c. Penrose or closed-system drainage output should be measured every 4-8 hours and if large may require replacement fluids; report drainage to physician.

10. Blood pressure must continue to be monitored closely throughout the postoperative period. Hypotension is a recurrent problem as lymph fluid may be continuously lost.

   a. Plasma protein or volume expanders may be necessary to maintain BP equilibrium.

   b. Continual assessment of peripheral perfusion is necessary to detect subtle changes. If any of the following symptoms are present, report these to a physician:

      i. Decreased capillary refill

      ii. Pale color

     iii. Mottling of the extremities

11. Observe suture-line integrity:
    a. Note and report any skin breakdown.
    b. Observe for increasing separation of skin flaps.
    c. Observe for increasing swelling or discoloration.
    d. Observe for excessive, purulent, or frankly bloody drainage.
    e. Cleanse suture line with hydrogen peroxide and sterile applicator every 4 hours to promote skin integrity and prevent infection.

12. Gastrostomy tube may have been placed during surgery for feeding purposes as oral feedings may be contraindicated for long periods of time. See Gastrostomy Care (pp. 347-349) in Chapter 12.

13. Infant should be weaned from ventilator support as respiratory function improves:
    a. Gradually reduce the ventilator settings while evaluating closely arterial blood gases.
    b. To promote adequate ventilation, observe for recurrence of respiratory difficulty.

14. Start feedings as condition improves and baby is at or near extubation:
    a. Feedings should be started with nipple (if extubated) or gastrostomy tube.
    b. Start feedings with Pedialyte® or sterile water every 2 hours; advance to formula and increase in amount as tolerated.
    c. For specific guidelines, see Chapter 9.

15. Position infant with head of bed elevated after feedings to prevent gastroesophageal reflux.

PARENT CARE

The nursing goal for discharging the baby from the hospital is to educate parents regarding the infant's need for follow-up and to promote home management.

1. Teach parents about the possibility of recurrence of the mass.

2. Teach parents the symptoms of respiratory distress.

3. Encourage them to report any feeding difficulties or signs of infection as this is indicative of a return of the mass.

4. Teach gastrostomy care, if one is present: see Gastrostomy Care (pp. 347-349) in Chapter 12 for specific guidelines

5. See Chapter 3 for specific guidelines.

REFERENCES

Choanal Atresia

Sadler, T.W. (1985). *Langman's medical embryology* (5th ed.) (p. 303). Baltimore: Williams & Wilkins.

Schaffer, A. J., Avery, M. E., & Taeusch, H. W. (1984). *Schaffer's diseases of the newborn* (5th ed.). Philadelphia: W. B. Saunders.

Cleft Palate and Lip

Goldberg, R. B., & Shprintzen, R. J. (1981). Hirschsprung megacolon and cleft palate in two sibs. *Journal of Craniofacial Genetics and Developmental Biology, 1*,185-189.

Guzzetta, P. C., Randolph, J. G., Anderson, K. D., Boyajian, M., & Eicchelberger, M. (1987). Surgery of the neonate. In G. B. Avery (Ed.), *Neonatology: Pathophysiology and management of the newborn* (3rd ed.) (pp. 944-984). Philadelphia: J. B. Lippincott.

Jorgenson, R. J., Sharpiro, S. D., & Odinet, K. L. (1984). Studies on facial growth and arch size in cleft lip and palate. *Journal of Craniofacial Genetics and Developmental Biology, 4*, 33-38.

Williams, M. A., Shprintzen, R. J., & Goldberg, R. B. (1985). Male-to-male transmission of the velo-cardio-facial syndrome: A case report and review of 60 cases. *Journal of Craniofacial Genetics and Developmental Biology, 5*, 175-180.

Esophageal Atresia Without Tracheoesophageal Fistula

Schreiner, R. L. (Ed.) (1982). *Care of the newborn.* (pp. 182-195). New York: Raven.

BIBLIOGRAPHY

Adzick, N. S., Harrison, M. R., Glick, P. L., Nakayama, D. K., Manning, F. A., & De Lorimier, A. A. (1985). Diaphragmatic hernia in the fetus: Prenatal diagnosis and outcome in 94 cases. *Journal of Pediatric Surgery, 20*, 357-361.

Arvystas, M., & Shprintze, R. J. (1984). Craniofacial morphology in the vel-car-dio-facial syndrome. *Journal of Craniofacial Genetics and Developmental Biology, 4*, 39-45.

Avery, G. B. (Ed.) (1987). *Neonatology: Pathophysiology and management of the newborn* (3rd ed.). Philadelphia: J. B. Lippincott.

Cassani, V. (1984). Tracheoesphageal anomalies. *Neonatal Network, 3,*(2) 20-27.

Dixon, A. G. (1986). Jeff's story: A unique approach to the care of an infant with esophageal atresia and a cervical esophagostomy. *Neonatal Network, 4*(6) 7-12.

Dykes, E. H., Rlaine, P. A. M., Arthur, D. S., Drainer, L. K., Young, D. G. (1985). Pierre Robin syndrome and pulmonary hypertension. *Journal of Pediatric Surgery, 20,* 49-52.

Edwards, N. S., & Millay, C. (1981). Persistent fetal circulation. In R. H. Perez (Ed.), *Protocols for perinatal nursing practice* (pp. 404-421) St Louis: C. V. Mosby.

Filston, H. C., & Izant, R. (1985). *The surgical neonate: Evaluation and care* (2nd ed.) (pp. 136-164). New York: Appleton-Century-Crofts.

Ford, W. D. A., Freeman, J. K., & Martin, A. J. (1985). Supraclavicular approach to cervical esophageal atresia with tracheoesophageal fistula. *Journal of Pediatric Surgery, 20,* 242-243.

Martin, L. W., Cox, J. A., Cotton, R., & Oldham, K. T. (1986). Transtracheal repair of recurrent tracheoesophageal fistula. *Journal of Pediatric Surgery, 21,* 402-403.

Moore, K. L. (1974). *Before we are born: Basic embryology and birth defects.* Philadelphia: W. B. Saunders.

Moore, K. L. (1982). *The developing human: Clinically oriented embryology* (3rd ed.). Philadelphia: W. B. Saunders.

Mott, S. R., Fazekas, N. F., & James, S. R. (1985). *Nursing care of children and families. A holistic approach.* Reading, MA: Addison-Wesley.

Muraji, R., & Mahour, G. H. (1984). Surgical problems in patients with VATER-associated anomalies. *Journal of Pediatric Surgery, 19,* 550-554.

Nakayama, D. K. Harrison, M. R., Chinn, D. H., Callen, P. W., Filly, R. A., Golbus, M. S., & De Lorimier, A. A. (1985). Prenatal diagnosis and natural history of the fetus with a congenital diaphragmatic hernia: Initial clinical experience. *Journal of Pediatric Surgery, 20,* 118-124.

Otte, J. B., Gianello, P., Wese, F. X., Claus, D., Verellen, G., & Moulin, D. (1984). Diverticulum formation after circular myotomy for esophageal atresia. *Journal of Pediatric Surgery, 19,* 68-71.

Purt, P., & Gorman, F. (1984). Lethal nonpulmonary anomalies associated with congenitial diaphragmatic hernia. Implications for early intrauterine surgery. *Journal of Pediatric Surgery, 19,* 29-32.

Rangecroft, L., Bush, G. H., Lister, J., & Irving, I. M. (1984). Endoscopic diathermy obliteration of recurrent tracheoesophageal fistulae. *Journal of Pediatric Surgery, 19,* 41-43.

Reynolds, M., Luck, S. R., & Lappen, R. (1984). The "critical" neonate with diaphragmatic hernia. A 1-year perspective. *Journal of Pediatric Surgery, 19,* 304-369.

Schaffer A. J., Avery, M. E., & Taeusch, H. W. (1984). *Diseases of the newborn* (5th ed.). Philadelphia: W. B. Saunders.

Smith, M. J., Goodman, J. A., Ramsey, N.S., & Pasternack, S. B. (1982). *Child and family: Concepts of nursing practice.* New York: McGraw-Hill.

Chapter 5

Alterations in the Gastrointestinal System

Jeanne Harjo   *Carole Kenner*
          Ann Brueggemeyer

Intestinal obstructions and alterations in the gastrointestinal (GI) system can occur for many reasons. Various atresias or stenoses such as pyloric stenosis or duodenal or jejunal atresia happen due to early embryological development. Meconium or mucus plugs also result in obstruction seen in cystic fibrosis and meconium-plug syndrome. Hirschsprung's disease is a functional obstruction characterized by aganglionic segments of bowel with resulting failure of bowel to empty. Necrotizing enterocolitis, most commonly occurring in premature and/or stressed infants results in a functional obstruction from anoxic bowel. The presence of a herniation of bowel through the abdominal wall, gastroschisis and omphalocele, can be with or without obstruction. Early recognition and medical or surgical intervention are essential for a favorable long-term prognosis.

SYMPTOMS

1. Vomiting, especially bilious, is suggestive but not diagnostic of obstruction.

2. Failure to pass meconium is also suggestive of obstruction, but passage of one or more meconium stools does not rule out obstruction, especially in proximal obstructions.

3. Abdominal distention, poor appetite and emesis may be present.

4. Polyhydramnios may be present in upper GI obstruction, including duodenal obstruction.

TRANSPORT

The nursing goal for transporting infants with alterations of the GI system is to promote gastric decompression and to prevent respiratory compromise and fluid losses.

1. Neonatal transport protocol: See Appendix A.

2. Gastric decompression: to prevent aspiration and respiratory compromise.
   a. Insert, either orally or nasally, a double-lumen suction catheter into the stomach.
   b. Secure the tube to the infant's face with tape to prevent accidentally dislodging tube.
   c. To prevent aspiration and facilitate gastric decompression, connect to straight drainage and suction stomach contents every 15-30 minutes. This frequency may not be necessary and should be tailored to fit each infant's needs.

ADMISSION SETUP

1. See Appendix B.

2. In addition to regular suction setup, suction equipment for gastric decompression is needed.
   a. Vacuum source with regulator head should be set at low-intermittent or continuous suction with the use of double-lumen tubes.
   b. To maintain accurate estimation of fluid loss, a drainage collection bottle is needed.
   c. Double-lumen catheters, sizes 8 and 10 F.
   d. Sterile water or normal saline solution (0.9 percent) for irrigation according to hospital protocol; may also use air for irrigation.

3. Diagnostic/lab work:
   a. Abdominal ultrasound.
   b. Upper and lower GI series.
   c. Radiographs: flat plate, left-lateral decubitus, and Wangenstein-Rice positions. (The left-lateral decubitus radiograph is useful for determining the presence of free air in the intestines or peritoneal cavity. For this radiograph the infant is placed supine on top of the radiograph plate. Next the infant and plate are rotated, as a unit, onto the infant's left side. This step ensures proper alignment of the infant with the plate. Next the radiograph cone is rotated horizontally so that the beam passes horizontally. The purpose of this position is to allow any free air to rise to the right side of the infant and be highly visible on the radiograph. The Wangenstein-Rice radiograph is taken to determine the bowel ends in relation to an imperforate anus. The infant is placed prone in a head-down position. With the

neonate's buttocks higher than the head, lateroabdominal and pelvic radiographs are taken. In this position the bowel end can be identified on film).

   d. Rectal exam: to examine directly intestinal tissue for ganglion cells, in the case of Hirschsprung's disease, and to determine the presence of an obstruction.

      i. Strip or suction biopsy of intestinal mucosa

     ii. Manual or digital examination

   e. Evaluate stool cultures to determine if there is an infection.

   f. Evaluate stool for trypsin and albumin levels. Alterations in these levels may occur with certain types of intestinal obstructions.

   g. To determine any alterations in trypsin levels, blood for trypsin should also be drawn.

   h. See Chapter 11 for more specific guidelines on general diagnostic studies.

PREOPERATIVE CONSIDERATIONS

Alterations in the GI system are so varied that general considerations are not very helpful. The goal preoperatively is to maintain or restore fluid and electrolyte status, to maintain gastric decompression, and to prevent infection if not already present. Another consideration is respiratory compromise. Since intra-abdominal pressure may be increased and there may be a shift in the placement of the diaphragm in many GI problems, respiratory insufficiency can result. Adequate ventilation and gas exchange is the goal preoperatively to place the infant in the best possible state for surgery. Specific considerations are addressed in the following sections.

POSTOPERATIVE CONSIDERATIONS

Enteral feedings are restarted as the GI function resumes. Based upon the return of bowel sounds, decreased gastric output, and stool formation, feedings are gradually progressed from clear liquids to elemental feedings like Pregestimil® (at first ¼ strength, then ½ strength, then full strength). Pregestimil® is composed of easily digested proteins and amino acids. Fats are in the form of medium chain triglycerides that make digestion easier even for infants who have had GI problems. This progression is determined by the infant's tolerance to the feeding and depends on bowel loss or severity of the defect and the length of the ileus. Small frequent or continuous feedings may be offered first. Then amount or strength may be increased. Both the strength and amount are not increased simultaneously. Observation for feeding intolerances is necessary. Diarrhea, vomiting, abdominal distention, and the presence of reducing substances in the stool are all signs of intolerance. Advancement should be stopped if any of these signs occur.

Gastric reflux is another complication that often occurs postoperatively. It is the failure of the esophagogastric valve to keep the gastric content from flowing in a retrograde fashion up into the esophagus. The inherent problem with this reflux flow is that the gastric content is very acidic. Esophagitis can develop with associated bleeding. An infant experiencing reflux may show signs of failure to thrive (e.g., poor weight gain and weakness), esophagitis, dysphagia, poor appetite, or refusal to feed, anemia, vomiting, or respiratory difficulties manifested by chest retractions, nasal flaring, and apnea. To decrease the chance of reflux, place the infant in an upright position for feedings and elevate the head of the bed slightly (30° in prone position, slightly higher in supine position) for at least 2 hours after feedings. Offering less amounts of feedings more frequently may also decrease reflux. Some institutions offer thickened feedings (formula mixed with rice cereal); however, this should be done under medical supervision since the GI tract may not absorb cereal after surgery.

Duodenal Obstruction
Jeanne Harjo

DESCRIPTION

Duodenal obstruction is a complete or partial blockage of the duodenum. The obstruction can occur at any level in the duodenum but most occur at the ampulla of Vater, the entrance from the stomach into the duodenum. Atresia is a complete blockage, whereas stenosis is a partial blockage. Often, annular pancreas is found, with the pancreas surrounding the second part of the duodenum causing the obstruction.

ETIOLOGY AND EMBRYOLOGY

Early gestational development of the gut produces a proliferation of cells. During tubule development in the middle of the first trimester, blockage occurs. It may be associated with other congenital anomalies, especially Down's syndrome.

INCIDENCE

Occurs in almost 1 out of every 5000 live births. It occurs more commonly in female newborns.

SYMPTOMS

1. Atresia:
   a. Bilious emesis and nasogastric aspirate.

   b. Meconium may or may not be passed.

   c. Visible left upper quadrant mass.

   d. Elevated bilirubin levels.

2. Stenosis:
   a. Emesis is intermittently bilious.
   b. Meconium is usually passed.
   c. Distention, if present, is minimal.
   d. Bilirubin levels are greater than normal.

3. Maternal polyhydramnios is noted in 40-50 percent of the cases.

DIAGNOSIS

1. To determine if a duodenal obstruction is present, obtain anteroposterior (AP) and lateroabdominal radiographs. A classic "double bubble" will be seen. The stomach and proximal duodenum is dilated to several times normal size and distal bowel is very narrow.

2. Perform a barium enema to rule out multiple atresias, malrotation, Hirschsprung's disease or meconium ileus.

TRANSPORT

A goal for transporting an infant suspected to have duodenal obstruction is to decompress the bowel and prevent aspiration. Prior to transport a double- or single-lumen nasogastric, gavage tube or suction catheter may be placed to straight drainage as a temporary measure. Assessment for any increasing abdominal distention should be done. Place infant on side or with head to the side to prevent aspiration.

1. See Appendix A.

2. Place a nasogastric tube, size 10 double lumen, to decompress the bowel. Suction every 15-30 minutes to maintain tube's patency.

3. Intravenous access: See Chapter 9 for specific guidelines. The goal is to maintain adequate hydration and preserve electrolyte balance. This balance is essential since a large amount of fluids may be lost through gastric suction and vomiting.

4. Parental support: see Chapter 3 for specific guidelines.

ADMISSION EQUIPMENT

1. Normal admission setup: see Appendix B.

2. Nasogastric decompression.

a. Size 10 double-lumen nasogastric tube.
b. Suction machine or wall unit with regulator, in addition to the regular suction setup.

PREOPERATIVE STABILIZATION

The preoperative goal is to maintain gastric and intestinal decompression and to prevent aspiration and respiratory compromise. If obstruction is large or gastric suctioning is resulting in a great amount of secretions, the infant may be losing significant fluids and electrolytes. Then the goal is to maintain fluid and electrolyte balance.

1. To detect any changes in status, monitor vital signs (temperature, heart rate, respiration, and BP) every 2 hours:
   a. To determine the presence of or any changes in the degree of abdominal distention, measure abdominal girth and report any distention or firmness.
   b. Observe respiratory effort and skin color to determine if respiratory compromise is occurring.

2. Insert nasogastric tube, size 10 double lumen:
   a. Place to low-intermittent or continuous suction to facilitate decompression.
   b. To maintain the tube's patency, irrigate every 2 hours with 2 cc of air.
   c. To determine the amount of fluid losses, measure, record, and discard output every 4-8 hours.
   d. Replace nasogastric output every 4-8 hours with dextrose 5 percent in 0.9% NaCl solution with 10 mEq potassium chloride/L. Replace cc for cc every 4–8 hours. See Chapter 9 for more details.

3. Parental support:
   a. See Chapter 3 for specific parent-care guidelines.
   b. Verify consent for surgery.

SURGERY

1. Duodenoduodenostomy requires an end-to-end anastomosis after resection of the area of atresia.

2. Duodenojejunostomy requires an end-to-end anastomosis after resection of the area of atresia

3. The trend is not to insert a gastrostomy tube for gastric decompression as readily has been done in the past. Some surgeons, however, still place a gastrostomy tube for this purpose.

4. Insertion of a central venous line provides adequate nutrition and maintains electrolyte balance. This procedure may not be performed if the infant will

resume oral feedings a few days postoperatively. Peripheral total parenteral nutrition is an acceptable alternative in short-term IV therapy if supported by hospital protocol.

POSTOPERATIVE STABILIZATION

The nursing goal in the postoperative period is to maintain fluid and electrolyte balance and to prevent disruption or infection of the suture line.

1. To determine any changes in status, close monitoring of vital signs and urine output is necessary:
   a. Check temperature, heart rate, respiratory rate, and BP every 15 minutes four times, every 30 minutes four times, every hour four times, every 2 hours until stable, and then every 4 hours.
   b. Report any urine output <1 cc/kg/hr.

2. Maintain IV access (see Chapter 9 for specific guidelines):
   a. Bowel resection may require total parenteral nutrition for hydration and electrolyte balance. This total parental nutrition may be given either by central venous line or peripheral line if supported by hospital protocol.
   b. To maintain serum electrolyte levels (especially sodium and potassium levels), replace any gastric losses every 4-8 hours with appropriate fluid and electrolyte solution via IV access.
   c. Administer broad-spectrum antibiotics: ampicillin 100 mg/kg/d IV in divided doses is given along with gentamicin 5 mg/kg/d IV in divided doses. These guidelines must be adapted to each infant and each hospital protocol.

3. Maintain patency of gastrostomy tube:
   a. Irrigate the gastrostomy tube every 2 hours with 2 cc of air.
   b. Connect gastrostomy tube to gravity drainage.
   c. To maintain hydration and replace electrolyte losses, record, discard, and replace output every 4-8 hours according to hospital policy. The general replacement fluid is dextrose 5 percent in 0.9% NaCl solution with 10 mEq potassium chloride/L. Replace all output cc/cc every 4-8 hours.

4. Observe for complications that would be indicative of infection, impaired skin integrity, or intestinal obstruction.
   a. Note and report any redness, drainage, swelling, or separation of suture line.
   b. Observe and report any abdominal distention or vomiting.

5. To prevent respiratory compromise, give respiratory support as needed.
   a. Neonate may require oxygen by oxygen hood or positive-pressure ventilator.
   b. Monitor breath sounds, color, and respiratory effort every 1-2 hours to detect any respiratory changes.

6. Parental support: see Chapter 3 for specific guidelines.

7. Feedings:
   a. Begin in approximately 2 weeks when bowel function returns. This return of function is indicated by:
      i. Passage of stool from rectum.
      ii. Decreased gastric output.
      iii. Gastric output changing from green to cloudy.
      iv. Bowel sounds in all four quadrants.
   b. Before starting enteral feedings, elevate the gastrostomy tube for 24 hours, unclamped. This action is taken to promote gastric motility and passage of gastric secretions from the stomach to the bowel.
      i. Measure gastric aspirate every 4 hours to determine the intestinal absorption of the stomach contents
      ii. Record and reinsert aspirate to preserve the electrolytes present in the gastric juices
      iii. If aspirate is clear and <5-10 cc every 4 hours, feedings can begin, as intestinal motility and absorption is occurring
   c. Advance feedings slowly to prevent gastric distention and malabsorption. Fluid tolerance is determined by advancing feedings from simple to complex fluids and monitoring each change. The more easily digested solutions are offered first and advanced according to each infant.
      i. Start with Pedialyte® every 2 hours for 24 hours.
      ii. Increase to ¼-strength formula and increase to full strength as tolerated.
      iii. Gauge tolerance of feedings by the following indicators:
         a) Check aspirate before each feeding. It should be <10-15 cc. This amount of aspirate indicates good tolerance of feeding.
         b) Note stool amounts and consistency. Check every 8 hours for reducing substances in the stool. If reducing substances are present (especially if >0.5 percent) or if the stool is watery, the formula is not being properly absorbed.
         c) To prevent intolerance of feedings and malabsorption, stop advancement if
            • aspirate is green or amount is >15 cc.
            • Diarrhea occurs.
            • Reducing substances in stool is >0.5 percent
            • If abdominal distention or vomiting occurs.
         d) To maintain fluid and electrolyte balance, parenteral nutrition is required until full feedings are tolerated.

PARENT CARE

1. See Chapter 3 for specific guidelines.

2. Discharge teaching: the goal of parent education is to prepare the parents for

home management and to recognize signs of the return of an intestinal obstruction. After bowel surgery, scar-tissue formation, adhesions, and other inflammatory processes may lead to the return of an intestinal blockage. Parents must be alert to the signs of complications to prevent long-standing compromise to bowel integrity. Alert the parents to signs of potential problems:
   a. Poor appetite
   b. Vomiting
   c. Abdominal distention
   d. Diarrhea or constipation

3. Teach the parents how to perform gastostomy care and feedings if required: see Gastrostomy Care (pp. 347-351) in Chapter 12 for specific guidelines.

4. Teach the parents the signs of gastric reflux. Parents need to know that an infant experiencing reflux may show signs of:
   a. Failure to thrive
   b. Esophagitis, dysphagia, poor appetite, or refusal to feed
   c. Anemia (infant may be pale)
   d. Vomiting
   e. Respiratory difficulties such as chest retractions, nasal flaring, or apnea

5. Remind the parents to report any of signs of gastroesophageal reflux to the physician immediately to prevent malnutrition, malabsorption, aspiration, and respiratory compromise.

6. Teach the parents to place the infant in an upright position for feedings and to elevate the head of the bed slightly (30° in prone position, slightly higher in supine position) for at least 2 hours after feedings if reflux is present. Offering less amounts of food more frequently is another suggestion to decrease reflux. Some institutions offer thickened feedings (formula mixed with rice cereal); however, this should be done under medical supervision since the GI tract may not absorb cereal after surgery. See Postoperative Considerations (pp. 123-124) in the introduction to this chapter for a discussion of reflux.

Omphalocele and Gastroschisis
Jeanne Harjo

DESCRIPTION

Omphalocele and gastroschisis are abdominal defects that allow internal organs to herniate through the abdominal wall and be externalized. A membranous covering may or may not be present. An omphalocele is the herniation of the abdominal contents through the umbilical cord. The defect is covered with an amniotic membrane. This membrane often ruptures at delivery. This defect is often associated with an increased incidence of other anomalies. Beckwith's syndrome is an example of a common syndrome that has an omphalocele as part of the characteristic features. Infants with trisomy 13 or 18 also may have an omphalocele. Infants with large omphaloceles may have Cantrell's pentalogy: epigastric omphalocele, lower sternal cleft, anterior diaphragmatic and pericardial defects, ectopia cordis, and intracardiac defects (Hershenson et al., 1985, p. 349). In gastroschisis the abdominal contents have herniated through the abdominal wall adjacent to the umbilical cord. There is no membrane present. The umbilical cord is intact.

ETIOLOGY AND EMBRYOLOGY

Omphalocele and gastroschisis result from the failure of the abdominal contents to return to the abdomen when the wall begins to close during the end of the first trimester. The protrusion can occur at the site of the umbilicus or along the central portion of the abdominal wall.

INCIDENCE

Either omphalocele or gastroschisis occurs in approximately 1 of every 6000-7000 births.

DIAGNOSIS

These defects are obvious and no diagnostic procedures are required. Prenatal ultrasound can often identify these defects but is not always accurate when the umbilical cord is long and tortuous.

TRANSPORT

The goal is to prevent excessive fluid loss and shock. Maintenance of adequate ventilation and gas exchange is another important transport consideration for these infants. Prevention of infection and cold stress during transport is also important. These goals should be implemented by the Level 1 or 2 nursery prior to the transport team's arrival.

1. There is an extreme risk of sepsis; maintain sterile technique:
   a. Place sterile gauze dressings over defect. Moisten with warmed saline solution. Next wrap the defect in plastic to prevent evaporative heat losses.
   b. Position infant supine on sterile barrier to prevent contamination of the defect. Bowel bags may be used to encircle the defect in place of a sterile barrier.

c. Use gloves and sterile technique when handling defect. To prevent infection and unnecessary heat loss, do not unwrap or attempt to reinspect the defect once it has been wrapped.

d. Begin antibiotic therapy according to orders or hospital policy. Generally ampicillin 100 mg/kg/d IV in divided doses and gentamicin 5 mg/kg/d IV in divided doses are prescribed.

2. Heat loss is quick and severe due to the large amounts of exposed bowel:
   a. Keep the newborn in a warmed isolette, at least 35° C. Monitor temperature frequently to avoid overheating, as this would only further stress the infant.
   b. Wrap defect in warm normal saline solution dressings, avoiding burns to the exposed, sensitive bowel.
   c. Cover wrapped defect with plastic to decrease heat loss.

3. Place a size 10 double-lumen nasogastric tube for decompression.

4. Position newborn slightly on side, avoiding kinking of the bowel. If pressure is being placed on bowel, position infant on back.

5. To support ventilation and gas exchange, give warmed, humidified oxygen to keep baby pink and allow for easy respiration.

6. Intravenous access: see Chapter 9, Parenteral Nutrition: Peripheral and Total Nutrition (pp. 280-285).

7. Give parental support:
   a. See Chapter 3 for specific guidelines.
   b. Allow the parents to touch the infant, but the infant should not be moved or held, in order to prevent trauma to bowel.

ADMISSION EQUIPMENT

1. Admission setup:
   a. See Appendix B.
   b. Nasogastric suction for gastric decompression in addition to regular suction setup:
      i. Size 10 double lumen tube.
      ii. Intermittent or continuous suction.

2. Dressing care:
   a. Warmed normal saline solution for irrigation.
   b. Gauze rolls or gauze dressings.
   c. Sterile gloves.
   d. Sterile barriers to drape scale and place in isolette.

PREOPERATIVE STABILIZATION

Preoperatively the nursing goal is to prevent hypovolemic shock by maintaining fluid and electrolyte balance. Prevention of infection and heat loss are also priority concerns in this period.

1. Maintain IV access; See Chapter 9 for specific guidelines.
   a. To maintain a normal fluid and electrolyte balance, give maintenance fluids such as dextrose 10 percent with sodium chloride and potassium chloride (determined by individual serum electrolyte results). In addition it may be necessary to administer up to two times the maintenance fluids in the form of an osmotic fluid such as dextrose 5 percent Ringer's lactate (do not administer a hypotonic solution for replacement of these losses as it will only lead to greater fluid shifts) to compensate for the third spacing of fluids in the bowel. Sodium and potassium levels should be evaluated to determine the amount of extra fluids and electrolytes needed to maintain adequate balance.
   b. To prevent circulatory collapse, volume expanders or extra fluid may be necessary for hypovolemic shock. Third spacing of fluids can be dramatic in a short period of time with these defects.

2. Give antibiotics to prevent the occurrence of infection. Many institutions will not give antibiotics unless an infection is actually present, so hospital protocol should be consulted. Generally ampicillin 100 mg/kg/d IV in divided doses and gentamicin 5 mg/kg/d IV in divided doses are prescribed.

3. Assess vital signs every 1–2 hours to detect any changes in status: (temperature, heart rate, blood pressure, and respiratory rate).
   a. Blood pressure: if hypotension occurs due to a tremendous loss of fluid from the bowel, administer plasma protein fraction 5 percent as a volume expander at 10 cc/kg. This dose may be repeated if needed.
   b. Measure and record urine output every hour. Report an output <1 cc/kg/h. Renal failure can occur easily due to dehydration or if extensive pressure is being placed on the renal arteries from the dislodged bowel; therefore, circulation is compromised to the kidneys. If BP is adequate and urine output low, attempts may be made to shift the infant's position to decrease the pressure of abdominal organs on the abdominal aorta.

4. Moisten dressing over the defect with warm normal saline solution every 2 hours to prevent excess drying.
   a. Change dressing only if necessary, using sterile technique.
   b. Observe color of the bowel every hour.
      i. Position baby on side to prevent kinking.
      ii. Any bluish-grey color of bowel requires repositioning infant to improve circulation to bowel.

5. Maintain nasogastric decompression:
   a. Insert a nasogastric tube, size10 double lumen.
   b. Irrigate with 2 cc of air every 2 hours.
   c. Connect to low-intermittent or continuous suction.
   d. Measure, record, and discard drainage every 4-8 hours.
   e. Replace nasogastric drainage, 1 cc of output with 1 cc of replacement fluids. Dextrose 5 percent in 0.9% NaCl with10 mEq potassium chloride/L

is a usual solution used. See Chapter 9, Fluid and Electrolyte Status: pre-op-/intra-op/post-op (pp. 269-272) for guidelines.

6. Respiratory support:
   a. Use oxygen hood or positive-pressure ventilator with oxygen as needed.
   b. Monitor color, breath sounds, and respiratory effort every 1-2 hours.

SURGERY

There are several surgical procedures that may be used to accomplish repair of an omphalocele or gastroschisis. The determination of which procedure to use is made based on (1) the surgeon's preference; (2) the size of the defect: a large defect if closed in one procedure increases the intra-abdominal pressure and displaces the diaphragm thus compromising ventilation, gas exchange, and cardiac circulation; and (3) the infant's preoperative condition.

1. Primary closure of the defect may involve the use of skin grafts, placement of synthetic patches, or stretching of the skin that surrounds the defect. Primary closure often leads to severe respiratory distress due to pressure from the tightened skin pushing downward on the abdominal contents and upward on the diaphragm. The increase in intra-abdominal pressure combined with a displacement of the diaphragm upward compromise the infant's respiratory system. The result is potentially severe respiratory insufficiency. Another consideration is that an infant with a giant omphalocele, especially if the liver is involved, may have a smaller than normal thoracic cavity as well as cardiac anomalies. Severe impediment to blood flow into and from the systemic circuit may also result from this pressure.

2. Staged reduction:
   a. Application of Silastic pouch surrounding the abdominal contents: In this procedure a Silo or pouch is sutured in place at the edge of the defect to apply pressure to the bowel. The abdominal contents and bowel are placed in a suspended position within the pouch. This suspension raises the bowel off the diaphragm. Daily, if respiratory distress does not occur, the pouch is squeezed, lowering the bowel into the abdominal cavity and gradually reducing the size of the defect. Eventually, the defect is closed. This closure may occur in several days (Mulligan, 1986).
   b. Gastrostomy tube: Some surgical teams do not insert this tube as there is questionable stability of the abdominal wall. Gavage feedings, then, are used after repair.
   c. Central line placement for long-term hyperalimentation: If there is any suspicion that the infant may have a short gut after surgery or require a long rest of the GI system, a central venous line is the mode of choice for hyperalimentation and is usually placed at the time of surgical repair. See Chapter 9, Parenteral Nutrition: Peripheral and Total Nutrition (pp. 280-285) for guidance on hyperalimentation.

3. Skin flaps: The use of skin flaps to cover a large defect is an acceptable procedure in some institutions. It does lessen the amount of increase in intra-abdominal pressure, thus decreasing the incidence of respiratory insufficiency. This procedure results in a large ventral hernia.

The following postoperative stabilization can be used for any infant that has undergone surgical repair. Specific information regarding staged reduction is included.

POSTOPERATIVE STABILIZATION

The goal for postoperative management is to maintain or restore fluids, electrolyte levels, and nutritional balance and to prevent respiratory compromise. The overriding goal is to prevent infection. Infection can result in disruption of the suture line, failure of the skin graft to remain viable, and death.

1. Monitor vital signs: temperature, BP, heart rate and respiratory rate every 15 minutes four times, every 30 minutes four times, every 2 hours four times, and then every 4 hours when stable
   a. Temperature:
      i. Heat loss is less severe after the abdominal defect is dressed.
      ii. Adjust isolette temperature to keep axillary temperature between 36.5° and 37° C to maintain a neutral thermal environment.
   b. Blood pressure:
      i. Large amounts of fluids are lost from the bowel into the pouch. This results in decreased plasma proteins causing retention of fluid in the abdomen. See Chapter 9 for third spacing of fluids.
      ii. Circulating fluid volume is decreased due to the fluid shifts.
      iii. Administer volume expanders such as plasma protein fraction 5 percent if systolic BP <40-50 mm Hg to maintain BP and decrease the fluid shifts.
   c. Measure and record urine output every hour to determine infant's fluid status:
      i. Decreased circulation and BP may cause a decline in urine output.
      ii. Physiologic pressure from the abdominal organs resting on the vena cava or renal artery may occur. This pressure has the potential of causing a decline in circulating blood flow to kidneys and decreasing urine output.
   d. Measure urine-specific gravity every 4 hours; specific gravity >1.015-1.020 requires the evaluation of the state of hydration (normal range is 1.005-1.012).

2. Suspend an abdominal sac with Silastic pouch, "silo" or "chimney," from the top of the isolette with tension adjusted by the surgeon:
   a. Lower extremities may be discolored or puffy or have decreased pulses due to poor perfusion. Only the surgeon may alter the tension of the silo.

    b. Do not attempt to turn the infant or do procedures such as weighing or holding the baby for radiographs without a second person applying steady tension on the silo.

    c. Position the neonate supine to prevent disruption of the tension on the omphalocele and to promote ventilation:

        i. Observe for signs of respiratory compromise, as respiratory insufficiency is common during a staged reduction or after a primary closure of the omphalocele.

        ii. Infants with increased intra-abdominal pressure combined with a smaller thoracic cavity (seen in infants with giant omphaloceles or ones that involve the liver) are at greatest risk for respiratory compromise: monitor closely for status changes.

    d. To prevent infection, moisten silo with povidone-iodine every 8 hours. Do not drench it, as this solution may irritate the skin. Some institutions no longer use povidone-iodine as the iodine in the solution may be absorbed and result in elevated iodine levels. Thyroid function may also be affected (Mulligan, 1986).

    e. Some institutions use an antibacterial agent such as neomycin to irrigate the bowel and reduce the chances of infection (Mulligan, 1986).

3. Respiratory support as necessary:

    a. Pressure is exerted on all internal organs, including the diaphragm, which is displaced upward; thus lungs are compressed and inadequate expansion occurs.

    b. Distress may develop at any point but is usually seen as the staged reduction progresses and intra-abdominal pressure increases.

    c. An infant may require oxygen by oxygen hood or positive-pressure ventilator:

        i. Administer oxygen to keep the baby pink and allow for easy respiration with adequate chest movement.

        ii. It is not unusual to require intubation and ventilation if (1) the abdomen is closed; (2) if arterial blood gases demonstrate hypoxemia; (3) respiratory acidosis develops; or (4) hypercarbia develops. Infants are usually first placed in oxygen hoods; if respiratory distress (cyanosis, nasal flaring, deteriorating blood gases) continues the infant may then be intubated based on the physician's judgment.

        iii. Use a transcutaneous oxygen monitor (TCM) or oximeter to monitor respiratory status during a staged reduction.

4. Intravenous access (see Chapter 9 for specific guidelines):

    a. Maintain the central line: Hyperalimentation is administered until the abdomen is closed and bowel function returns. Several weeks to several months of hyperalimentation may be required.

    b. Maintain the peripheral line:

        i. Administer antibiotics.

        ii. Administer replacement fluids for gastric losses.

5. Maintain patency of gastrostomy tube:
   a. To maintain patency, irrigate tube every 2 hours with 2 cc of air.
   b. Connect the tube to gravity drainage.
   c. To maintain fluid balance, measure, record, and empty gastric drainage; give replacement IV fluids every 4-8 hours as identified under Preoperative Stabilization in this section (pp. 132-133).
6. Parental support: see Chapter 3.
7. Feeding: To restore and maintain nutritional status without stressing the healing GI system of infant.
   a. Begin feeding when abdominal defect has been closed and bowel has begun to function; otherwise, absorption of nutrients will be compromised. Return of GI function is indicated when
      i. Gastric output has decreased and color is clear or cloudy.
      ii. Infant begins to form stool.
      iii. Bowel sounds are present.
   b. Begin with small, frequent feedings with gastrostomy tube open and elevated; if no gastrostomy tube is in place proceed in the same manner with gavage or nipple feedings by bottle. Feedings for some infants may need to be continuous with an elemental diet (like Pregestimil®), depending on bowel loss or severity of the defect and length of the ileus.
      i. Offer clear liquids: 5-10 cc every 2 hours; this allows an easily digested substance to be attempted before formulas are introduced.
      ii. If clear liquids are tolerated, advance to diluted formula:
         a) Increase the amount of feedings every 24-48 hours.
         b) Increase the strength of formula every 24-48 hours.
         c) Do not change both amount and strength at same feeding as both changes may stress the GI system and lead to malabsorption or abdominal distention.
      iii. Stop advancement if not tolerated; indications of intolerance are:
         a) Aspirate: check before feeding, if greater than half of the previous feeding, stop advancement.
         b) Stool: check for reducing substances every 8 hours. If >0.5%, or if amount of stool is increasing, stop advancement. If an elemental formula such as Pregestimil® is used, a paper strip indicator may be used instead of reducing substance tablets to detect reducing substances in the stool.
         c) Stool pH: check every 8 hours. A pH level of < 6 is indicative of the presence of reducing substances (Mulligan, 1986).
      iv. Gastric reflux: may occur due to an impediment to the flow of gastric contents into and through the intestines. This impediment may be the result of the surgical intervention itself through manipulation of the bowel. It may be linked with other associated intestinal problems, such as malrotation or volvulus that are present in addition to the original omphalocele or gastroschisis. See Postoperative Considerations (pp. 123-124) in this chapter for more specific information.

PARENT CARE

1. See Chapter 3 for specific guidelines.
2. Discharge planning: the goal of parent education is home management. Parents must be alert to the potential for complications. The major concern is the development of intestinal obstruction or malabsorption.
   a. Teach parents to be alert to complications such as:
      i. Poor appetite
      ii. Vomiting
      iii. Abdominal distention
      iv. Constipation or diarrhea
   b. Teach parents the need for follow-up care to prevent the development of complications and to ensure normal growth and development.

Hirschsprung's Disease
Carole Kenner

DESCRIPTION

In congenital Hirschsprung's disease there is an absence of ganglion cells in the bowel, aganglionosis. Skip areas have been found where one or two zones of aganglionic bowel may be separated by innervated or "normal" bowel. A transition zone can sometimes also be identified where aganglionosis and ganglion cells are interspersed.

ETIOLOGY AND EMBRYOLOGY

The primitive gut in the embryo is divided into three parts: foregut, midgut, and hindgut. It is from the hindgut that the sigmoid and descending colons arise. The neural-crest-cell peripheral nervous system leads to a conduction failure and resultant ineffective peristaltic action. As fecal matter is slowed in its propulsion down the intestine, an outpouching occurs. This eventually results in a functional obstruction, usually occurring in the rectosigmoid area; however, it can extend to the small intestine. As the obstruction progresses, more and more fecal material distends the bowel above the functional aganglionic segment. This distention is called megacolon or large colon. If this functional obstruction is allowed to persist, enterocolitis may occur. This condition can ultimately lead to peritonitis and septic shock with a 25 percent associated mortality rate. Hirschsprung's disease may not become obvious until after several days of feeding and bacterial formation in the gut has occurred. It is at this time that fecal matter will form and begin to cause obstructive symptoms.

In the first few weeks of embryological development, neural-crest cells migrate to the intestines, innervating the bowel. This innervation occurs at approximately the same time as the formation of oral and facial structures (including the palate). Thus, newborns with cleft lips or a palates should be watched for the development of Hirschsprung's disease. In the skip-zone or double-zone Hirschsprung's disease as it may be called, the suspected cause is anoxia to the bowel caused by regression and atrophy of neural cells. This anoxic insult could explain the discovery of normal-abnormal-normal segments. Most at risk for this type of Hirschsprung's disease would be the premature, stressed infants.

INCIDENCE

Hirschsprung's disease occurs in 1 of every 5000 live births. It is most common in full-term male newborns.

RISK FACTORS

1. Familial history: 3.6 percent risk for siblings of a child with Hirschsprung's disease.

2. Anoxic episode prior to birth.

3. Occasionally associated with Down's syndrome.

4. Associated with the occurrence of cleft lip or palate, may be autosomal recessive linkage.

5. Imperforate anus.

COMPLICATIONS

1. Malnutrition.

2. Fluid and electrolyte imbalance.

3. Enterocolitis.

4. Septic shock.

5. Death.

SYMPTOMS

1. Delayed passage of meconium, from 24 to 48 hours.

2. Meconium may be passed initially, followed by alternating constipation and diarrhea.

3. Abdominal distention, progressing if obstruction is not alleviated.

4. Vomiting, may or may not be bilious.

5. Feedings may be tolerated for several days before vomiting and distention occurs.

6. Enterocolitis may develop at any time and presents with diarrhea, dehydration, acidosis, sepsis, presence of blood either obvious or occult, and rapid deterioration of the baby's condition. This is the most common complication.

DIAGNOSIS

1. Rectal exam may appear normal or show slight tightening of the rectal canal. Explosive stools usually occur following the exam. This occurrence is indicative of Hirschsprung's disease. This explosive stool follows the exam because stool may not be present in the rectum itself, as with other constipation problems. The fecal matter is trapped up in the area of aganglionosis until pressure of the rectal exam propels it downward.

2. Abdominal radiographs, AP and lateral, will show air-filled, dilated bowel. There may be no air in the rectum.

3. Barium (this should be used first if Hirschsprung's disease is suspected) or water-soluble contrast enema will show a dilated portion of the bowel followed by a narrow atrophied distal bowel. The pigtail sign or funnel appearance is a characteristic usually not present for the first few days or weeks of life as atrophy must take place to narrow the bowel.

4. Enema solution will not be expelled after 24 hours.

5. Rectal biopsy—suction biopsy—demonstrating aganglionic areas in the rectal mucosa.

6. A negative biopsy does not completely preclude the diagnosis of Hirschsprung's disease. A strip biopsy may show a transition zone.

7. Positive neonatal history of delayed meconium, vomiting, constipation, and increasing abdominal distention.

8. Manometric measurement indicative of a negative rectoanal reflex.

TRANSPORT

The goal in transporting an infant with Hirschsprung's disease is to maintain gastric decompression and to prevent aspiration. Measures should be instituted by the transferring hospital prior to the transport team's arrival. If no double-lumen tube is available, a single-lumen nasogastric tube, gavage tube, or suction catheter may be placed to straight drainage as a temporary measure for gastric decompression. See Appendix A.

1. Insert a size 10 double-lumen tube for nasogastric decompression and to prevent aspiration.

2. Intravenous access:
   a. See Chapter 9 for a discussion of fluid management.
   b. Antibiotic coverage is needed if enterocolitis is suspected.

3. Parent care: see Chapter 3.

ADMISSION EQUIPMENT

1. Regular unit setup: see Appendix B.

2. Nasogastric suction equipment to maintain gastric decompression:
   a. Double-lumen nasogastric tube size 10
   b. Intermittent or continuous suction to facilitate gastric drainage

PREOPERATIVE STABILIZATION

Surgery includes exploratory laparotomy and probable colostomy. If the infant has enterocolitis, it must be treated with broad-spectrum antibiotics. If the enterocolitis has progressed to septic shock, volume expanders and resuscitation efforts may be necessary. Treatment of dehydration and acidosis is essential before testing for Hirschsprung's disease.

1. Abdominal assessment:
   a. To detect any abdominal distention or sudden changes in distention that may indicate enterocolitis, measure abdominal girth every 4 hours.
   b. Palpate abdomen over left lower quadrant for a loop of dilated bowel. Usually, however, the physical exam is normal.

2. Maintain IV fluids: see Chapter 9 for specific guidelines. This fluid balance is especially critical if fluroscopic contrast studies using dye have been done. The dye may cause a shift of fluid into the bowel. Diuresis may take place and increase the need for IV fluids. Continually assess the newborn for signs of dehydration, sunken fontanelles, poor skin turgor, or dry skin; a rule of thumb is 40 mL/kg/d of urine output.

3. Administer broad-spectrum antibiotics to prevent infection. Some institutions will not give antibiotics as a precautionary measure, so consult hospital protocol. See Chapter 9 for specific antibiotics.

4. Insert a nasogastric tube, size 10 double-lumen, and connect to low, continuous, or intermittent suction for gastric decompression.

a. Irrigate every 2 hours with 2 cc of air to maintain patency.
b. Measure, record, and discard output every 4-8 hours.
c. Replace nasogastric output, 1 cc replacement fluids for every 1 cc of gastric drainage, every 4-8 hours. See Chapter 9, Gastric Losses and Replacement (pp. 271-272) for specific information.
d. During the rectal exam be prepared for loose, explosive stool. If stool is expelled, do not assume that infant is cured. Assess infant carefully and make sure that if discharge from the hospital is imminent follow-up is arranged.

5. Obtain AP and lateroabdominal radiographs to determine the exact location and extent of Hirschsprung's disease.

6. Assist with administering barium or water-soluble contrast enemas; carefully assess the infant during this procedure, as fluid shifts can occur causing respiratory compromise and circulatory collapse. It may be necessary to give dextrose 5 percent Ringer's lactated solution with 5 g/100 mL salt-poor albumin following the contrast enema to raise the oncotic pressure and prevent fluid shifts into the bowel (Filston & Izant, 1985). An isotonic enema is also given preoperatively to cleanse the bowel, decrease the bacterial flora present, and prevent infection.

7. Assist with administering the rectal suction biopsy:
a. Verify informed parental consent for biopsy.
b. Use a suction biopsy tray with 35-cc syringe and Lubrafax®.
c. Hold infant to restrain.
d. Observe for signs of perforation after biopsy:
   i. Bleeding
   ii. Decreased hematocrit level
   iii. Increasing abdominal girth
   iv. Change in vital signs

8. Monitor vital signs every 2 hours to detect status changes due to perforation, infection, or obstruction:
a. Temperature, heart and respiratory rates, and BP.
b. Abdominal girth, noting distention and firmness.
c. Color, breath sounds, and respiratory effort.

9. Parent care: see Chapter 3.

SURGERY

Initial surgery is for the creation of a colostomy. A transverse colostomy is the most common. This colostomy must be performed in an area of bowel with ganglion cells proximal to the aganglionic segment. Corrective surgery is done at 12-18 months of age. It involves a rectal pull-through procedure with colostomy closure. The most common corrective procedures are (1) Duhamel's posterior colorectostomy (modification of Swenson's, involving the removal of the aganglionic bowel with an anastomosis of the colon to the rectum; the rectum is surgically closed with the creation of a new rectal segment); (2) Swenson's endorectal pull-through procedure (involves the disection of the rectum and sigmoid colon; the upper portion of healthy bowel is pulled down through a sleeve of abnormal bowel to create a functional intestinal surface); and (3) Soave's endorectal pull-through procedure (two-step procedure involving removal of rectal mucosa with a pull-down of the normal colon extending beyond the anus; within the next few weeks this extra skin is trimmed).

POSTOPERATIVE STABILIZATION

The postoperative goal is to restore GI function and to prevent infection.

1. Closely monitor vital signs and urine output to maintain a stable infant:
   a. Check temperature, heart and respiratory rates, and BP every 15 minutes four times; every 30 minutes four times; every hour four times; every 2 hours until stable, and then every 4 hours.
   b. Report any urine output <1 cc/kg/h.

2. Maintain IV access: see Chapter 9 for specific guidelines regarding fluid and antibiotic management.

3. Nasogastric decompression:
   a. Connect a size 10 double-lumen tube to low-intermittent or low-continuous suction.
   b. Irrigate the tube every 2 hours with 2 cc of air to keep tube patent.
   c. To maintain fluid balance, measure, record, and discard gastric output.
   d. Replace gastric output every 4-8 hours to keep infant in fluid balance. See Chapter 9, Gastric Losses and Replacement (pp. 271-272) for guidelines.

4. Colostomy care (see Chapter 12, Colostomy Care):
   a. Apply petroleum jelly gauze to stoma and cover with gauze dressing. Replace every 4 hours to prevent skin breakdown and infection.
   b. Record and report any bleeding or discoloration of stoma that may indicate impaired healing.
   c. Initially, the stoma will be dark, crusted, and bleed slightly. As healing occurs, the crusts will slough and the stoma becomes pink. The stoma should not bleed excessively, be prolapsed or retracted, or remain dark after 24 hours.

5. Observe and report any complications that indicate the development of an intestinal obstruction, respiratory compromise, or infection:
   a. Intestinal obstruction:
      i. Vomiting
      ii. Constipation or diarrhea
      iii. Abdominal distention

       iv. Change in vital signs (increased heart and respiratory rates, increased or decreased BP)

  b. Infection:
       i. Abscesses
       ii. Leakage or dehiscence of wound
       iii. Change in vital signs (fever, increased heart and respiratory rates)

  c. Respiratory distress:
       i. Increased respiratory rate
       ii. Substernal retractions
       iii. Lung congestion by auscultation

  d. Enterocolitis:
       i. Vomiting
       ii. Abdominal distention
       iii. Lethargy
       iv. Fever, increased heart and respiratory rates, and decreased BP
       v. Explosive, foul-smelling diarrhea (*Clostridium difficile* has been implicated in the development of enterocolitis)

6. Feedings:
  a. Begin when colostomy begins to function, 7-10 days.
  b. To decrease the stress on the newly functional bowel, begin with Pedialyte® (Ross Labs, Columbus, OH) by mouth every 2 hours. Advance to formula as tolerated:
       i. To ensure adequate absorption and tolerance of feedings, observe and record amount of stool every 8 hours. Slow advancement of feedings if stool output is more than half of intake during an 8-hour period.
       ii. If vomiting occurs, stop advancement.

PARENT CARE

1. See Chapter 3.

2. See Chapter 12, Colostomy Care.
  a. Make sure that parents are comfortable with changing colostomy bags and in applying dressings if these are to be used in place of colostomy bags.
  b. Supply parents with equipment and arrange for continued supply.
  c. Teach parents about the potential colostomy problems to prevent long-term complications, infection, and skin breakdown:
       i. Diarrhea
       ii. Constipation
       iii. Skin breakdown
       iv. Bleeding, prolapse, or retraction of stoma

3. Teach parents to be alert to symptoms of complications that indicate intestinal obstruction or gastric reflux:
  a. Poor appetite.

b. Vomiting.

c. Abdominal distention.

Imperforate Anus
Jeanne Harjo

DESCRIPTION AND EMBRYOLOGY

Normally, in the eighth week of embryonic life, the membrane that separates the rectum from the anus is absorbed and a continuous canal is formed. If this does not occur and union does not take place, then an imperforate anus results.

Classifications of imperforate anus are related to the placement of the distal end of the colon. In a low defect, the rectum ends near the surface of the external anal site. The defect is below the level of the levator musculature, indicating intact rectal muscles. Continence is possible in these infants. The term *atretic* or blind pouch is used in describing low defects to indicate an intact anal sphincter. A stenotic, or narrowed, anal canal further describes low defects that end in a smaller than normal anus. The anal defect may also be described as membranous, meaning that the tissue covering exists at or near the anus. In the intermediate defect, the bowel ends above the external site, but within the distance to correct the defect fairly easily. The puborectalis sling or muscle and the levator musculature along with the anal sphincter is usually intact, leading to continence after surgery. The high lesion ends well above the external anal site, above the puborectalis area of the levator muscle. It may be difficult to achieve a correction for the high lesion. It is this type of defect that is the most complicated. Determination of the presence of the end of the rectum in relation to the musculature is necessary to attempt to restore continence in the postoperative period. If the anal sphincter or musculature function is not restored, continence is not possible. The term *agenetic* is sometimes used in association with a high lesion to indicate that the bowel ending is located somewhere above the puborectalis.

Along with an imperforate anus, the following may also be present:

1. In the female neonate, a fistula may be present between the rectum and vagina or perineum.

2. The male neonate may present with a fistula between the rectum, and the urinary tract, at the scrotum or perineum.

The infant should be examined for the Vacterl syndrome:

V   Vertebral anomalies

A   Anal, imperforate anus

C   Cardiac, multiple defects possible

T   Tracheal, trachealesophageal fistula

E   Esophageal, atresia

R   Renal anomalies

L   Limb, deformities and dysplasia

ETIOLOGY

As development occurs, there is a failure of the cloaca and urogenital sinus to close. In some cases, an abnormal closure may occur, causing a fistula.

INCIDENCE

Imperforate anus occurs in 1 of every 15,000-20,000 births.

SYMPTOMS

1. Inability to insert rectal thermometer.
2. No meconium passed.
3. Meconium passed through a fistula or a misplaced anus.
4. Gradual distention and bowel obstruction present if there is no fistula.

DIAGNOSIS

1. Radiographs should include the following:
   a. The Wangenstein-Rice method: Head-down position while lateral abdominal and pelvic radiographs are taken. Any gas in the colon will rise and show the outline of the end of the rectum in relation to the anus. Radiograph markers may be taped to the external rectum to identify length of sealed tissue. Some physicians question the accuracy of this method and may not recommend its use since the rectum may contain meconium that will not allow the air to pass through; in this case the rectal area cannot be accurately identified. Abdominal ultrasound may be more useful in determining the rectal pouch.
   b. Flat-plate abdominal films to rule out any bowel obstructions.
2. Urinalysis may show evidence of stool or urinary tract infection, indicating a fistula.

TRANSPORT

The goal is to promote gastric decompression and maintain fluid balance. Prior to transport, the referring nursery can place a double-lumen nasogastric tube (if available), a single-lumen nasogastric tube, or a suction catheter to straight drainage to facilitate gastric decompression. If needed, an IV infusion may be started. The infant should be closely monitored for signs of increasing abdominal distention and dehydration.

1. See Appendix A.

2. Insert a size 10 double-lumen nasogastric tube if there is no fistula present. If draining fistula is present, distention and obstruction may not be present
   a. Connect to low-intermittent or continuous suction to facilitate gastric decompression.
   b. Irrigate every 2 hours with 2 cc of air to maintain tube's patency.

PREOPERATIVE STABILIZATION

The preoperative goal is to prevent dehydration and abdominal distention.

1. Monitor vital signs every 2 hours: include axillary temperature, apical pulse, respiratory rate and effort, color, and peripheral BP.

2. Measure abdominal girth every 2-4 hours to detect abdominal distention or the worsening of present distention.

3. Keep a strict record of intake and output, including stool, to maintain fluid and electrolyte balance. A large volume of stool may be expelled after a fistula is dilated and may cause dehydration.

4. To prevent abdominal distention and possible aspiration, maintain nasogastric decompression:
   a. Connect size 10 double-lumen catheter to continuous-low suction.
   b. Irrigate with 2 cc of air or normal saline solution every 2 hours to maintain tube's patency.
   c. To restore or maintain fluid balance, measure, record, and discard output every 4-8 hours. See Chapter 9 for specific replacement guidelines.

SURGERY

The goal for surgical intervention is to restore the anal canal and to promote continence of urine and stool.

1. Low defect:
   a. Rupture of a covered anal membrane may be all the repair needed.
   b. Locally dilating fistula promotes the formation of stools and delays a peripheral repair of the anus or anoplasty for 3-4 months.
   c. Most often a peripheral anoplasty is performed in the neonatal period.

2. Intermediate defect:
   a. If a fistula is present it is dilated and a sacroperineal pull-through is performed later, at 9-12 months. This usually applies only to female infants with low vaginal fistulas.
   b. If no fistula is present, a colostomy is performed and later a sacroperineal pull-through at the age of 9-12 months is performed

3. High defect: All of these lesions require a colostomy with a sacroperineal or abdominal pull-through usually done at 9-12 months of age. Recently, some surgeons have been treating high defects with a sigmoid-loop colostomy and then waiting only 1-14 days before a sacroperineal or abdominosacroperineal pull-through procedure is completed. The colostomy is then closed at 3-4 months of age if the infant is experiencing no intestinal or nutritional problems. The success rate of this quick repair is reported to be 70 percent with good results (Freeman & Bulut, 1986).

POSTOPERATIVE STABILIZATION FOR ANOPLASTY

1. Closely monitor vital signs and urine output:
   a. Check temperature (axillary), pulse, respiration, and BP every 15 minutes four times; every 30 minutes four times; every hour four times; every 2 hours until stable, and then every 4 hours.
   b. To maintain fluid balance, report any urine output <1 cc/kg/h.

2. Maintain IV access. See Chapter 9 for guidelines.
   a. Administer broad-spectrum antibiotics to prevent infection. Some institutions, however, will not recommend use of precautionary drugs and will only give antibiotics if an infection is present; consult hospital protocol.
   b. Give replacement fluids to maintain fluid and electrolyte balance. Since nasogastric secretions contain large amounts of sodium and potassium, these need to be replaced with dextrose 5 percent and 0.9% NaCl with 10 mEq of potassium chloride/L; 1 cc of replacement fluids for 1 cc of gastric drainage is the usual dosage.

3. Maintain nasogastric decompression: see Preoperative Stabilization in this section (p. 146).

4. Anoplasty care:
   a. Irrigate exterior anoplasty with antimicrobial cleansing solution every 4 hours and after every stool. Do not wipe or rub area as this may break down the suture line.
   b. Do not fasten diapers.
   c. Do not take the rectal temperature, give rectal medications, or perform any rectal examination.
   d. Avoid tension on suture line. Position baby on side or abdomen, not on back.

5. Observe for complications indicative of impaired skin integrity or recurrence of intestinal obstruction.
   a. Note and report any drainage, redness, or breakdown of anoplasty.
   b. Observe and report any abdominal distention or vomiting.

6. Feedings:

   a. Wait at least 24 hours after surgery before starting feedings to minimize
      stooling until incision is healing. Some surgeons even suggest waiting 5
      days.
   b. Discontinue nasogastric tube for 24 hours before attempting feedings.
      Report any abdominal distention or vomiting that may result from the dis-
      continuation of the gastric decompression and retention of gastric
      secretions in the stomach.
   c. Advance feedings as tolerated starting with simple solutions and moving to
      more complex formulas to allow intestinal absorption:
        i. Start with clear fluids every 2-3 hours for 24 hours.
       ii. Change to ½-strength formula or breast milk every 2-3 hours for 24
           hours.
      iii. Advance to full-strength formula or breast milk and increase the
           amount as tolerated. Any increase in stooling or suture-line breakdown,
           vomiting, or abdominal distention may indicate the need to stop advance-
           ment of the feedings.

PARENT CARE

1. See Chapter 3 for specific guidelines.

2. Discharge planning to promote home management and prevent complications
   once the infant is home:
   a. Teach parents the importance of medical follow-up to prevent com-
      plications.
   b. Teach parents the signs of intestinal obstruction, poor tolerance of feedings,
      and impaired healing processes to prevent long-term complications. Signs
      that should be reported are:
        i. Diarrhea or constipation
       ii. Redness or breakdown of anal area
      iii. Poor appetite
       iv. Vomiting
   c. Schedule anal dilation to be performed 2-3 weeks after discharge from
      hospital, to achieve elasticity of the anal sphincter and to prevent stricture
      and scar formation.

POSTOPERATIVE STABILIZATION FOR COLOSTOMY

   The goal for the infant with a colostomy is to prevent skin breakdown and to
restore normal bowel function.

1. Closely monitor vital signs and urine output:
   a. Check and record temperature (axillary), pulse, respiratory rate, and BP
      every 15 minutes four times; every 30 minutes four times; every hour four

times; every 2 hours until stable and then every 4 hours to detect any changes in infant's status.

   b. Report any urine output <1 cc/kg/h that might be indicative of fluid and electrolyte imbalance.

2. Maintain IV access. See Chapter 9 and Postoperative Stabilization for Anoplasty in this section (p. 147).

3. Maintain nasogastric decompression: See Preoperative Stabilization (p. 146).

4. Colostomy care:

   a. Initially the stoma is dark, crusted, and bleeds easily. Apply petroleum jelly gauze to the stoma. A red rubber catheter or glass rod may be inserted through the loop of bowel to allow the stoma to remain above the skin. Support the catheter with gauze dressings and change at least every 4 hours to prevent skin breakdown and preserve integrity of stoma.

   b. After bleeding stops, apply a protective ointment to skin area around the stoma. Continue to support the catheter and change the dressings at least every 4 hours. The catheter will be removed in 7-10 days.

   c. When stool formation begins, apply a colostomy pouch. See Chapter 12 Colostomy Care.

   d. Empty colostomy bag every 8 hours. Change bag as needed to prevent leakage.

5. Observe for complications:

   a. Note and report any redness, drainage, swelling, or separation of suture line or skin around the stoma.

   b. Observe and report any abdominal distention or vomiting that might indicate intestinal obstruction.

6. Give feedings to promote adequate nutrition without inducing hypermotility and diarrhea:

   a. Begin feeding when bowel begins to function (usually 3-5 days), as indicated by:

      i. Passage of stool from colostomy

      ii. Decreased nasogastric output

      iii. Nasogastric output changing from green to cloudy

   b. Discontinue nasogastric tube 24 hours before attempting feedings and report any distention or vomiting.

   c. Advance feedings as tolerated: see Postoperative Stabilization for Anoplasty in this section (p. 147). Any increase in stool formation or any skin breakdown around stoma, vomiting, or distention indicates the need to stop the advancement of feedings.

PARENT CARE

1. See Chapter 3 for specific guidelines.

2. For instructions on colostomy care, see Chapter 12 Colostomy Care.

Malrotation and Volvulus
Jeanne Harjo

DESCRIPTION

Malrotation is a failure of the rotation and fixation of both the small and large bowel. The small bowel is positioned on the right side of the abdomen and the cecum rests in the right upper quadrant. The colon is fixed into the left side of the abdomen.

Volvulus is an infarction of part or all of the small and large bowel due to obstruction of mesenteric blood supply. Ladd bands are peritoneal bands that form abnormal attachments and resulting obstruction.

ETIOLOGY AND PATHOPHYSIOLOGY

Malrotation and volvulus is a congenital failure of the intestines to rotate counterclockwise as they return to the abdomen in embryologic formation. The result is a twisting of the bowel (malrotation) and subsequent intestinal obstruction that may result in a volvulus.

EMBRYOLOGY

The intestines form outside the abdominal cavity. By 10-12 weeks of gestation they return to the abdomen, rotating in a counterclockwise direction. The duodenum adheres to the right upper quadrant. The cecum rests in the right lower quadrant. Large intestines adhere into ascending and descending positions. A failure of this process results in malrotation with possible obstruction and ensuing volvulus.

INCIDENCE

An exact incidence is not usually reported since volvulus may be associated with many different intestinal obstructions.

SYMPTOMS

1. The neonate may appear healthy before symptoms appear from 3 days to several weeks. It is presumed that the dilatation of the bowel by food and gas precipitates the symptoms.

2. Abdominal distention.
3. Vomiting:
   a. Usually bilious.
   b. May be intermittent or persistent.
   c. Occurs after feeding.
4. Dehydration and electrolyte depletion and shock:
   a. Can occur rapidly due to vomiting.
   b. Fever usually follows.
5. Changes in stool usually associated with volvulus and infarction of the bowel:
   a. Scanty stools.
   b. Diarrhea.
   c. Bloody stools.
6. Rapid deterioration with volvulus:
   a. Distention.
   b. Lethargy.
   c. Mottled skin with poor perfusion.
   d. Dehydration from bilious vomiting.
   e. Bloody stools.

DIAGNOSIS

1. Abdominal films showing gas-filled dilated stomach and duodenum indicate malrotation but are inconclusive for indicating volvulus.
2. Upper GI series may show the following:
   a. Stomach is larger than normal.
   b. First part of the duodenum is dilated.
   c. The point of obstruction is marked by a minute amount of contrast passing below this area.
3. Barium enema or contrast studies may show the following:
   a. Abnormal positioning of the cecum and the ascending colon, usually with the cecum in the upper right instead of lower right quadrant.
   b. The point of obstruction of the colon where volvulus has occurred.

TRANSPORT

The infant must be rushed to a center for immediate surgical intervention. Any delay in treatment may compromise the chances for saving large segments of bowel. Referring nurses should closely assess the infant's status while waiting for the transport team. If gastric decompression is needed, a single or double-lumen nasogastric tube or suction catheter may be placed to straight drainage as a temporary measure. An IV infusion should be started, if possible, for IV access.

1. See Appendix A.

2. Insert a nasogastric tube for decompression to prevent abdominal distention and aspiration.
   a. Use a size 10 double-lumen tube.
   b. Connect tube to low-continuous suction as available to facilitate drainage.

3. Intravenous access: see Chapter 9 for specific guidelines. Antibiotics may be given as a precautionary measure to prevent infection; however, not all institutions recommend the use of broad-spectrum antibiotics unless an infection is present.

4. Parental support: see Chapter 3 for specific guidelines.

ADMISSION EQUIPMENT

1. Normal admission setup: see Appendix B.

2. Nasogastric suction equipment for gastric decompression:
   a. Size 10 double-lumen tube.
   b. Intermittent or continuous suction.

PREOPERATIVE STABILIZATION

The preoperative goal is to stabilize infant's fluid and electrolyte status, to prevent abdominal distention, and to promote comfort.

1. Monitor vital signs every 2 hours to determine baseline changes:
   a. Check temperature, heart and repiratory rates, and BP.
   b. Measure abdominal girth and report any distention or firmness.
   c. Observe breath sounds, respiratory effort, and color.

2. Maintain IV access: see Chapter 9 for specific guidelines.

3. Administer antibiotics, usually ampicillin and gentamicin: see Chapter 9 for specific guidelines.

4. Maintain nasogastric decompression to prevent abdominal distention. See Preoperative Stabilization (p. 146) in the section Imperforate Anus in this chapter.

5. Parental support:
   a. See Chapter 3 for specific guidelines.
   b. Verify informed surgical consent.

SURGERY

Volvulus necessitates emergency surgery as the entire bowel may infarct rapidly. The Ladd procedure involves dividing the numerous adhesions that hold the bowel in a malrotated position and lysis of the bands obstructing the duodenum. The duodenum is placed into the right lower quadrant. Transverse and ascending colons are placed into the left side of the abdomen. Necrotic bowel is resected. Appendectomy may be done. A gastrostomy tube is inserted and a central line may be inserted if necrotic bowel will necessitate long-term hyperalimentation.

POSTOPERATIVE STABILIZATION

The postoperative goal is to promote gastric decompression, restore fluid and electrolyte balance, and to promote nutrition for growth.

1. Closely monitor vital signs and urine output:
   a. Check temperature, heart rate, respiratory rate, and BP every 15 minutes four times, every 30 minutes four times, every hour four times, every 2 hours until stable, and then every 4 hours.
   b. Report any urine output <1 cc/kg/h; this is essential after any abdominal surgery, since third spacing of fluids may occur. See Chapter 9 for a discussion of third spacing of fluids (p. 271).

2. Maintain IV access, see Chapter 9 (pp. 280-285) for specific guidelines:
   a. Bowel resection requires total parenteral nutrition for hydration and electrolyte balance.
   b. Central line care if indicated.
   c. Replace gastric losses every 4-8 hours. See Gastric Losses section (pp. 271-272) of Chapter 9.
   d. Administer antibiotics (ampicillin and gentamicin); specific guidelines may be found in Chapter 9.

3. Maintain patency of nasogastric tube to ensure decompression:
   a. See preoperative stabilization (p. 146) in this section.
   b. Discontinue tube in 3-5 days or when gastrostomy tube begins to function adequately.

4. Maintain patency of gastrostomy tube:
   a. Irrigate tube every 2 hours with 2 cc of air to keep open.
   b. Connect tube to gravity drainage system.
   c. Record and discard output and give replacement fluids every 4-8 hours. See Chapter 9 for Gastric Losses and Replacement (pp. 271-272).

5. Observe and report any abdominal distention or vomiting:
   a. Note and report any redness, drainage, swelling, or separation of suture line.
   b. Observe and report any abdominal distention or vomiting which may indicate an intestinal obstruction.

6. Provide respiratory support as needed:
   a. Infant may require an oxygen hood or positive-pressure ventilator.

    b. Adjust oxygen by monitoring breath sounds, color, and respiratory effort every 1-2 hours.

7. Parent Care: See Chapter 3.

8. Feedings: The time to start feedings may vary according to the amount of ischemia the bowel has suffered due to strangulation by the volvulus:

    a. Begin feedings when the bowel begins to function, usually in 7-10 days, as indicated by:

        i. Passage of stool.

        ii. Decreased gastric output.

        iii. Gastric output changing from green to cloudy.

    b. Elevate gastrostomy tube for 24 hours to determine the adequacy of intestinal absorption of gastric secretions:

        i. Measure gastric aspirates every 4 hours.

        ii. Record and reinsert aspirates to maintain electrolyte balance as gastric secretions contain sodium and potassium in particular.

        iii. If aspirate is clear and <5-10 cc every 4 hours, feedings can begin.

        iv. If aspirate is green and >10 cc, wait another 24 hours to start feedings.

    c. Advance feedings slowly to decrease the chance of hypermotility, malabsorption, and diarrhea with resultant fluid loss:

        i. Start with clear liquids every 2 hours for 24 hours.

        ii. Increase to ¼-strength formula and increase by ¼ strength every 24 hours as tolerated.

        iii. Gauge tolerance of feedings:

            a) Check aspirate before each feeding, record, and reinsert.

            b) Check stool for reducing substances every 8 hours.

            c) Stop advancement if aspirate is green or >10-15 cc, vomiting occurs, abdominal distention is noted, or stool reducing substances are >0.5 percent.

9. Parenteral nutrition is required until full feedings are tolerated and weight gain is steady.

PARENT CARE

1. See Chapter 3 specific guidelines.

2. Alert parents to potential problems that would indicate intestinal obstruction or feeding intolerance; the goal is to prevent long-term complications, malnutrition, and dehydration:

    a. Diarrhea or constipation.

    b. Poor appetite.

    c. Vomiting.

    d. Abdominal distention.

e. Skin breakdown or leakage around gastrostomy tube, may be indicative of an intestinal obstruction.

3. Gastrostomy care and feedings: See Chapter 12, Gastrostomy Care (pp. 347-351).

Intussusception
Carole Kenner

DESCRIPTION AND PATHOPHYSIOLOGY

Intussusception is a telescoping of one segment of the intestines into another segment of bowel, thus creating an obstruction. This obstruction may occur anywhere in the intestinal tract, with the terminal ileum and ascending colon being the most common sites. The obstruction and pressure of the one segment of intestines pressing upon the other decreases circulation within the affected bowel. The result is bowel ischemia and bleeding from the intestinal wall. The stool then may be described as mucoid and bloody, "currant jelly"-like in appearance.

ETIOLOGY

The exact etiology can only be determined in about 5 percent of the cases. It is found in infants with cystic fibrosis, Meckel's diverticulum, and congenital intestinal atresias. In each of these instances there may be an effort by the body to attempt to move stool through a narrowed or blocked segment of bowel. The result is increased peristaltic activity. Exactly how this increased activity causes the sliding of one intestinal segment into another is not understood.

INCIDENCE

An exact incidence is difficult to determine since it occurs after many other medical conditions. It is more common in male than female neonates. It is generally found in those infants with cystic fibrosis or a history of gastroenteritis or celiac disease. It usually occurs between the ages of 2-24 months; however, in the neonatal period, intussusception may follow the development of an atresia that arose in utero.

SYMPTOMS

The symptoms are directly related to the intestinal obstruction and the decrease in blood supply to the bowel.

1. Severe colicky abdominal pain.

2. Intermittent retraction of infant's legs to decrease painful spasms.

3. Irritable, high-pitched crying.

4. Intermittent bilious vomiting initially, but as obstruction progresses bilious vomiting and pain increase in frequency.

5. Abdominal distention with associated guarding.

6. Currant-jelly appearance of stool: bloody and mucoid as obstruction progresses; initially stool may appear normal.

7. Increasing lethargy and eventual shock.

DIAGNOSIS

The diagnosis is made from the neonate's history as well as objective data. The intermittent colicky pain, bilious vomiting, and currant-jelly stool are highly indicative of intussusception. A mass may be palpated in the right upper quadrant or in the epigastric region. A barium enema will reveal the site of the obstruction, which is described as having a "coil-spring" appearance in the area of the intussusception (Rockenhaus, 1985).

TRANSPORT

Generally these infants will not be transported for intussusception but for another problem. Therefore, the referring nursery and transport management should be geared towards the stabilization of the condition of the infant and should vary depending on the underlying problem. If a neonate is transported for intussusception, the goal is to promote abdominal decompression and infant comfort and to prevent dehydration, shock, and peritonitis. See Appendix A for specific guidelines for neonatal transport.

ADMISSION EQUIPMENT

1. See Appendix B for admission setup

2. Nasogastric decompression equipment:
   a. Size10 double-lumen tube for gastric decompression.
   b. A second suction setup for nasogastric decompression.

PREOPERATIVE STABILIZATION

The preoperative goal is to prevent dehydration and the development of peritonitis, promote infant comfort, facilitate gastric decompression, and to prevent aspiration. The overriding concern is to treat the intussusception as quickly as possible to prevent the development of either bowel ischemia or peritonitis. The infant's bowel integrity and survival are dependent upon early intervention.

1. Assess the infant's status for an accurate description of episodic pain.

2. Observe infant's stool for the appearance of mucus or blood.

3. Measure the abdominal girth and recheck every 4 hours to detect any changes.

4. Insert a nasogastric tube, size 10 double lumen, for gastric decompression; this tube may be connected to low-intermittent or low continuous suction.

5. Palpate abdomen for the presence of a mass in the right upper quadrant or epigastric area.

6. Observe for vomiting and note whether it is bile-stained or not.

7. Observe for signs of dehydration such as sunken fontanelles; decreased skin turgor; dry, flaky skin; skin warm to the touch; or decreased urine output, <1 cc/kg/h.

8. Closely monitor vital signs including the BP at least every 2 hours to detect early the onset of fever—a sign of infection or the beginning of shock.

9. Do a complete blood cell count (CBC) especially for the hemoglobin and hematocrit levels, since anemia may result from intestinal bleeding.

10. Explain to parents the possibility of treating the condition through the use of a barium enema and change in hydrostatic pressure; however, they need to know that surgical intervention may be required.

11. Start an IV infusion for maintenance of fluids, replacement of fluids to restore the electrolytes and fluids lost through nasogastric suction, and for access in case of shock.
    a. Antibiotics may be given if pneumonia due to aspiration, or peritonitis is present.
    b. See the section Fluid and Electrolyte Status (pp. 263-293) in Chapter 9 for specific guidelines regarding fluid replacement, maintenance, and antibiotic therapy.

NONSURGICAL TREATMENT

An attempt may be made to treat intussusception by hydrostatic reduction; however, surgical intervention may still be necessary. The infant is made NPO. A nasogastric tube is placed to decompress the GI tract and to prevent aspiration. A Foley catheter is placed in the infant's rectum and the balloon is inflated. Leakage of barium may occur around the catheter. It may be necessary to tape the buttocks together to prevent this reflux from the rectum. Next the infant is given a barium enema very slowly. The enema bag should be placed approximately 30 inches above the bed. This height increases the pressure within the bowel. As the bowel fills, the barium causes the bowel to reduce and return to its normal position. This movement should be verified by several radiographs taken at different points during the procedure.

The success rate is 75 percent in older infants and children but not reported in the neonate (Rockenhaus, 1985). The infant should be observed closely after this procedure for reintussusception that is most likely to occur in the first 24-48 hours following the initial reduction. The symptoms present prior to reduction would return if intussusception recurred. Feedings may be resumed as soon as bowel sounds are present. This may be only 24 hours after the procedure. If the infant tolerates feedings and the return of normal stool formation occurs, the infant may be discharged safely from the hospital.

It should be remembered that this procedure is most often conducted in an older infant. The surgeon's discretion and hospital policy should be followed regarding its use in the neonate. This procedure should also not be done in the presence of shock or peritonitis (Rockenhaus, 1985).

SURGERY

Intussusception is corrected by transabdominal reduction. This procedure involves pressing the bowel together to squeeze the telescopic segment to return to its normal position. A resection of a segment of the bowel may also be necessary if bowel ischemia and resultant necrosis are present. The goal is to preserve as much of the bowel as possible and to return or restore normal bowel function.

POSTOPERATIVE STABILIZATION

The postoperative goal is to promote fluid balance and positive nutrition and to correct alterations in bowel elimination.

1. Monitor vital signs closely: temperature, heart and respiratory rates, along with BP every 15 minutes four times, every 30 minutes four times, every hour four times, every 2 hours until stable, and then every 4 hours.

2. Nasogastric decompression may be necessary postoperatively to relieve abdominal distention and prevent aspiration:
   a. Connect a size 10 double-lumen tube to low-intermittent or continuous suction.
   b. Irrigate tube every 2 hours with 2 cc of air to maintain patency.
   c. Record, discard, and replace nasogastric output every 4-8 hours to maintain fluid balance. Replacement fluids are usually dextrose 5 percent in 0.9%

NaCl solution with 10 mEq of potassium chloride/L, with 1 cc of replacement fluid given for every 1 cc of gastric output.

d. Discontinue nasogastric suction, under a physician's supervision, as soon as bowel sounds resume and oral feedings may begin.

3. Assess infant closely for signs of infection (fever, tachycardia, subtle color changes, increasing abdominal distention) as peritonitis in the postoperative period is a concern.

4. Give broad-spectrum antibiotics, ampicillin 100 mg/kg/d IV in divided doses along with gentamicin 5 mg/kg/d IV in divided doses; some institutions do not recommend the use of antibiotics unless an infection is present, so consult hospital protocol.

5. If the infant has peritonitis or has undergone extensive surgery, ventilatory support may be necessary:

a. Assess color, respiratory effort, and breathing patterns.

b. If infant is experiencing cyanosis, labored respiration, or ineffective breathing patterns, notify the physician immediately.

c. Check levels of arterial blood gases to determine the presence of hypoxemia, hypercapnia, or respiratory acidosis.

d. A transcutaneous oxygen monitor or pulse oximeter may be placed on the infant for continuous monitoring of the oxygen status; if either of these parameters is low, TCM indicating PaO_2 between 50 and 70 is normal for a full-term or near-term infant (this value may vary, consult infant's preoperative baseline and compare) and oximeter indicating <90 percent saturation, notify the physician.

e. Supplemental oxygen may be needed as well as ventilatory support with a positive-pressure ventilator if hypoxemia is present; give oxygen to maintain pink skin color and arterial blood gases within normal limits (see Appendix D, Blood Gases).

6. Maintain fluid balance with intravenous fluids (see the section Parenteral Nutrition: Peripheral and Total Nutrition (pp. 280-285) in Chapter 9 for specific guidelines) until oral feedings can be resumed.

a. Check intake and output every 8 hours, including nasogastric drainage, to maintain fluid status.

b. Check urine-specific gravity every 8 hours to assess for signs of dehyration or overhydration.

7. Begin oral feedings slowly, offer clear fluids every 2 hours, then gradually advance as tolerated to full-strength feedings:

a. Assess for abdominal distention, vomiting, or alterations in stool formation: diarrhea or constipation; any of these may indicate malabsorption, intolerance of feedings, or an intestinal obstruction. If problems arise, stop advancement and notify physician.

b. If the infant has undergone extensive bowel resection, hyperalimentation may be necessary; feeding progression may be quite slow depending upon the amount of bowel that remains. See Necrotizing Enterocolitis with Intestinal Perforation, Postoperative Section (pp. 176-177) in this chapter for a description of this feeding.

8. Assess suture line at least every 4 hours for signs of infection, separation, or drainage to ensure adequate wound healing. Any problem with healing should be reported to the physician immediately as this infant is at risk for infection postoperatively.

The postoperative course may vary if another underlying problem, such as cystic fibrosis or gastroenteritis, has been the causative factor in the development of intussusception. In these cases, the postoperative course will depend on the treatment of that particular disease or surgical problem.

PARENT CARE

1. See Chapter 3 for specific guidelines

2. If parents are taking the infant home after medical treatment with no surgical intervention, teach them to look for signs of intestinal obstruction to promote health maintenance once home. Signs of complications are:
   a. Abdominal distention.
   b. Vomiting.
   c. Stool alterations, diarrhea or constipation.
   d. Poor appetite.

3. Teach parents the need to report immediately to the physician any feeding or stool formation problems once the infant is home. Parents need to understand the importance of the prevention of complications. These complications can occur whether or not the infant has undergone surgery.

Meconium Ileus Associated with Cystic Fibrosis (Mucoviscidosis)

Carole Kenner

DESCRIPTION

Meconium ileus is a congenital mechanical intestinal obstruction resulting from thickened meconium collecting in the terminal ileum. The thickened meconium is often a result of cystic fibrosis. There is a form of meconium ileus that may be familial in nature; however, this form is rare.

ETIOLOGY AND PATHOPHYSIOLOGY

Meconium ileus is literally an ileum filled with meconium resulting from a viscous meconium that builds up due to mucoviscidosis or production of thickened secretions. This meconium eventually mechanically obstructs the intestines at the level of the ileum. The colon, which is unused, will atrophy and become narrowed and small. At the level of the ileocecal valve, meconium collects and distention occurs. Intestinal loops may be visible or palpated in the lower right quadrant. On a radiograph, especially on an upright film, a soap-bubble appearance will be noted due to the trapped air that results from the thick meconium. If the distention has become too great, and bowel ischemia, necrosis, and finally perforation has occurred, the upright film will demonstrate free air in the peritoneal cavity.

INCIDENCE

Approximately 10 percent of infants with cystic fibrosis will have meconium ileus (Guzzetta, Randolph, Anderson, Boyajian, & Eichelbergen, 1987). It usually occurs in full-term infants.

SYMPTOMS

1. Abdominal distention.

2. Bilious vomiting.

3. Distended bowel loops in right lower quadrant with resultant soap bubble appearance on radiograph.

4. Atrophied colon shown on radiograph or following barium enema.

DIAGNOSIS

1. History of abdominal distention.

2. Presence of bilious vomiting.

3. Upright radiograph depicting soap-bubble or ground-glass appearance in right lower quadrant.

4. Barium enema demonstrating atrophied colon, must be distinguished from Hirschsprung's disease and meconium-plug syndrome.

5. Distended loops of bowel in right lower quadrant on upright radiograph.

6. Upright x-ray film will also show if there is free air in peritoneal cavity; left lateral decubitus x-ray film may also show free air.

7. Meconium ileus may be the first suggestion of cystic fibrosis, so positive familial history of cystic fibrosis is suggestive of diagnosis.

8. Failure to pass meconium or passage of meconium plug is suggestive.

9. Meconium testing for trypsin and amylase levels, which are decreased if cystic fibrosis is present; trypsin levels in cystic fibrosis are 0-450 µg/kg/50 min, and amylase levels in cystic fibrosis are 0-117 IU/kg/50 min (Wallach, 1983). (Trypsin levels will also be decreased in complete intestinal obstruction.)

10. Perform sweat chloride test if cystic fibrosis is suspected. A level >60 mEq/L is considered abnormal (Filston & Izant, 1985). The sweat chloride test is not always accurate until about 8-12 weeks of age. The reason for the inaccuracy is that an infant does not effectively produce sweat in the initial newborn period.

TRANSPORT

The transport goal is to promote gastric decompression and hydration and to prevent aspiration. These measures should be instituted if possible in the referring hospital.

1. See Appendix A.

2. Position infant with head elevated slightly and turned to the side, if vomiting, to decrease chance of aspiration.

3. If abdominal distention is present, place a nasogastric tube to straight gravity for decompression.

4. Start an IV if the infant appears dehydrated from vomiting.

ADMISSION EQUIPMENT

1. See Appendix B.

2. Nasogastric tube size 10 double lumen.

PREOPERATIVE STABILIZATION

1. Assess infant for abdominal distention:
   a. Measure abdominal girth to determine baseline measurement.
   b. Palpate abdomen, especially right lower quadrant, for distended bowel loops.

c. Place nasogastric tube, size 10 double lumen, for decompression if distention is present:

    i. Put nasogastric tube to straight drainage or to intermittent-low suction to prevent aspiration.

    ii. Irrigate nasogastric tube every 2 hours with 2 cc of air to keep tube patent.

    iii. To maintain fluid and electrolyte balance, measure and record output from nasogastric tube every 4-8 hours.

2. Check vital signs for baseline measurements, including BP as perforation may have occurred; be especially aware of hypotension, tachycardia, and shock if a perforation is present.

3. Start IV fluids for maintenance and make infant NPO pending results of diagnostic tests; see Chapter 9 for specific guidelines on fluids.

4. Obtain the neonatal history to determine if meconium has ever been passed or if a meconium plug has been noted.

5. To attempt to produce stool defecation, rectal stimulation may be attempted if no meconium has been passed; if meconium ileus is present, no stool will usually be obtained in this manner.

6. Assess infant for signs of dehydration if vomiting has occurred:
   a. Skin turgor.
   b. Sunken fontanelles.
   c. Sunken eyeballs.
   d. Dry skin.
   e. Check urine-specific gravity every 8 hours.
   f. Measure intake and output, including nasogastric drainage every 8 hours.

7. To assist in determining location of a possible obstruction, observe vomitus for bile.

8. Assist with diagnostic radiographs and contrast studies:
   a. Position infant with head of bed elevated and infant's head turned to the side between tests to protect against aspiration.
   b. To prevent cold stress, maintain neutral thermal environment as much as possible during testing; keep the infant under a warmer or in an isolette during tests, wrap the infant in blankets if a warming unit cannot be used.
   c. Constantly assess infant during testing for changes in color and respiratory effort or pattern, as such testing may be stressful to the infant.

9. Broad-spectrum antibiotics may be started prior to a definitive diagnosis, for specific guidelines see Antibiotics (pp. 290-293) in Chapter 9. Some institutions do not recommend starting antibiotics as a precautionary measure, so consult hospital protocol.

10. Obtain serum electrolyte levels and a CBC for baseline measurements.

11. Notify parents of the possibility of surgery.

NONSURGICAL TREATMENT

1. A barium enema should be administered to determine if colon is small and atrophied from disuse.

2. Next a hyperosmotic solution may be instilled. Meglucamine diatrizoate is most often used. This contrast material will moisten the meconium and cause the meconium to be expelled.

3. If this treatment successfully relieves the obstruction, surgery may not be necessary; however, the infant will need to be assessed for dehydration secondary to fluid shifts that may occur from the instillation of a hyperosmolar fluid.

4. Installation of a hyperosmolar solution should never be attempted if perforation is suspected.

5. If this treatment is unsuccessful, surgery is necessary.

SURGERY

The surgery involves relieving the intestinal obstruction and reestablishing a useful colon. A Bishop-Koop anastomosis may be done or a Mikulicz enteroenterostomy. Each relieves the mechanical obstruction, removes the meconium, evacuates the air, and reestablishes bowel function.

Bishop-Koon anastomosis involves a resection of the affected ileum and an anastomosis from the proximal ileum to the distal portion of the ileum. An ileostomy is created in the distal segment. This ileostomy can be used for irrigations of Mucomyst to dissolve any meconium that remains.

Mikulicz surgery involves a resection of affected ileum and removal of all the meconium. A double-barrel colostomy or ileostomy is created. The proximal ileum is anastomosed to the distal ileum. With the two segments of the colostomy, the proximal end serves to decompress the intestine while the distal segment allows intestinal irrigations. A Mikulicz clamp is then placed 5 days postoperatively to destroy the web between the two segments of the colostomy. The colostomy is usually temporary.

POSTOPERATIVE STABILIZATION

The postoperative goal is to prevent the recurrence of intestinal obstruction or the development of infection, especially enterocolitis, and to promote hydration and nutritional balance. Promotion of adequate respiratory gas exchange and ventilatory patterns is equally important. Concern initially is with the prevention of abdominal distention and promotion of wound healing, particularly at the stoma site.

1. To detect any changes in status, closely monitor vital signs and urine output:
   a. Measure temperature, heart and respiratory rates, and BP every 15 minutes four times, every 30 minutes four times, every hour four times, every 2 hours until stable, and then every 4 hours.
   b. Report any urine output <1 mL/kg/h.
   c. Measure intake and output at least every 8 hours since an infant's fluid status may change rapidly.

2. Maintain hydration via an IV; see Chapter 9 for specific guidelines.

3. Give broad-spectrum antibiotics, usually ampicillin and gentamicin in divided doses; see Antibiotics (pp. 290-293) in Chapter 9 for specific guidelines.

4. Nasogastric decompression may be necessary postoperatively to relieve abdominal distention and potential pressure on the suture line:
   a. See Preoperative Stabilization (p.163) in this section for specific instructions.
   b. Discontinue nasogastric suction when no signs of distention are present and a small amount of drainage is being obtained.

5. Colostomy care:
   a. See Chapter 12 for specific guidelines.
   b. Apply petroleum jelly gauze to stoma and cover with gauze dressing. If Mikulicz clamp is present, wrap petroleum jelly gauze carefully around the clamp.
   c. Change gauze and/or dressing every 4 hours.
   d. Initially, the stoma will be dark, crusted and bleeding slightly. As healing occurs, the crusts will slough off and the stoma become pink. The stoma should not bleed excessively, prolapse, retract, or remain dark after 24 hours. If a clamp is in place, observe for excessive bleeding or signs of bowel perforation that can occur.

6. To prevent or at least reduce any long-term problems from intestinal obstruction, infection, or respiratory compromise observe and report any signs of complications:
   a. Signs of intestinal obstruction include the following:
      i. Vomiting
      ii. Constipation or diarrhea
      iii. Abdominal distention
      iv. Changes in vital signs, especially tachycardia or tachypnea, and hypertension
   b. Signs of infection include the following:
      i. Leakage or dehiscence of wound
      ii. Changes in vital signs especially fever, tachycardia or tachypnea
      iii. Inflammation around stoma
   c. Respiratory distress may be detected by the following:
      i. Assessing the respiratory status for ineffective breathing patterns or increased chest retractions

    ii. Auscultating the chest for adventitious sounds and to determine the need for suctioning; this is especially important for the infant with cystic fibrosis who has thickened secretions. Tracheal suctioning is sometimes necessary to remove very viscous secretions. To promote airway clearance, suction as needed, usually every 2-4 hours in the first 24-48 hours postoperatively.

  d. Enterocolitis, a potentially life-threatening complication, may present with the following signs:
    i. Vomiting
    ii. Abdominal distention
    iii. Lethargy
    iv. Fever, tachycardia, tachypnea, or hypotension
    v. Explosive, foul-smelling diarrhea

7. Respiratory support as needed:
  a. Provide an oxygen hood if infant is breathing independently and only needs supplemental oxygen, or provide a positive-pressure ventilator if ventilatory assistance is needed.
  b. Monitor breath sounds, color, and respiratory effort every 1-2 hours to quickly detect any changes in respiratory status.

8. Feedings:
  a. Begin when colostomy begins to function and bowel sounds have returned, usually 7-10 days postoperatively.
  b. Pancreatic enzyme supplements are necessary if the diagnosis of cystic fibrosis has been made.
  c. Begin feeding with Pedialyte® (Ross Laboratories, Columbus, OH) by mouth every 2 hours. Advance to formula as tolerated. If the infant is diagnosed as having cystic fibrosis, elemental formulas may be preferred. Pregestimil® (Mead-Johnson Laboratories, Evansville, IN) consists of medium-chain triglycerides and easily absorbed fat, which facilitates digestion in severe GI disorders, especially where fat absorption is impaired.
    i. To detect any signs of malabsorption, observe and record amount of stool output every 8 hours. If there is an intolerance, stool output will be greatly increased.
    ii. To facilitate absorption, slowly advance feedings if stool output is less than half of intake during an 8-hour period.
    iii. If vomiting occurs, stop advancement to increase the chances of feeding tolerance. Offer a smaller amount; if vomiting stops, then gradually increase amount of feedings over next several feedings.

PARENT CARE

1. See Chapter 3 for specific guidelines.
2. Encourage the parents to express their feelings. If cystic fibrosis is the underlying cause, parents may feel guilty because it is autosomal recessive in inheritance.

3. Encourage the parents to meet with physicians on a regular basis, especially if cystic fibrosis is suspected.
4. Refer the parents to the Cystic Fibrosis Foundation or a cystic fibrosis clinic if cystic fibrosis is suspected.
5. Begin early teaching the parents how to care for their baby at home, especially regarding colostomy care. Promote comfort and confidence in the parents to care for their infant. Health maintenance will be enhanced for the infant if the parents can manage the care effectively at home.
   a. Colostomy care (see Chapter 12):
      i. Make sure that the parents are confident in applying dressings as well as colostomy bags.
      ii. Determine a resource for their medical supplies.
   b. Teach parents the signs of complications:
      i. Feeding problems:
         a) Poor appetite
         b) Vomiting
         c) Abdominal distention
         d) Diarrhea
      ii. Colostomy problems:
         a) Diarrhea
         b) Constipation
         c) Skin breakdown
         d) Bleeding, prolapse, or retraction of stoma
      iii. Long-term care will be necessary for the infant with cystic fibrosis; referral and follow-up should be done through a cystic fibrosis clinic or center:
         a) For respiratory care, chest physiotherapy and suctioning may be necessary; humidification may be used at home.
         b) Digestive enzymes and fat-soluble vitamin supplementation will be necessary.

The parents must thoroughly understand the importance of following the prescribed medical regimen to prevent respiratory compromise and malnutrition. A multidisciplinary team effort is needed: respiratory therapist, physician, nurse, and social worker—especially for the child with cystic fibrosis facing a life-long disease. A public-health nurse or home visiting by a cystic fibrosis clinic nurse may be beneficial to promote parent understanding of cystic fibrosis.

Meconium-Plug Syndrome
Carole Kenner

DESCRIPTION

Meconium-plug syndrome is an intestinal obstruction resulting from the presence of one or more meconium plugs.

ETIOLOGY AND PATHOPHYSIOLOGY

Meconium-plug syndrome is a congenital intestinal obstruction that is the result of an immature bowel and associated small left colon. Due to the functional immaturity of the bowel and the smallness of the colon, the meconium does not move through the intestines. Instead, the meconium fills the intestine, usually resulting in multiple plugs in a stringlike formation, causing distention and eventual obstruction. Another speculated cause of this entity is a spasm of the ileum due to high glucagon levels in an infant of a diabetic mother (Filston & Izant, 1985). The term *small left colon syndrome* is sometimes used interchangeably with meconium-plug syndrome, but they are really separate complications.

INCIDENCE

Meconium-plug syndrome is usually associated with premature infants and infants of diabetic mothers; however, the exact rate of incidence is not reported.

SYMPTOMS

1. Abdominal distention

2. Bile-stained vomitus

DIAGNOSIS

1. Contrast enema with a water-soluble material usually demonstrates multiple plugs. Repeating the instillation of contrast material usually results in expelling of the plugs. Obstruction is completely relieved when no more plugs are expelled and instillation of material is accomplished easily. Repeated use of a water soluble material can result in fluid shifts into the bowel and a vascular hypovolemic state. An isotonic IV fluid is suggested to counteract this effect (Filston & Izant, 1985). Another potential hazard of this material is perforation of the bowel following an inflammatory process resembling enterocolitis.

2. This syndrome should be differentiated from meconium ileus or small left colon syndrome or Hirschsprung's disease.

TRANSPORT

The goal for transport is to prevent abdominal distention and aspiration.

1. See Appendix A for specific guidelines.

2. Position infant with head elevated slightly and turned to the side, if vomiting, to decrease chance of aspiration.

3. If abdominal distention is present, place a nasogastric tube to straight gravity for decompression.

4. Start an IV influsion if infant appears dehydrated from vomiting.

ADMISSION EQUIPMENT

1. See Appendix B.
2. Nasogastric tube size10 double lumen.

PREOPERATIVE STABILIZATION

Nursing concerns for this infant are (1) maintaining gastric decompression, (2) promoting hydration, (3) preventing aspiration, and (4) assessing for signs of infection.

1. No surgery is usually necessary to correct this intestinal obstruction;

2. See Preoperative Stabilization (p. 162-163) in Meconiium Ileus associated with Cystic Fibrosis, in this Chapter.

TREATMENT

1. Rectal stimulation is sometimes all that is necessary for treatment.

2. Contrast enema with a water-soluble material usually demonstrates multiple plugs. Repeating the instillation of contrast material usually results in the expelling of the plugs. Obstruction is completely relieved when no more plugs are expelled and instillation of material is accomplished easily.

POSTTREATMENT CARE

1. To prevent hypovolemia, infection, or perforation, monitor vital signs closely, every 1-2 hours for the first 12 hours. This infant is at risk for the development of hypovolemia secondary to fluid shifts, enterocolitis, and perforation; any changes in baseline measurements of vital signs should be reported immediately.

2. Observe for signs of dehydration, since the use of contrast materials for the enema, being hyperosmolar, may result in fluid shifts, dehydration, and hypovolemia.

3. To prevent intestinal obstructions from recurring observe infant for stool formation pattern. Failure to defecate or alterations in the stooling pattern or consistency (diarrhea, constipation, hard, or ribbon-like) may indicate an obstruc-

tive process. Repeat contrast studies should be done to rule out Hirschsprung's disease. Even if the infant is discharged from the hospital with no alterations in stool formation and defecation, a repeat contrast study with barium should be done at about 4 weeks of age to determine if Hirschsprung's disease is present (Filston & Izant, 1985). Hirschsprung's disease may have been the underlying cause of the initial meconium-plug syndrome.

PARENT CARE

1. See Chapter 3 for specific guidelines.
2. To promote home management and to prevent life-threatening complications, teach parents the signs of complications:
   a. Bowel obstruction (feeding problem):
      i. Poor appetite
      ii. Vomiting
      iii. Abdominal distention
   b. Enterocolitis:
      i. Vomiting
      ii. Abdominal distention
      iii. Lethargy
      iv. Fever, tachycardia, tachypnea, hypotension
      v. Explosive, foul-smelling diarrhea

Necrotizing Enterocolitis
Jeanne Harjo

DESCRIPTION

Necrotizing enterocolitis (NEC) is a condition involving necrosis of the bowel caused by anoxia or trauma at birth or during the early neonatal period. It involves a loss of the protective mucosal barrier of the bowel as a result of this hypoxic injury. This simplistic explanation does not discount the complexity of this condition. It is multifactorial in nature, as any stress-producing event either prenatally or postnatally can potentially result in NEC.

ETIOLOGY

Necrotizing enterocolitis is the result of an insult to the bowel producing hypoxia within the bowel. Areas of the bowel become inflamed and die, ultimately leading to perforation of the bowel and peritonitis if untreated.

Prematurity may predispose the infant to periods of anoxia, resulting in bowel ischemia and finally NEC. Maternal diabetes, intrauterine infection, multiple births, and maternal bleeding late in pregnancy have the potential for fetal stress. Thus NEC may develop. It is also associated with functional obstructions, such as Hirschsprung's disease, that also cause pressure on the bowel wall, bowel ischemia, and ultimately NEC. The exact mechanism however is unknown. Infectious processes may play a role in the development of NEC.

INCIDENCE

Necrotizing enterocolitis is the most common surgical emergency in the newborn intensive care unit (NICU). Up to 20 percent of all premature babies found in an NICU will potentially develop NEC (Schreiner, 1982).

RISK FACTORS

No baby should be considered "just a grower." This condition can occur at any point in the neonatal period and does affect the full-term as well as the premature infant. There are certain conditions that appear to predispose an infant to NEC:

1. Prematurity and/or birth weight <1500 g.

2. Maternal diabetes, multiple births, third-trimester bleeding, and intrauterine infection (Filston & Izant, 1985).

3. Any stress that results in ischemia of the bowel: birth asphyxia, severe respiratory distress, and sepsis.

4. Conditions contributing to decreased blood flow to the bowel: patent ductus arteriosus, umbilical-artery catheterization, anemia, polycythemia, and shock.

5. Feedings: special attention must be paid when infants are started on oral feedings. Formula provides the perfect environment for bacterial invasion in an already compromised bowel.

SYMPTOMS

1. Early signs of the development of NEC include:
   a. Poor appetite with emesis and gastric aspirates.
   b. Apnea and bradycardia.
   c. Loose, seedy, guaiac-positive stools or visible blood in stools.
   d. Unstable temperature.
   e. Irritability.
   f. Abdominal distention.

Medical treatment must begin at the first occurrence of these signs to prevent the progression of this condition.

2. Late signs, indicating actual or impending bowel perforation:
   a. Lethargy.
   b. Increasing apnea and bradycardia.
   c. Pallor and shock with dropping hematocrit levels and platelet counts and increasing WBC counts. Mottling of extremities may appear.
   d. Grossly bloody stools.
   e. Hypothermia.
   f. Unstable glucose levels.
   g. An increase in abdominal distention. The abdomen becomes hard, red, and warm. It may also become discolored over the suspected area of perforation or around the umbilicus.

3. Abdominal radiographs showing the following:
   a. Pneumatosis intestinalis (gas in the bowel wall) or intramural air.
   b. Pneumoperitoneum (free air outside the bowel wall).
   c. Gas in the portal vein.
   d. Fixed dilated loops of bowel.

4. Need for surgical intervention:
   a. Worsening of condition despite medical treatment.
   b. Radiograph findings as above.
   c. Peritonitis.
   d. Thrombocytopenia.
   e. Abdominal-wall cellulitis with palpation of mass suggesting a walled-off perforation of the bowel.

DIAGNOSIS

1. Obtain abdominal radiographs every 6-8 hours to watch for progression or improvement of condition, including:
   a. Flat-plate abdominal film.
   b. Left lateral decubitus film of the abdomen. See Admission Setup (p. 122) in the introduction to this chapter for explanation of this film and how to position the infant.

2. Perform a CBC every 6-8 hours to detect a
   a. Change in hematocrit level.
   b. Decrease in platelet count.
   c. Increase in WBC count

TRANSPORT

The infant should be transferred to a regional center for evaluation as quickly as possible. The secondary-care units and outlying hospitals need to assess and monitor the infant for subtle signs of status changes that may indicate the development of NEC.

1. The transfer should occur with the onset of early symptoms—when the infant is more stable and before surgical intervention is required.

2. See Appendix A.

3. See Transport (p. 122) in the introduction to this chapter.

ADMISSION EQUIPMENT

1. See Appendix B.

2. See Admission Setup (pp. 122-123) in the introduction to this chapter.

PREOPERATIVE STABILIZATION

The goal is to allow for bowel rest in an attempt to avoid surgery.

1. To promote abdominal decompression keep infant NPO with nasogastric tube to low-continuous or intermittent suction:
   a. Use a size10 double-lumen tube; insert orally or nasally.
   b. Irrigate the tube every 1-2 hours to keep patent. Use normal saline solution (0.9 percent), water, or air to irrigate according to hospital policy.
   c. To promote fluid balance, measure, record, and discard output every 4-8 hours.
   d. Give replacement fluids IV as required. See Chapter 9 for specific replacement fluids. The fluid of choice is dextrose 5 percent in 0.9% NaCl solution with 10 mEq potassium chloride/L. Every 1 cc of output is replaced by 1 cc of replacement fluids given IV during a 4 -8 hour period.

2. Intravenous therapy: see Fluid and Electrolyte Status (pp. 280-285) and Parenteral Nutrition: Peripheral and Total Parenteral (pp. 280-285), in Chapter 9 for a discussion of fluid requirements.
   a. Fluids for hydration and nutrition: Due to the need for prolonged bowel rest, the infant will require hyperalimentation.
   b. Antibiotics for treatment of sepsis: Broad-spectrum antibiotics, especially ampicillin and gentamicin, are usually given to treat gram-negative intestinal infections and anerobic bacteria.

3. To monitor closely any progression in NEC, including the development of pneumoperitoneum or pneumatosis, abdominal radiographs every 6-8 hours are indicated.

4. Abdominal assessment:
   a. Measure abdominal girth every 4 hours to detect changes in abdominal distention.
   b. Check for signs of perforation and observe and record distention, color of abdomen, any tenseness, or palpable mass.
   c. Test all stools for occult blood.

5. Assess CBCs and arterial blood gas every 4-8 hours to detect any of the following:
   a. Shock and sepsis.
   b. Respiratory or metabolic acidosis or respiratory compromise. Acidosis may be demonstrated by a drop in pH level, a decrease in serum bicarbonate level, or a rise in $PaCo_2$.

6. To detect early signs of perforation or any status changes, monitor vital signs and assess respiratory effort and color every 1-2 hours.

7. Parental care:
   a. See Chapter 3.
   b. Verify informed surgical consent.

SURGERY

1. Ostomy in area of the perforation is performed. The enterostomy may be a colostomy, ileostomy, jejunostomy or multiple ostomies, to allow:
   a. The damaged bowel to rest.
   b. Resection of perforation and/or necrotic bowel. If a small area of NEC is found, primary resection and reanastomosis of the bowel may be performed; however, some physicians prefer an ostomy procedure to allow the complete healing of any damaged bowel. Primary closure has been implicated in the development of postoperative intestinal strictures, anastomotic leaks, and fatal enterocolitis (Pokorny, Garcia-Prats, & Barry, 1986).

2. Gastrostomy tube may be inserted by some physicians to facilitate gastric decompression during the initial postoperative period to:
   a. Decompress the stomach.
   b. Facilitate feedings.

3. A central line is inserted for hyperalimentation.

POSTOPERATIVE STABILIZATION

The goal postoperatively is to promote bowel healing, adequate ventilation and gas exchange, and nutritional status.

1. To detect subtle changes in status, closely monitor vital signs and urine output:
   a. Check temperature, heart rate, respiratory rate and BP every 15 minutes four times, every 30 minutes four times, every hour four times, and every 2 hours until stable, and then every 4 hours.
   b. Report any urine output <1 cc/kg/h.

2. Allow complete bowel rest for at least 2 weeks:
   a. Maintain NPO status.

    b. To facilitate gastric decompression, insert a nasogastric tube for 3-5 days or for 2 weeks if no gastrostomy tube has been inserted. See Preoperative Stabilization in this section (p. 173) for details on nasogastric decompression.

3. Connect the gastrostomy tube catheter, to gravity drainage:
    a. Irrigate every 2 hours with 2 cc air to keep patent.
    b. Empty, record, discard, and replace output every 4-8 hours.

4. To maintain hydration give IV fluids (for maintenance and replacement); hyperalimentation may be warranted if large segments of bowel have been removed or if infant is to be NPO for several weeks:
    a. Insert a peripheral or central line: see Central Venous Line Care (pp. 351-357).
    b. To prevent further infection and aggressively treat existing infection, give broad-spectrum antibiotics. Ampicillin and gentamicin IV in divided doses are the drugs of choice. Antibiotics that treat gram-negative and anerobic bacteria are needed for intestinal infections.
    c. See Chapter 9 for specific fluid management and hyperalimentation guidelines.

5. Colostomy care:
    a. Initially, the stoma will be dark and crusty and will bleed easily. As healing and toughening occurs, crusts slough off, bleeding decreases, and stoma becomes pink to red.
    b. Use colostomy dressings (gauze dressings, rolls, or squares) until stoma is healed and stool is present. Change dressing every 4 hours. See Colostomy Care (pp. 364-365).
    c. Apply colostomy bag as soon as the stoma is healed and stool is being formed.
        i. Use premie pouches with stoma adhesive ring.
        ii. Change pouch if it is leaking or loose.
        iii. Empty the colostomy bag and measure, record, and discard stool output every 8 hours.
    d. Chart the amount, color, and consistency of the stool. Test for the presence of reducing substances in the stool.
        i. Report stool output greater than half of the food intake. After bowel surgery, the infant can dehydrate easily as detected by increased stool output.
        ii. Report any sugar or reducing substances >0.5 percent. Feeding intolerance is also common due to the damaged intestinal mucosa and decreased intestinal absorption. If feeding intolerance is present, increased reducing substances (e.g., sugars) will appear in the stool.

6. Complications:
    a. To monitor skin integrity, record and report any redness, drainage, swelling, or separation of suture line.

b. To prevent potential severe intestinal obstruction, observe and report any abdominal distention or vomiting.

c. A lack of stool after 5-7 days following surgery may indicate an obstruction.

7. Respiratory support: postoperatively an infant with NEC may suffer severe respiratory compromise, especially if a perforation or severe peritonitis was present preoperatively.

   a. To promote adequate ventilation and gas exchange, the infant may require an oxygen hood for supplemental oxygen or positive-pressure ventilator.

   b. See Chapter 10 for respiratory assessment and oxygen adjustment guides.

8. Parent care: See Parent Care (Chapter 3).

9. Feedings (many infants following bowel resections may develop malabsorption; a long period of trial-and-error feeding is needed to determine the type, amount, and strength of formula that is required):

   a. Begin feedings when bowel begins to function in 7-10 days. Return of bowel function is signified by:

      i. Passage of stool from colostomy.

      ii. Decreased gastric output.

      iii. Gastric output changing from green to cloudy.

      iv. Return of bowel sounds.

   b. To promote gastric fluid absorption and motility, elevate gastrostomy tube for 24 hours.

      i. Measure, record, and reinsert gastric aspirate every 4 hours to determine absorption of secretions.

      ii. If gastric aspirate is clear and <5-10 cc every 4 hours, feedings can begin.

      iii. If gastric aspriate is green and/or >10 cc, wait another 24 hours to start feedings.

   c. Advance feedings slowly:

      i. Start with Pedialyte® (Ross Laboratories, Columbus, OH) every 2 hours for 24 hours.

      ii. Increase to ¼-strength formula and increase by ¼ strength as tolerated. To facilitate absorption of fats and nutrients an elemental formula such as Pregestimil® (Mead-Johnson, Evansville, IN) may be used. Such a formula contains easily digested amino acids and proteins along with medium chain triglycerides that promote intestinal absorption.

   d. To gauge tolerance of feedings:

      i. Check aspirate before each feeding, record, and reinsert.

      ii. Measure and record the amount of stool every 8 hours.

      iii. Check stool for reducing substances every 8 hours.

      iv. Stop advancement if:

         a) Aspirate is green or is >10 cc.

         b) Vomiting occurs.

         c) Abdominal distention is noted.

    d) Stool output is greater than half the intake every 8 hours.

    e) Stool-reducing substances or sugar >0.5 percent.

  e. Parenteral nutrition is required until full feedings are tolerated. See Parenteral Nutrition: Peripheral and Total Nutrition (pp. 280-285) for specific guidelines on hyperalimentation.

PARENT CARE

1. See Chapter 3.

2. To promote home management, teach parents to be alert to the following potential problems:

  a. Diarrhea or constipation.

  b. Poor appetite.

  c. Vomiting.

  d. Abdominal distention.

  e. Skin breakdown around colostomy.

  f. Drainage or skin breakdown around gastrostomy.

3. Colostomy care: See Chapter 12 (pp. 364-365).

4. Gastrostomy care and feeding: See Chapter 12 (pp. 347-351).

Pyloric Stenosis
Jeanne Harjo

DESCRIPTION

Pyloric stenosis is an obstruction at the outlet of the stomach in the form of a stiff ringlike muscular structure. Initially, spasm of the circular muscle around the pylorus occurs followed by a progressive hypertrophy, which develops in 24-48 hours. Often, it does not manifest itself until the infant if 6 weeks old.

ETIOLOGY

Exact etiology is unknown. Hypertrophy of the pyloric muscle occurs with spasmodic episodes following feedings.

INCIDENCE

Pyloric stenosis is one of the most common surgical problems for the newborn. It occurs in approximately 4-5 live births of every 1000. Incidence is highest in first-born males.

SYMPTOMS

1. An otherwise healthy baby who is normal at birth and continues to be asymptomatic for 2-8 weeks postnatally.

2. Vomiting:
   a. Occasional vomiting of feedings.
   b. Increased frequency and severity of vomiting.
   c. Vomiting becomes forceful and may be projectile.
   d. Emesis may contain mucus but is never bilious.
   e. Infant is eager to refeed after vomiting.
   f. Becomes irritable and is excessively hungry.

3. Dehydration may occur if untreated. Signs of dehydration are:
   a. Decreased stool with progressive constipation.
   b. Scant urine output.
   c. Electrolyte imbalance.
   d. Weight loss.

DIAGNOSIS

1. A thorough history should be completed that describes the episodes of vomiting, including the times and nature of the emesis.

2. Palpation of an olive-shaped mass in the right upper quadrant of the abdomen when the abdomen is relaxed.

3. As the obstruction progresses, the stomach becomes so hyperactive in response to its outlet obstruction that visible peristaltic waves can be seen across the abdomen after feedings.

4. Abdominal radiographs show a dilated, gas-filled stomach with little gas in the intestines beyond the pylorus.

5. Upper GI series show:
   a. An enlarged stomach with a rounded end.
   b. Increased gastric peristalsis, noted under fluoroscopy.
   c. A markedly narrowed pylorus that never opens normally.

TRANSPORT

It is likely that an infant with pyloric stenosis will be transported for another neonatal problem. Since this surgical defect does not appear in the immediate neonatal period, the transport consideration should be based on other problems.

1. See Appendix A.

2. See the beginning of this chapter for specific considerations with GI problems (p. 122).

ADMISSION EQUIPMENT

1. See Appendix B.

2. See Admission Setup (p. 122-123) in the introduction to this chapter for specific admission needs for infants with GI complications.

PREOPERATIVE STABILIZATION

The nursing concern in the preoperative stage is to restore or maintain fluid and electrolyte status.

1. Monitor vital signs according to routine, usually every 2–4 hours.

2. Maintain IV access for adequate hydration and to correct any electrolyte imbalance occurring from vomiting. Severe losses of sodium, potassium, and chloride ions occur with vomiting. Metabolic alkalosis is a by-product of this electrolyte imbalance and dehydrated state. For severe dehydration dextrose 5 percent and 0.9% NaCl solution with at least 10 mEq potassium chloride/L may be used for replacement of electrolytes. Filston and Izant (1985, p. 172) recommend using as much as 30 mEq potassium chloride/L in dextrose 5 percent and 0.9% NaCl solution to equal at least 1 ½ times the usual amount of maintenance fluid when the infant shows signs of extreme dehydration.

3. Maintain nasogastric suction to prevent gastric distention and persistent emesis
   a. Place size 10 double-lumen nasogastric tube.
   b. Connect nasogastric tube to low-continuous suction.
   c. Irrigate nasogastric tube every 2 hours with 2 cc of saline solution or air to maintain tube's patency.

SURGERY

Fredet-Ramstedt pyloromyotomy may be performed. The hypertrophic muscle at the pylorus is split, leaving the mucosa and the submucosa intact so that the lumen of the duodenum is not entered.

POSTOPERATIVE STABILIZATION

The nursing concerns in the postoperative period are (1) promotion and restoration of the fluid and electrolyte balance, (2) prevention of infection, (3) promotion of wound healing, and (4) promotion of the resumption of oral feedings.

1. Closely monitor vital signs to determine baseline status and detect any changes in the infant's condition. Usually temperature and BP are checked every 15 minutes four times, every 30 minutes four times, every 1 hour four times, every 2 hours until stable, and then every 4 hours.

2. To promote hydration and electrolyte balance, maintain IV access until feedings are tolerated.

3. To promote gastric decompression and return of intestinal function, maintain nasogastric suction for 4-24 hours postoperatively:
   a. To promote intestinal motility, discontinue nasogastric suction when infant is fully awake.
   b. To ready infant for feedings, discontinue nasogastric tube when bowel sounds are heard.

4. Observe for complications to prevent dehydration and impaired skin integrity as well as infection. Signs of problems are:
   a. Resumption of persistent vomiting.
   b. Suture-line breakdown.

5. Parental support: see Chapter 3.

6. Feedings:
   a. Begin slow feedings at 6-24 hours of age.
   b. Begin with clear liquids; advance the strength and amounts of formula daily.
   c. Maximum feedings should be reached by 3-5 days postoperatively.

PARENT CARE

1. See Chapter 3.

2. To promote home infant management, review feeding schedule and instruct parents to be alert to complications. Tell the parents the importance of immediately reporting to a physician the following signs:
   a. Vomiting.
   b. Suture-line breakdown.

Small-Bowel Atresia
Jeanne Harjo

DESCRIPTION

Small-bowel atresia occurs as a complete obstruction within the passage of the small bowel. The most common site is the ileum, followed by the jejunum. In some instances, multiple areas of atresia are found.

ETIOLOGY AND EMBRYOLOGY

In small-bowel atresia, one or more portions of bowel end in blind pouches. It is commonly believed that hypoxia during fetal life is responsible for the atretic areas. Malrotation that occurs in utero is another suspected cause. Intussusception may also result in small-bowel atresia. In over one third of all infants with small-bowel atresia, multiple atretic areas are found.

INCIDENCE

Incidence rates are difficult to calculate since other obstructions may simultaneously occur: malrotation, volvulus, or intussusception.

SYMPTOMS

1. Lack of gastric emptying:
   a. Large amount of bilious fluid suctioned from stomach with initial assessment.
   b. Vomiting which may or may not occur for 24 hours but will be bilious.
2. Elevated bilirubin levels may be present due to the enterohepatic and biliary obstruction.
3. Meconium may be passed but will stop being passed after 24 hours.
4. Visible and palpable bowel loops.
5. Variable amounts of distention.

DIAGNOSIS

1. Abdominal radiographs:
   a. Flat plate of the abdomen showing numerous loops of dilated bowel.
   b. An upright film showing fluid levels in the bowel.
2. Barium enema to:
   a. Help distinguish between small and large bowel obstruction; however, a clear determination may not be possible as it is difficult to determine small and large intestinal differences in the neonate.
   b. Determine if colon is unused or microcolon is present.
   c. Determine if malrotation is present.

TRANSPORT

Prior to transport, stabilization in an outlying hospital should involve monitoring respiratory status, especially if acute abdominal distention is present. Attention should be paid to promoting gastric decompression, preventing aspiration, and maintaining fluid balance.

1. Insert a nasogastric tube, size 10 double lumen, to allow intermittent or continuous suction and facilitate gastric decompression.
2. See Appendix A for transport considerations.

ADMISSION EQUIPMENT

1. Nasogastric suction equipment:
   a. Size 10 double-lumen tube
   b. Intermittent or continuous suction
2. Regular unit setup: See Appendix B.

PREOPERATIVE STABILIZATION

The overriding consideration is to facilitate early surgical intervention. If malrotation and volvulus are present, bowel ischemia and necrosis can occur resulting in loss of large amounts of the intestines if surgery is unnecessarily delayed (Filston & Izant, 1985). Promotion of nasogastric decompression and prevention of aspiration is important. Maintenance of nutritional status may call for hyperalimentation if infant is to be NPO for a long period.

1. Assess infant and monitor vital signs every 2 hours to detect any status changes:
   a. Measure temperature, heart rate, respiratory rate, and BP.
   b. Measure abdominal girth and report any distention or firmness that may be indicative of progressive intestinal obstruction or perforation.
   c. Observe breath sounds, respiratory effort, and color since the infant is at risk for respiratory compromise secondary to abdominal distention and perforation.
2. To promote hydration, maintain IV access: see Parenteral Nutrition: Total and Peripheral Nutrition (pp. 280-285) in Chapter 9 for specific information.
3. Administer broad-spectrum antibiotics to prevent gram-negative and anerobic intestinal infections. Some institutions do not recommend precautionary antibiotics, so check hospital protocol. See Antibiotics (pp. 290-293) in Chapter 9 for specific information.
4. Insert a nasogastric tube, size 10 double lumen, if not already in place.
   a. To promote gastric decompression, place at low-intermittent or continuous suction.
   b. Irrigate tube every 2 hours with 2 cc of air or saline solution to maintain patency.

c. To maintain adequate hydration, measure, record, and discard gastric output every 4-8 hours.

d. Dextrose 5 percent in 0.9% NaCl solution with 10 mEq potassium chloride/L should be used as a replacement fluid every 4-8 hours. This solution will replace the sodium, chloride, and potassium ions that are lost in gastric suctioning. For every 1 cc of gastric output 1 cc of replacement fluid should be administered via IV access to maintain fluid volume.

5. Parental support:
   a. See Chapter 3.
   b. Verify informed surgical consent.

SURGERY

The surgery that is performed is determined by what is found during the exploratory laparotomy. Commonly, the extent of the procedure is as follows:

1. Resection of the areas of atresia with end-to-end anastomosis.

2. Exteriorization procedure: proximal and distal bowel loops are brought out through the abdominal wound forming a double-barrel colostomy. Cautery is performed to open a passage between the two bowel loops.

3. A central line for hyperalimentation is inserted.

4. Gastrostomy tube may be used to provide long-term gastric decompression. Some physicians no longer routinely use gastrostomy tubes.

POSTOPERATIVE STABILIZATION

The nursing care postoperatively centers on maintaining hydration and gastric decompression, preventing infection, and facilitating a return to oral feedings.

1. Closely monitor vital signs and urine output; this is essential since this infant may have had a lengthy surgical procedure.
   a. Check temperature, heart rate, respiratory rate, and BP every 15 minutes four times, every 30 minutes four times, every hour four times, every 2 hours until stable, and then every 4 hours.
   b. Report any urine output <1cc/kg/h.

2. To promote and maintain fluid balance, maintain IV access. See Parenteral Nutrition: Peripheral and Total Nutrition (pp. 280-285) in Chapter 9 for additional guidelines.
   a. Long-term IV access will be needed to provide fluid and nutrition to give rest to the intestines.
   b. Replace gastric losses every 4-8 hours; see Preoperative Stabilization in this section (pp. 182-183) for nasogastric decompression and replacement fluids.

   c. Administer broad-spectrum antibiotics as described under Preoperative Stabilization section in this section (p. 182).

3. Maintain patency of gastrostomy tube, if present:
   a. Irrigate gastrostomy tube every 2 hours with 2 cc of air.
   b. Connect tube to gravity drainage to facilitate gastric decompression and prevent vomiting.
   c. Record gastric output, discard, and give replacement fluids every 4-8 hours in the same manner as nasogastric replacement described in the Preoperative Stabilization section in this section (pp. 182-183).

4. Colostomy care. see Chapter 12 (pp. 364-365):
   a. Initially the stoma is dark, crusted, and bleeds easily. Apply petroleum jelly gauze to the stoma.
   b. Empty colostomy bag and record output every 8 hours. Change bag if leaking.

5. Observe for complications to promote skin integrity and intestinal motility:
   a. Note and report any redness, drainage, swelling, or separation of the suture line.
   b. Observe and report any abdominal distention or vomiting suggestive of a possible intestinal obstruction.

6. Parental support: see Chapter 3.

7. Feedings (Many infants with extensive bowel resections may develop "short gut syndrome," malabsorption; a long period of trial-and-error feedings is required to determine the type, amount, and strength of formula appropriate):
   a. Begin feedings when bowel begins to function (7-10 days), as indicated by:
     i. Passage of stool from colostomy
     ii. Decreased gastric output
     iii. Gastric output changing from green to cloudy
   b. To promote gastric motility and intestinal absorption, elevate gastrostomy tube for 24 hours, do not clamp at this time.
     i. Measure gastric aspirate every 4 hours.
     ii. Record and reinsert aspirate to prevent loss of essential electrolytes (sodium, chloride, and potassium).
     iii. If aspirate is clear and <5-10 cc every 4 hours, feedings can begin.
     iv. If aspirate is green and >10 cc, wait another 24 hours to start feeding.
   c. Advance feedings slowly:
     i. Start with clear liquids every 2 hours for 24 hours.
     ii. Increase to ¼-strength formula and increase by ¼ strength as tolerated. Infant may tolerate a change every 24 hours. (An elemental formual such as Pregestimil® may be used since it contains medium-chain triglycerides and easily digestable proteins and amino acids. This is an important consideration when an infant's intestinal absorption of nutrients and fats may be altered due to GI surgery.)

iii. Gauge tolerance of feedings:
   a) Check aspirate before each feeding, record, and reinsert to preserve electrolytes present in gastric aspirate.
   b) Measure and record amount of stool every 8 hours to prevent dehydration secondary to fluid losses through the stool.
   c) Check stool for reducing substances every 8 hours.
   d) Stop advancement if:
      • Aspirate is green
      • Vomiting occurs
      • Abdominal distention is noted
      • Stool output is >60 cc every 8 hours
      • Stool reducing substances or sugar content >0.5 percent
   e) Parenteral nutrition is required until full feedings are tolerated

PARENT CARE

1. See Chapter 3.

2. Teach parents the need to report any signs that may be indicative of malabsorption or an intestinal obstruction. Signs of complications are:
   a. Diarrhea or constipation
   b. Poor appetite
   c. Vomiting
   d. Abdominal distention
   e. Skin breakdown around colostomy or gastrostomy

3. Colostomy care: see Colostomy Care (pp. 364-365) in Chapter 12.

4. Gastrostomy care and feedings: see Gastrostomy Care (pp. 347-351) in Chapter 12.

REFERENCES

Omphalocele and Gastroschisis

Anderl, H., Menardi, G., & Hager, J. (1986). Closure of gastroschisis by mesh skin grafts in problem cases. *Journal of Pediatric Surgery, 21*, 870-872.

Brueggemeyer, A. (1979). Omphalocele: Coping with a surgical emergency. *Pediatric Nursing, 5*(4), 54-56.

Canty, T. G. & Collins, D. L. (1983). Primary fascial closure in infants with gastroschisis and omphalocele: A superior approach. *Journal of Pediatric Surgery, 18*, 707-712.

Hershenson, M. B., Brouillette, R. T., Klemka, L., Raffensperger, J. D., Poznanski, A. K. & Hunt, C. (1985). Respiratory insufficiency in newborns with abdominal wall defects. *Journal of Pediatric Surgery, 20*, 348-353.

Mulligan, K. S. (1986). Gastrointestinal disorders, in N. S. Streeter (Ed.), *High-risk neonatal care* (pp. 315-351). Rockville, MD: Aspen.

Schwartz, M. Z., Tyson, K. R. T., Milliorn, K., & Lobe, T. E. (1983). Staged reduction using a Silastic sac is the treatment of choice for large congenital abdominal wall defects. *Journal of Pediatric Surgery, 18*, 713-717.

Imperforate Anus

Carson, J. A., Barnes, P. D., Tunell, W. P., Smith, I., & Jolley, S. G. (1984). Imperforate anus: The neurologic implication of sacral abnormalities. *Journal of Pediatric Surgery, 19*, 838-842.
Freeman, N. V., & Bulut, M. (1986). "High" anorectal anomalies treated by early (neonatal) operation. *Journal of Pediatric Surgery, 21*, 218-220.

Intussusception

Filston, H. C., & Izant, R. (1985). *The surgical neonate: Evaluation and care* (2nd ed.). New York: Appleton-Century-Crofts.
Rockenhaus, J. M. (1985). Ingestion, digestion, and elimination: Implications of inflammation and obstruction. In S. R. Mott, N. F. Fazekas, & S. P. James (Eds.), *Nursing care of children and families: A holistic approach* (pp. 1295-1360). Reading, MA: Addison-Wesley.

Meconium Ileus Associated with Cystic Fibrosis

Filston, H., & Izant, R. (1985). *Surgical neonate: Evaluation and care* (2nd ed.). New York: Appleton-Century-Crofts.
Guzzetta, P. C., Randolph, J. G., & Anderson, K. D., Boyajian, M., & Eichelberger, M. (1987). Surgery of the neonate. In G. B. Avery (Ed.) *Neonatology: Pathophysiology and management of the newborn* (2nd ed.) (pp. 944-984). Philadelphia: J. B. Lippincott.
Wallach, J. (1983). *Interpretation of pediatric tests: A handbook synopsis of pediatric, fetal, and obstetric laboratory medicine* (pp. 160-161). Boston: Little, Brown.

Necrotizing Enterocolitis

Filston, H. C., & Izant, R. J. (1985). *The surgical neonate: Evaluation and care* (2nd ed.) (pp. 222-227). Norwalk, CT: Appleton-Century-Crofts.
Pokorny, W. J., Garcia-Prats, J. A., & Barry, Y. N. (1986). Necrotizing enterocolitis: Incidence, operative care, and outcome. *Journal of Pediatric Surgery, 21*, 1149-1154.
Schreiner, R. L. (1982). *Care of the newborn* (pp. 175-181). New York: Raven Press.

Pyloric Stenosis

Filston, H. C., & Izant, R. J. (1985). *The surgical neonate: Evaluation and care* (2nd ed.) (p. 172). Norwalk, CT: Appleton-Century-Crofts.

BIBLIOGRAPHY

Behrman, R. E., & Vaughan, V. C. (Eds.) (1983). *Nelson's textbook of pediatrics.* Philadelphia: W. B. Saunders.

Billingham, K. A. (1982). *Developmental psychology for the health care profession, Part 1: Prenatal through adolescent development* (pp. 19-58). Boulder, CO: Westview.

Carson, J. A., Barnes, P. D., Tunell, W. P., Smith, E. I., & Jolley, S. G. (1984). Imperforate anus: The neurologic implication of sacral abnormalities. *Journal of Pediatric Surgery, 19*, 838-842.

Chadarevian, J. P., de Sims, M., & Akel, S. (1982). Double zone aganglionosis in long segment Hirshsprung's disease with a "skip area" in transverse colon. *Journal of Pediatric Surgery, 17*, 195-197.

Cloherty, J. P., & Stark, A. R. (1985). *Manual of neonatal care (2nd ed.).* Boston: Little, Brown.

Cram, R. W. (1982). Hirschsprung's disease: Long-term follow-up of 65 cases. *anadian Journal of Surgery, 25*, 435-437.

Cropley, C. (1986). Assessment of mothering behaviors. In S. H. Johnson (Ed.), *High-risk parenting: Nursing assessment and strategies for the family at risk* (2nd ed.) (pp. 13-40). Philadelphia: J. B. Lippincott.

Davis, D. W. (19XX). Congenital duodenal obstruction. *Neonatal Network, 3*(6), 9-13.

Dimler, M. (1981). "Acquired" Hirschsprung's Disease. *Journal of Pediatric Surgery, 16*, 844-845.

Dykes, E. J., Gilmour, W. H., & Azmy, A. F. (1985). Prediction of outcome following necrotizing enterocolitis in a neonatal surgical unit. *Journal of Pediatric Surgery, 20*, 3-5.

Filston, H., & Izant, R. J. (1986). Congenital anomalies presenting with obstructive gastrointestinal symptoms. In M. H. Klaus & A. A. Fanaroff (Eds.), *Care of the high-risk neonate* (3rd ed.) (pp. 135-137). Philadelphia: W. B. Saunders.

Filston, H. C. (1982). *Surgical problems in children, recognition and referral.* St. Louis: C. V. Mosby.

Filston, H. C., & Izant, R. J. (1985). *The surgical neonate: Evaluation and care.* (2nd ed.) (pp. 180-184). Norwalk, CT: Appleton-Century-Crofts.

Goldberg, R. B., & Shprinzer, R. J. (1981). Hirschsprung megacolon and cleft palate in two sibs. *Journal of Craniofacial Genetics and Developmental Biology, 1*, 185-189.

Greenholz, S. K., Lilly, J. R., Shikes, R. H., & Hall, R. J. (1986). Biliary atresia in the newborn. *Journal of Pediatric Surgery, 21*, 1147-1148.

Hirschsprung, H. (1887). Stuhltragheir Neugeborener in Folge, von Dilation und hypoertrophie des colons. *Jahrbuck Kinderh., 27*(1).

Hirsig, J., Baals, J., Tuchschmid, P., Spitz, L., & Stauffer, U. G. (1984). Dumping syndrome following Nissen's fundoplication: A cause for refusal to feed. *Journal of Pediatric Surgery, 19*, 155-157.

Kenner, C., & Brueggemeyer, A. (1984). Hirschsprung's disease: Current trends and practices. *Neonatal Network, 3*(1), 7-16.

Kimura, K., Nishijima, E., Muraji, T., Tsugawa, C., & Matsumoto, Y. (1981). A New surgical approach to extensive aganglionosis. *Journal of Pediatric Surgery, 16*, 840-843.

Kisloske, A. M., Ball, W. S., Umland, E., & Skipper, B. (1985). Clostridial necrotizing enterocoliitis. *Journal of Pediatric Surgery, 20*, 155-159.

Lemons, P. K. M. (1981). The family of the high-risk newborn. In R. H. Perez (Ed.), *Protocols for perinatal nursing practice* (pp. 440-449). St. Louis: C. V. Mosby.

MacMahon, R. A., Moore, C. C. M., & Cussen, L. Y. (1981). Hirschsprung-like syndromes in patients with normal ganglion cells on suction rectal biopsy. *Journal of Pediatric Surgery, 16*, 835-839.

Miyano, T., & Suruga, K. (1985). New operative technique for Hirschsprung's disease. *Journal of Pediatric Surgery, 20*, 160-163.

Moore, K. L. (1974). *Before we are born: Basic embryology and birth defects.* Philadelphia: W. B. Saunders.

Page, E. W., Villee, C. A., & Villee, D. B. (1981). *Human reproduction: Essentials of reproductive and perinatal medicine (3rd ed.).* Philadelphia: W. B. Saunders.

Passarge, E. (1967). The genetics of Hirschsprung's disease: Evidence for heterogenous etiology and a study of sixty-three families. *New England Journal of Medicine, 276*, 138-143.

Pokorny, W. J., Garcia-Prats, J. A., & Barry, Y. N. (1986). Necrotizing enterocolitis: Incidence, operative care, and outcome. *Journal of Pediatric Surgery, 21*, 1149-1154.

Porth, C. M. (1986). *Pathophysiology: Concepts of altered health status.* Philadelphia: J. B. Lippincott.

Quintero, H., & Quinter, J. (1976). Modified surgical technique for the treatment of congenital megacolon. *International Surgery, 61*, 529-531.

Schreiner, R. L. (1982). *Care of the newborn.* New York: Raven Press.

Schwoebe, M. G., Jirsig, J., Schinze, A., & Stauffer, U. G. (1984). Familial incidence of congenital anorectal anomalies. *Journal of Pediatric Surgery, 19*, 179-182.

Short, K., Groff, D. B., & Cook, L. (1985). The concomitant presence of gastroschisis and prune belly syndrome in a twin. *Journal of Pediatric Surgery, 20*, 186-187.

Sieber, W. K. (1976). Hirschsprung's disease. *Annals of Surgery, 1*, 1035-1058.

Sugar, W. C. (1981). Hirschsprung's disease. *American Journal of Nursing, 81*, 2065-2067.

Swenson, O., & Bill, A. H. (1959). Resection of rectum and rectosigmoid with preservation of the sphincter for benign spastic lesions producing megacolon: An experimental study. *Surgery, 45*, 690.

Takada, Y., Aoyama, K., Goto, T., & Mori, S. (1985). The association of imperforate anus and Hirschsprung's disease in siblings. *Journal of Pediatric Surgery, 20*, 271-273.

Tam, P. K. H., Saing, H., Koo, J., Wong, J., & Ong, G. B. (1985). Pyloric function five to eleven years after Ramstedt's pyloromytomy. *Journal of Pediatric Surgery, 20*, 236-239.

Thomas, D. F. M., Malone, M., Fernie, D. S., Bayston, R., & Spitz, L. (1982). Association between *Clostridium difficile* and enterocolitis in Hirschsprung's disease. *Lancet,* 78-79.

Vaillant, C., Bullock, A., Dimaline, R., & Dockray, G. J. (1982). Distribution and development of peptidergic nerves and gut endocrine cells in mice with congenital aganglionic colon and their normal littermates. *Gastroenterology, 82*, 291-300.

Vestal, K., & McKenzie, C. A. (1983). *High risk perinatal nursing: The American association of critical-care nurses.* Philadelphia: W. B. Saunders.

Wijesinha, S. S., & Steer, H. W. (1982). Observations on the immunocytes and macrophages in megacolon. *Diseases of the Colon and Rectum, 25*, 312-320.

Chapter 6

Alterations in the Genitourinary System

Ann Brueggemeyer

Alterations in the genital system may not be evident in the neonatal period and may not pose a significant problem in the first few weeks of life. Neonates experiencing alterations in the urinary system will usually exhibit symptoms of acute renal failure. These symptoms may be mild or severe depending upon the specific urinary disorder.

Acute Renal Failure

Ann Brueggemeyer

DESCRIPTION

Acute renal failure occurs as the kidneys fail to maintain or regulate fluid and electrolyte balance. The newborn is expected to void within the first 24 hours of life. About 90 percent of all infants fall into this category (Vestal, 1983). Another 10 percent void within the first 48 hours of life and can often be considered normal. The very small percentage of infants who are born with oliguria or anuria experience acute renal failure due to a variety of factors. Perinatal factors that may lead to neonatal renal failure include maximal dehydration, hemorrhage, and the ingestion of nephrotoxic drugs (Vestal, 1983). Newborn factors include a wide variety of causes, often classified as prerenal, renal, and postrenal.

Prerenal factors include hydration problems, renal artery obstructions, and poor perfusion. Renal factors can include aplastic kidney (Potter's syndrome), cystic disease, renal necrosis, or nephrotoxic agents. Postrenal factors include the potentially correctable surgical anomalies such as ureteropelvic junction obstruction, prune belly syndrome (Eagle-Barrett syndrome), Vacterl syndrome also known as

VATER (Vertebral, Anal-imperforate, Cardiac, Tracheoesophageal fistula, Renal, and Limb deformities), and neurogenic bladder.

Commonly associated with renal-tract disorders are a variety of defects and disorders including low-set ears, single umbilical artery, hypoplastic lungs, and gastrointestinal (GI) defects. A thorough analysis of renal functioning should be made prior to repair of other disorders. A decision may be made not to begin repair of defects if renal function is not sufficient to support life.

TRANSPORT

See Appendix A and subsections of this chapter for the specific renal problem resulting in acute renal failure and the transport information therein. Nursing goals during transport are to maintain fluid and electrolyte balance and thermoregulation.

PREOPERATIVE STABILIZATION

1. Assist with admission diagnostic workup; see Appendix B:
   a. Blood tests: serum electrolyte and renal group (blood urea nitrogen [BUN] and creatinine) levels
   b. Urinalysis and urine culture
   c. Chest and abdominal radiographs
   d. Abdominal ultrasonogram
   e. Voiding cystogram
   f. Intravenous pyelogram

2. Assess balance of fluid and electrolyte levels:
   a. Observe and record fluid intake and output.
   b. Measure urine output by indwelling catheter, ostomy appliance, or pediatric urine drainage bags (diaper weights are not as reliable when accurate measurements must be attained).
   c. See Fluid Requirements (pp. 263-280) in Chapter 9. Maintain IV access to provide fluid and electrolyte replacement. Potassium should not be administered IV until appropriate renal functioning has been determined.
   d. Measure urine specific gravity at least every 4 hours or after every void.

3. Provide respiratory support as needed: hypoplastic or dysplastic lungs are often associated with renal anomalies. The increase in abdominal pressure due to expanding kidneys places pressure on the thoracic cavity, which inhibits the growth of lung tissue (Inturrisi, Perry, & May, 1985). It is unclear why lung hypoplasia occurs in conjunction with renal agenesis.
   a. Assess respiratory status.
   b. Provide humidified oxygen through mask or head hood as needed.
   c. If ventilation is required, use minimal pressure to oxygenate, thus decreasing risk of a pneumothorax.

4. Maintain proper thermoregulation: see Thermoregulation (p. 51) in Chapter 2 for specific guidelines.

SURGERY

Acute renal failure can occur for a variety of reasons; therefore, no one type of surgery is performed. Each of the sections of this chapter describes renal problems and the associated surgeries.

GENERAL RENAL POSTOPERATIVE STABILIZATION

1. Maintain adequate aeration and oxygenation:
   a. Provide humidified oxygen if needed.
   b. Turn and reposition newborn at least every 2 hours.
2. Maintain patency of tubes and lines:
   a. Place urinary drainage tube to closed system drainage (e.g., Foley catheter, nephrostomy tubes, suprapubic tubes, and stints).
   b. Do not irrigate lines.
   c. To prevent kinking of tubes, position drainage bags for gravity drainage.
3. Maintain clean incision sites:
   a. Keep dressings clean and dry.
   b. Observe for and report any drainage on dressings or around urinary tubes.
   c. Urine leakage may occur through some incision sites depending on the type of surgery performed. Dressings should be changed when damp or to prevent buildup of urine on skin.
4. Prevent skin breakdown:
   a. Observe dressings frequently for drainage. It is important to assess the dressings for dampness as visual assessment may not detect clear drainage.
   b. Change dressings frequently, cleaning skin area to prevent build up of irritating chemicals on skin.
   c. When possible, use barrier products to protect skin. Incision sites should be well healed before application of appliances or barriers. Stomas or leaking fistulas may be protected with ointments or Stomahesive® before applying dressings or appliances.
5. Maintain fluid and electrolyte balance; see Chapter 9 for specific information.
   a. Provide maintenance fluids per guidelines in Fluid Requirements and General Considerations (pp. 263-280).
   b. Provide fluids to replace urine output; replace 1 cc of urine output with 1 cc of replacement fluid.

PARENT CARE

See Chapter 3 for specific guidelines. Begin early preparing parents to care for the infant at home. Teach them the following:

1. The long-term effects of renal disease, including frequent medical follow-up, implications for growth and development, and potential changes in diet.

2. The observation for and prevention of urinary tract infections.

3. The administration of prophylactic and therapeutic medications.

Hydronephrosis
Ann Brueggemeyer

DESCRIPTION AND PATHOPHYSIOLOGY

Hydronephrosis is relatively common in infants. It usually follows some congenital obstruction at the ureteropelvic junction (UPJ) or at the ureterovesical valve. Proximal to this obstruction, fluid accumulates. The urine that is continually formed in the fetal kidney has no avenue for drainage. The kidney then becomes fluid-filled and distended. This can occur in one or both kidneys. Significant buildup of fluid can lead to permanent kidney damage.

Hydronephrosis can easily be detected in the fetal stage through maternal ultrasonography. When hydronephrosis is caused by UPJ obstruction with posterior urethral valve obstruction, fetal surgery may be performed in several instititutions nationwide. Current surgical techniques attempt to bypass or relieve the obstructions to prevent permanent renal damage. Although many times successfully performed, these techniques have not always been in time to prevent permanent damage. By 16-18 week's gestation, renal damage may have already occurred (Inturrisi, Perry, & May, 1985). Progressive renal enlargement in the fetus can lead to abdominal wall defects and hypoplasia of the lungs (Harrison, Ross, Noall, & de Lorimier, 1983; Inturrisi et al., 1985). Early recognition and prompt treatment may prevent permanent renal and lung damage.

Current treatment for obstructive hydronephrosis includes the use of a catheter that is inserted through the maternal abdominal wall and to the fetus's bladder. The end of the catheter is left to drain within the amniotic sac (Harrison et al., 1983; Inturrisi et al., 1985).

ETIOLOGY

Hydronephrosis occurs when a congenital malformation occurs with resulting obstruction of urinary flow from the kidneys. Little is known about the causes of hydronephrosis when obstructive uropathies are not present (Harrison et al., 1983).

INCIDENCE

The incidence of hydronephrosis is difficult to determine since it occurs secondary to various forms of obstructive uropathies.

SYMPTOMS

1. Abdomen with palpable mass, sometimes felt as a solid mass.
2. Often accompanied by fever and discomfort. These symptoms are often associated with a urinary tract infection.
3. Decreased urine output during the first several days of life. Actual amount is dependent on the amount of functioning kidney mass.

DIAGNOSIS

1. Often can be determined by palpation.
2. If physical findings are doubtful, other diagnostic studies may include IV pyelogram, retrograde pyelogram, ultrasonography, or computed tomographic (CT) scan.
3. Evidence of recurrent urinary tract infections.

TRANSPORT

See Appendix A for general guidelines. The nursing goal is to maintain thermoregulation, fluid and electrolyte balance, and to prevent respiratory compromise.

ADMISSION EQUIPMENT

1. Regular admission set up: see Appendix B.
2. Obtain parental consent for renal studies and radiographs.

PREOPERATIVE STABILIZATION

1. Assist with routine admission work up: see Appendix B.
2. Assist with determination of baseline data:
   a. Urine culture specimen may be obtained by clean catch, sterile catheterization, or by suprapubic tap, to prevent contamination of specimen.

b. Blood tests to include electrolyte group and renal group, including BUN and creatinine levels.

c. Abdominal girth measurement for baseline measurement to observe for distention.

d. Abdominal radiograph, IV or retrograde pyelogram, ultrasonogram or CT scan. Assist with procedure and careful observation of the infant as needed.

3. Maintenance of fluid and electrolyte balance: see Fluid Requirements and General Nutritional Considerations (pp. 263-280) in Chapter 9 for specific guidelines.

4. Treatment of current infection as prescribed by physician: see Antibiotics in Chapter 9 for specific guidelines.

POSTOPERATIVE STABILIZATION

The surgical treatment for hydronephrosis is relief of the obstruction and drainage of the kidney. This is usually accomplished by pyeloplasty with nephrostomy drainage. Nursing care focuses on assessment of fluid and electrolyte balance and maintenance of skin integrity.

1. Maintain fluid and electrolyte balance: See Fluid Requirements and General Nutritional Considerations (pp. 263-280) in Chapter 9 for specific guidelines.

2. Maintenance and patency of tubes and stints:
   a. Nephrostomy tube should be in place to drain the kidney:
      i. Place this tube to closed system drainage collector.
      ii. Avoid kinking of the tube or pulling of the tube.
      iii. Do not attempt to irrigate this tube since it is inserted into the kidney pelvis. Pink-tinged urine or bloody streaks in urine are not uncommon.
      iv. A dry dressing should secure this tube in place. Some leakage of urine around this tube occurs at times.
      v. When the tube is removed, a dry dressing must cover the site. Urine leakage may occur for up to 48 hours.
   b. Often a stint is placed in the ureter to splint the anastomosis.
      i. This tube generally does not drain but must be connected to a closed, sterile drainage system to prevent infection.
      ii. This tube should be well protected to prevent trauma to the ureter or dislodgement of the tube.
   c. A Foley catheter may be in place. Place the catheter to closed drainage system.

3. Monitor vital signs postoperatively according to hospital protocol; usually every 15 minutes four times, every 30 minutes four times, every 1 hour four times, and every 2 hours until stable.

4. Monitor and record urine output every hour for the first 24 hours, every 4 hours for the next 24 hours, and then every 8 hours.

5. Monitor and record characteristics of urine, such as color, specific gravity, dipstick results, pH, and mucus and blood streaks.

6. Weigh newborn twice a day on the same scale and record to watch for dramatic shifts in water balance.

7. Prevent tissue breakdown, especially at edematous sites, by turning and repositioning the newborn at least every 2 hours.

8. Administer oral fluids as soon as tolerated postoperatively.

PARENT CARE

See Chapter 3 for general guidelines and the beginning of this chapter for specific care.

Polycystic Kidneys
Ann Brueggemeyer

DESCRIPTION AND PATHOPHYSIOLOGY

Polycystic kidney is the replacement of normal kidney tissue by numerous cysts. There is a wide variation in the severity of the problem, ranging from asymptomatic to severe renal failure. Atresia of the upper portions of the ureter often occurs along with polycystic kidney. If both kidneys are severely affected, death will occur. Permanent dialysis and organ transplant are potential solutions to permanent renal failure, but success in the neonate is not broadly accepted. Hepatic fibrosis may occur in the infantile form. If hepatic circulation is impeded, portal hypertension may result. It is most common in infants who have extremely enlarged abdomens with a concomitant increase in intra-abdominal pressure (Belman, 1987).

ETIOLOGY AND EMBRYOLOGY

Its mode of transmission can be autosomal recessive in some instances. Polycystic disease is usually due to an obstruction distal to the renal pelvis. This obstruction occurs by the middle of the first trimester. Cells in the ureter fail to develop into a tubular structure and the result is an obstruction or atresia.

INCIDENCE

The exact rate of occurrence is difficult to determine due to the various classifications of multicystic disease found in the newborn. Such classifications may include polycystic disease and hereditary renal disorders.

SYMPTOMS

1. Enlarged abdomen
2. A large, palpable mass felt in the midportion of the abdomen, often not easily identified as a kidney

TRANSPORT

See Appendix A. Nursing goals include maintenance of thermoregulation and fluid and electrolyte balance and prevention of respiratory compromise.

ADMISSION EQUIPMENT

Regular admission setup: see Appendix B.

PREOPERATIVE STABILIZATION

1. Assist with admission workup; see Appendix B:
   a. Blood tests to include renal group (BUN and creatinine) and serum electrolyte levels.
   b. Urinalysis and urine culture: the physician may wish to perform a suprapubic tap. A sterile bladder catheterization may be necessary for follow-up of accurate output.
2. Assess abdomen to include girth measurement at least every 8 hours.
3. Assist with diagnostic procedures: abdominal radiograph, IV or retrograde pyelogram, ultrasonogram, or CT scan may be performed.
4. Maintain proper fluid and electrolyte balance:
   a. Administer IV fluids as determined by renal function and electrolyte balance. See Fluid Requirements and General Nutritional Considerations (pp. 280-285) in Chapter 9 for specific guidelines.
   b. Obtain serum electrolyte, BUN, and creatinine levels at least every 24 hours and as needed.
5. Monitor for infection:
   a. Obtain a complete blood cell count (CBC) with differential within 24 hours prior to surgery.
   b. Obtain urinalysis and urine culture at least 24 hours before surgery is scheduled. If the infant has an indwelling catheter in place, hospital policy should be followed in regard to collection of specimen.

c. Vital signs should be monitored every 2-4 hours and compared to baseline assessment. Any discrepancies should be reported to the physician.

6. Parent care: for specific parent care see General Care (pp. 57-63) in Chapter 3 and Acute Renal Failure in the beginning of this chapter.

SURGERY

An exploratory laparotomy is performed and the affected kidney is removed. Occasionally, if viable kidney tissue is found, a partial nephrectomy is performed.

POSTOPERATIVE STABILIZATION

1. Assessment and care of surgical wound site:
   a. Observe dressing for drainage. Bleeding is a common occurrence at the site but should not be extensive. Urine drainage on the dressing may indicate the need for revision of the operative site since a total nephrectomy should not have urine leakage from the site.
   b. Reinforce dressing as needed. Change dressing as indicated by physician's orders.

2. Maintain gastric decompression. Nasogastric tube may be in place to prevent distention and stress to the operative site. If nasogastric tube is not in place, frequent oral suctioning may be necessary to keep stomach empty and to prevent vomiting.
   a. Securely tape nasogastric tube to infant's face using porous tape. Do not allow tube to cause pressure on the infant's face.
   b. Irrigate the nasogastric tube using 2 cc of air or saline solution as indicated to insure patency and easy drainage.
   c. Connect nasogastric tube to low-intermittent suction.

3. Maintain skin integrity: turn and position the infant at least every 2 hours, especially if edema is present.

4. Maintain fluid and electrolyte balance:
   a. See Fluid Requirements and General Nutritional Considerations (pp. 263-290) in Chapter 9 for specific information.
   b. Obtain electrolyte and renal group levels at least every 24 hours and as ordered, until stable.

5. Maintain gastric decompression. The nasogastric tube may be discontinued within the first few days and oral feedings begun. Adequate bowel sounds must be heard before feedings begin.

6. Monitor vital signs as ordered. Pulse, respiration, BP, and respiratory effort should be recorded every 15 minutes four times, every 30 minutes four times, every hour two times, and every 2 hours until stable.

7. Monitor and record output at least every 4 hours. If output decreases, the level should be recorded every hour. Check urine specific gravity and dipstick for blood at least every 2 hours in the first 24 hours postoperative.

PARENT CARE

See Chapter 3 for general guidelines. Begin early teaching parents to observe for future problems including frequent urinary tract infections and their prevention, signs of decreased output, and signs of wound infection.

Potter's Syndrome
Ann Brueggemeyer

DESCRIPTION

Potter's syndrome is the association of bilateral renal agenesis with the typical appearance of the facies including low-set, malformed ears; wide-set eyes with prominent epicanthal folds; small chin (micrognathia); beaklike nose with a flattened tip; and a malnourished "senile" appearance. The infant is often stillborn or dies within the first 4 days of life. Corrective therapeutic interventions for complete renal failure have not been successful in the neonate. Hypoplastic lung, often occurring with Potter's syndrome, is often considered the cause of death in these infants.

ETIOLOGY AND EMBRYOLOGY

Potter's syndrome is a result of the failure of the uretic bud to divide or develop, leading to renal agenesis.

INCIDENCE

Potter's syndrome occurs in 1 of every 3000 births with almost half of these being stillborn.

DIAGNOSIS

1. The syndrome is suspected if oliguria or anuria is present within the first 48 hours of life.

2. Infant may have been stillborn with the diagnosis being made by appearance or on autopsy.

3. Presence of typical facies: see Description above.

4. Ultrasound or radiologic exam for presence of kidneys, to confirm diagnosis.

PARENT CARE

1. Since prognosis is very poor and the infant will die within the first few days of life, anticipatory grieving should be instituted with the parents. See Parent Care, Anticipatory Grief (p. 58), in Chapter 3.

2. Spiritual counseling may be beneficial at this time.

Exstrophy of the Bladder
Ann Brueggemeyer

DESCRIPTION AND PATHOPHYSIOLOGY

Exstrophy of the bladder is a defect in the abdominal wall resulting in an exteriorization of the bladder and ureters. The defect includes an opening in the anterior wall of the bladder. This defect then allows the posterior aspect of the bladder wall to push forward on the abdomen. In male neonates this defect is associated with a broad, short penis. In female neonates, the labia do not merge. Although other urinary tract structures may be intact, reflux and infection are common. Urine continuously drains over the abdomen making hygiene a problem.

Frequently associated problems include rectal prolapse and nonfusing pubic bones. Corrective surgery is required to maintain bowel function with prolapse. The degree of spread of the pubic bones determines whether or not surgery is required in the newborn period.

ETIOLOGY AND EMBRYOLOGY

At the end of the first month of gestation, the abdominal wall fails to fuse due to the lack of migration of the mesenchymal cells. A thin membrane that forms later ruptures producing the exposed bladder (Moore, 1982).

INCIDENCE

Exstrophy of the bladder occurs in 1 of every 30,000-40,000 live births (King, 1980) and occurs almost four times more often in male than female newborns (King, 1980).

SYMPTOMS

1. Opening in the continuity of the abdominal wall, below the umbilical stump.

2. Exposed bladder mucosa over the opening in the lower abdomen.

3. The presence of ureters visible in the posterior wall of the exposed bladder.

4. Continuous leakage of the urine from the ureters, often undetected visually but noted on dressings around the area.

5. Abnormal genitalia: broad, flattened penis in the male and nonmerging labia in the female newborn.

6. Presence of externalized bowel loop or rectal opening through the abdominal defect.

DIAGNOSIS

1. Visible defect at birth, with an open, exposed bladder on the lower abdomen.

2. Radiological studies as needed to determine extent of genitourinary (GU) defects.

3. Differentiate bladder tissue from bowel tissue, which may accompany the defect.

TRANSPORT

The goal during transport is to prevent trauma to the exposed abdominal defect and maintain thermoregulation.

1. See Appendix A.

2. Apply and maintain abdominal dressings to protect site and absorb urine drainage.
   a. Apply petroleum jelly gauze to cover defect, especially over mucosal areas to prevent dressing's adherence to delicate tissue.
   b. Apply dry, absorbent dressings over petroleum jelly gauze for absorption of urine.
   c. Loose-fitting diaper may be placed over dressings on infant.

ADMISSION EQUIPMENT

1. See Appendix B for general guidelines.

2. Maintain thermoregulation while preserving exposed tissue. An isolette may be preferred over a radiant warmer for infants of all sizes, since radiant heat may be too drying for exposed mucosal tissue.

3. Maintain skin integrity using dressing pack for aseptic dressing technique:
   a. Petroleum jelly gauze.
   b. Absorbent gauze or dressing material.
   c. Montgomery ties or disposable surgical ties and mask (with wire removed) to secure dressings in place over abdomen.

PREOPERATIVE STABILIZATION

1. Assist with admission workup; see Appendix B for general guidelines:
   a. Obtain urinalysis and urine culture (can often be obtained by placing sterile urine collection cup against side of infant and turning the infant in that direction).
   b. Obtain abdominal girth measurement above the level of the defect for baseline data.
   c. Assist with chest and abdominal films to rule out concurrent defects.
2. Maintain fluid and electrolyte balance through oral or IV fluids as needed. See Fluid Requirements and General Nutritional Considerations (pp. 263-280) in Chapter 9 for specific guidelines.
3. Prevent infection at the site:
   a. Use aseptic technique for dressing changes.
   b. Keep dressings as dry as possible without frequent handling of exposed surface.

SURGERY

Surgical treatment of the defect includes primary closure of bladder and abdominal site. Every attempt is made to retain as much normal structure and functioning as possible. Although early closure is recommended, immediate closure is not necessary. The proper technique during dressing changes can greatly reduce the risk of infection to delay surgery until the infant's optimal health has been reached. The nursing goal includes maintenance of fluid and electrolyte balance and assessment of adequacy of urinary drainage sites and output.

POSTOPERATIVE STABILIZATION

1. Maintain proper fluid and electrolyte balance. See Fluid Requirements and General Nutritional Considerations (pp. 263-280) in Chapter 9 for specific guidelines. Oral fluids may be initiated when the infant is stable postoperatively and adequate bowel functioning has been determined.
2. Maintain patency of Foley catheter. Intake and output must be closely monitored. Patency of the catheter is most important to prevent buildup of

urine in the bladder. The catheter should be connected to a closed system drainage bag to prevent infection.

3. Maintenance of tubes and stints:
   a. Suprapubic stints or drainage tubes may be in place depending on the extent of the surgery. Connect all open tubes to closed system drainage bags. Prevent kinking or pulling on tubes.
   b. Maintain dry sterile dressings around tube sites.

4. Assess for leakage of urine and record and report any leakage through suture site or on abdominal dressings.

5. Monitor vital signs frequently according to hospital protocol.

PARENT CARE

See Chapter 3 for general guidelines. Begin early teaching parents to observe for future problems:

1. Symptoms of urinary tract infection.

2. Signs of wound infection.

3. Observation of surgical site for leakage of urine.

4. Identification of decreased urine output or increased abdominal distention.

5. Observation of externally rotated hips, possibly requiring surgical correction before infant begins crawling.

Prune-Belly Syndrome
Ann Brueggemeyer

DESCRIPTION AND PATHOPHYSIOLOGY

Prune-belly syndrome is the congenital absence of abdominal musculature. It is also commonly known as the Eagle-Barrett syndrome and the triad syndrome. Although it affects males in 95 percent of the cases, females never acquire the true syndrome (Short, Groft, & Cook, 1985). The complete syndrome includes "deficiency or hypoplasia of abdominal musculature, varying degrees of dilation of the urinary tract, and undescended testes" (Griggs, 1982, p. 253). The abdomen is extremely round and distended or flabby and wrinkled, depending on the amount of urine distending the bladder. Bowel loops and bladder outline may be seen or felt.

Associated problems include renal damage ranging from normal to complete atresia. There may be obstructions of the ureters and urethra with concomitant hydronephrosis. In some cases, a patent urachus develops to allow urine drainage. Hypoplastic lung may develop as a result of increased abdominal pressure and oligohydramnios.

ETIOLOGY AND EMBRYOLOGY

The congenital malformation results from a failure of the abdominal musculature to form.

INCIDENCE

Prune-belly syndrome occurs in about 1 of every 35,000-50,000 live births. Approximately 95 percent are male (Griggs,1982).

SYMPTOMS

1. Flabby, distended abdomen, may be stretched or wrinkled.
2. Patent urachus, continuous urine drainage may be present.
3. May have no urine output through the urethra due to urethral obstruction, with grossly distended bladder.
4. Decreased urine output due to renal damage.
5. Palpable bladder, kidney, and bowel loops.

DIAGNOSIS

1. Visual inspection: further diagnostic techniques are necessary to determine extent of renal damage and concurrent anomalies.
2. Renal studies may include
   a. Abdominal radiographs.
   b. Abdominal ultrasonogram.
   c. Intravenous pyelogram.
   d. Voiding cystograms.
   e. BUN and creatinine analysis.
3. Chest radiograph to rule out hypoplastic lung.
4. Urine cultures to determine presence of infection and allow for early treatment.

TRANSPORT

Nursing care goals are to maintain thermoregulation, fluid and electrolyte balance, and to prevent distention by maintaining urinary drainage. See Appendix A for general information.

PREOPERATIVE STABILIZATION

1. Carefully assess renal status:
   a. Measure intake and output, including diaper and dressing weights. Credé's method may be necessary to evacuate the bladder. Many physicians, however, do not recommend this procedure as it may cause reflux leading to hydronephrosis. An indwelling catheter may be used but intermittent catheterization should be avoided due to increased risk of trauma and infection.
   b. Assist with testing, including radiographs, cystograms, IV pyelogram.
   c. Frequently analyze urine specific gravity, at least every 4 hours.
2. Provide skin care:
   a. Prevent urine accumulation on the skin, especially the abdominal wall and urachus openings:
      i. Change diaper and/or dressing frequently.
      ii. Wash area with mild soap and water with each change.
      iii. Apply ostomy appliance to urachus to maintain drainage.
   b. Turn infant every 2 hours to prevent pressure areas on sensitive skin.
3. Maintain adequate respiratory status:
   a. Frequently turn infant to prevent atelectasis.
   b. Use chest physiotherapy and postural drainage to open airways.
   c. Assess vital signs, including respiratory effort, color, and breath sounds at least every 2-4 hours.

SURGERY

In mild cases, surgery may not be necessary. If adequate output can be maintained and renal damage prevented, the use of abdominal binders may be sufficient to provide abdominal support. The patent urachus may be an advantage in maintaining an avenue for urine drainage. Large defects may be repaired. If obvious obstruction is present in the urethra or ureters, these are often surgically opened to allow normal drainage. When adequate urine drainage cannot be maintained, ureterostomies are often performed to allow continuous flow of urine for collection outside the body. If significant damage has occurred to one kidney, a nephrectomy is usually performed. No surgical correction of the abdominal-wall musculature is possible.

POSTOPERATIVE STABILIZATION

Postoperative care is directly dependent on what surgical needs the infant has at this time.

1. Maintain respiratory status because prune-belly syndrome is often associated with hypoplastic lungs. Careful attention must be paid to prevent complications:
   a. Frequently assess vital signs including color, respiratory effort, and breath sounds.
   b. Perform chest physiotherapy, postural drainage, and suctioning at least every 2 hours.
   c. Turn and reposition infant at least every 2 hours.
2. Provide skin care:
   a. Turn and reposition infant every 2 hours.
   b. Apply ostomy appliance to urachus, ureterostomies, or vesicostomy if possible.
   c. Use mild soap and water to wash skin if urine leakage occurs.
   d. Change dressings as needed.
3. Maintain gastric decompression:
   a. Nasogastric tube may be needed for gastric decompression:
      i. Connect to low-intermittent suction apparatus.
      ii. Irrigate with 2 cc of air or normal saline solution every 2 hours to ensure patency.
   b. Administration of glycerin suppositories may be necessary for bowel elimination.

PARENT CARE

See Chapter 3 for general guidelines. Prune-belly syndrome will provide a lifetime of stress for the family. Parents need to be aware of all immediate and long-term problems. They need to understand home management of the following:

1. Urinary tract care:
   a. Urachus.
   b. Vesicostomy.
   c. Ureterostomy.
2. Renal function:
   a. Assessment of adequate output.
   b. Prevention of urinary tract infection.
   c. Symptoms of urinary tract infection.
   d. Use of prophylactic antibiotics.
3. Prevention of constipation:
   a. Use of natural food.
   b. Use of suppositories.
4. Psychological support:
   a. Parental acceptance of long-term prognosis.
   b. Use of binders for functional control of bladder and for infant's appearance.

Hydrocele
Ann Brueggemeyer

DESCRIPTION AND PATHOPHYSIOLOGY

Hydrocele is described as the failure of the processus vaginalis testis (in the male newborn) or the processus vaginalis peritonei (in the female newborn) to close, thus allowing fluid to pass from the abdomen into the scrotal sac, or labia, respectively. If the opening is large, fluid readily passes back to the abdomen, causing a shift in the size of the hydrocele. A large opening may also allow the herniation of bowel loops through to the scrotal sac, causing an inguinal hernia. A small processus opening will readily allow fluid to pass from the abdomen into the scrotal sac. Because of increased abdominal pressure, the fluid will not be able to pass back into the abdomen causing the fluid-filled hydrocele. In the female newborn, the hydrocele may appear as edematous labia.

ETIOLOGY

It is a congenital malformation that results when the processus vaginalis fails to close, allowing peritoneal fluid to accumulate within the sac.

INCIDENCE

Hydrocele is more common in male than female newborns. No exact rate is reported.

DIAGNOSIS

1. Visual inspection: must be verified by other means.

2. Abdominal transillumination: fluid-filled sac will transilluminate.

3. Tumors or herniated bowel permits no transillumination.

4. Palpation of a solid mass or tumor rules out hydrocele.

5. Percussion of abdomen reflecting fluid versus air is indicative.

6. Observation for herniation of bowel must be routinely performed.

TRANSPORT

The nursing goal is to prevent secondary trauma and to maintain thermoregulation. See Appendix A for general considerations.

PREOPERATIVE STABILIZATION

No special nursing care is required other than thorough skin care and protection from trauma. Observe for and report pain, as discomfort is indicative of herniation.

SURGERY

Surgical intervention is often not attempted until after 1year of age. Bowel herniation or incarceration is considered to require immediate surgical intervention. Undescended testes may also require surgical treatment in the infant. Surgical intervention consists of drainage of the hydrocele and closure of the patent duct.

POSTOPERATIVE STABILIZATION

1. Prevent increased abdominal pressure:
   a. Infant may need nasogastric tube for gastric decompression.
   b. Provide comfort measures to keep infant's crying to a minimum, to prevent increased intra-abdominal pressure, which may place stress on the suture site.
   c. Do not elevate the head of the bed.
   d. Infant should not be placed on the abdomen in the immediate postoperative period.

2. Maintain infant's skin integrity by using waterproof occlusive dressing to prevent contamination. Wash area after void or defecation.

Inguinal Hernia
Ann Brueggemeyer

DESCRIPTION AND ETIOLOGY

Inguinal hernia is one of the most common problems requiring pediatric surgery. It occurs as a failure of the processus vaginalis to close, allowing bowel loops and gonads to enter the scrotal sac in the male or the soft tissue in the female newborn. Right-side hernias are more common than left. Incarceration occurs when bowel loops or gonads are caught within the processus, leading to obstruction. When blood supply is cut off from the herniated organs, gangrene can result. Within several hours, strangulation of herniated organs can occur.

INCIDENCE

There is a 10–42 percent incidence in the neonatal population with a 30-55 percent incidence in premature infants (Rescorla & Grasfeld,1984). Bilateral hernias are found in only 10-20 percent of the infants with hernias.

SYMPTOMS

1. The infant is often asymptomatic.
2. "Lump" or mass in groin or abdomen determined by palpation, or, if large, by observation.
3. Irritability (e.g., excessive crying).
4. Scrotum may be edematous or may appear larger with crying.
5. Groin lump or mass may increase in size with crying.
6. Obstructive signs include vomiting, abdominal distention, constipation, or no stool output.
7. Incarceration of organs leads to discoloration of hernia and surrounding area, increased irritability, and fever.

DIAGNOSIS

1. Observation of a lump in the groin.
2. Palpation of swelling and firmness in the scrotum.
3. Transillumination is not useful because of too many false-positive results due to air in the bowel.
4. Bowel obstruction may be a sign of incarceration.

TRANSPORT

Nursing care goals include prevention of tissue damage and maintenance of thermoregulation. See Appendix A for general considerations.

PREOPERATIVE STABILIZATION

Observation of the infant for strangulation of bowel is an ongoing process until the surgery is performed. Oral feedings may be given if obstruction of the bowel does not occur. In some cases, bowel loops are manually guided back into the abdominal cavity using gentle pressure. Crying or upright positioning of the infant may increase the size of the hernia due to an increase in intra-abdominal pressure.

SURGERY

Unless incarceration occurs, inguinal hernias are not always considered to require emergency surgery. Surgery is often delayed for 12-24 months. When surgery is performed, the herniated organs are returned to the abdomen and the processus vaginalis is closed. If incarceration has occurred, a bowel resection or gonadal removal is necessary. Surgery is not contraindicated in the neonatal period.

POSTOPERATIVE STABILIZATION

Because of the large population of premature and formerly premature infants as candidates for inguinal hernia repair, careful attention is paid to apnea after surgery. Although performed as "same-day surgery," premies operated on for inguinal hernias should be observed at least 24 hours after surgery for apnea and bradycardia. If bowel obstruction has occurred, see Small Bowel Atresia, in Chapter 5 for specific nursing care.

1. Maintain skin integrity.
   a. Clear, occlusive dressings may be used to protect the site yet maintain visibility of the wound.
   b. Wash area with mild soap and water after every void or defecation.
2. Observe for bleeding or swelling at the site and report it to physician.
3. Maintain adequate nutrition. If bowel trauma has not occurred, oral feedings may begin as soon as the infant has recovered from anesthesia.

PARENT CARE

See Chapter 3 for general considerations.

Undescended Testes
Ann Brueggemeyer

DESCRIPTION

The descent of the testes involves the differentiation of the inguinal region into the inguinal canal and the partitioning of the peritoneal cavity and tunica vaginalis. Once this communication is no longer open, the testes begin to descend through the inguinal canals, moving from within the peritoneal cavity, reaching their final position in the scrotal sac at around the 32nd to 34th week of gestation (Moore, 1982). It should be noted that the complete obliteration of the communication between the scrotal portion of peritoneal cavity and the vaginal process occurs several months postnatally.

ETIOLOGY

Descent of the testes occurs as a shift of positioning from abdominal cavity to scrotal sac with the closure of the canal wall.

INCIDENCE

Undescended testes occurs frequently, as the descent and canal closure do not completely occur for several months after birth. It may be more common in premature babies. No exact incidence is reported.

SYMPTOMS

May occur in the presence of hydrocele or hernia.

DIAGNOSIS

Absence of testes in the scrotal sac indicates either lack of descent, temporary regression of the testes into the abdomen, or lack of testes. Diagnosis is often not made in the neonatal stage as the testes may not descend for several months. Surgery is usually delayed until at least 2 years of age to allow for normal descent.

Torsion of the Testis
Ann Brueggemeyer

DESCRIPTION

Torsion of the testis is commonly described as a twisting or occlusion of the testis or spermatic cord. Left untreated, permanent damage may occur to the testis. When it occurs in the neonate, permanent damage may have already occurred, since infarction can be evident in 4 hours. Torsion may also occur in female new-borns as a torsion of the fallopian tube, constricting flow to the ovary.

ETIOLOGY

Torsion of the testis is a congenital malformation resulting in a problem with the descent of the testis into the scrotal sac. There usually is a twisting of the tunica vaginalis and its contents.

INCIDENCE

It is somewhat common in the neonatal period; however, an exact incidence rate is not reported.

SYMPTOMS

1. Scrotal enlargement and edema.

2. Scrotum is firm-to-hard to the touch.

3. Palpable mass, may be tender.

4. Mass does not transilluminate.

5. Scrotum may be discolored, either red or blue.

DIAGNOSIS

Diagnosis can be difficult as it can be easily confused with other defects such as hernias or hydroceles.

1. Transilluminate the scrotum, observing for fluid, air or mass. If torsion is present, scrotum will not transilluminate.

2. Surgical exploration may be required to provide a differential diagnosis.

TRANSPORT

The nursing goal is to maintain thermoregulation and prevent further tissue damage. See Appendix A for general considerations.

1. Maintain careful observation of the site to observe for any changes in color, size, and firmness.

2. Observe for abdominal distention. Vomiting may occur if obstruction occurs due to pressure on lower abdomen, peritonitis, or concurrent hernia.

3. Position infant on back to prevent further trauma to site.

ADMISSION EQUIPMENT

See Appendix B for general considerations.

PREOPERATIVE STABILIZATION

1. Assess abdomen:
   a. Measure, assess, and record abdominal girth, scrotum size, area of edema, and color and temperature of scrotum.
   b. If distention or vomiting is present, insert a nasogastric tube and place to low-intermittent suction for decompression.
   c. Assess and record vital signs at least every 2 hours.
   d. Place infant only on side or back.
2. Observe respiratory status. If distress is present, administer supportive oxygen.
3. Maintain adequate fluid and nutritional balance:
   a. Keep infant NPO for surgery.
   b. Provide appropriate IV fluids as ordered. See Fluid Requirements and General Nutritional Considerations (pp. 280-285) in Chapter 9 for specific guidelines.

POSTOPERATIVE STABILIZATION

1. Assess infant for baseline response to surgery.
   a. Measure vital signs and record every 15 minutes four times, every 30 minutes four times, every hour four times, and every 2 hours until stable.
2. Observe for respiratory compromise due to abdominal distention.
3. Assess abdominal and urinary tract status:
   a. Observe surgical area for edema, drainage, or bruising.
   b. Keep dressing or suture line clean and dry. Infant may need continuous urinary drainage bag to prevent contamination of site.
   c. Observe and record output of urine every hour. Examine specimen every 4 hours for specific gravity and examine dipstick every 4 hours for blood.
   d. Observe and record frequency and characteristics of stool output. Test for occult blood every 8 hours.
   e. Maintain nasogastric tube. Irrigate every 2 hours with air or saline solution to insure patency. Measure and record output.

4. Maintain adequate fluid and nutritional balance. See Fluid Requirements and General Considerations (pp. 263-290) in Chapter 9 for specific guidelines. Feedings can be initiated when the nasogastric tube is discontinued and bowel sounds are heard.

PARENT CARE

1. See Chapter 3 for general considerations.

2. Prepare parents for home care including observation of site, maintenance of clean suture line, and reporting of observations to the physician.

3. Identify future concerns of infant's fertility. Testis may have become necrosed prior to surgery, thus requiring removal. Assist parents in gaining appropriate information in relation to infant's surgery and outcome.

REFERENCES

Acute Renal Failure

Inturrisi, M., Perry, S., & May, K. (1985). Fetal surgery for congenital hydronephrosis. *Journal of Obstetric, Gynecologic, and Neonatal Nursing, 13,* 271-276.
Vestal, K., & McKenzie, C. (1983). *High risk perinatal nursing,* p. 443-451. Philadelphia: W. B. Saunders.

Hydronephrosis

Harrison, M., Ross, N., Noall, R., & de Lorimier, A. (1983). Correction of congenital hydronephrosis in utero. I. The model: Fetal urethral obstruction produces hydronephrosis and pulmonary hypoplasia in fetal lambs. *Journal of Pediatric Surgery, 18,* 247-256.
Inturrisi, M., Perry, S., & May, K. (1985). Fetal surgery for congenital hydronephrosis. *Journal of Obstetric, Gynecologic, and Neonatal Nursing, 14,* 271-276.

Polycystic Kidney

Belman, A. B. (1987). Abnormalities of the genitourinary system, in G. B. Avery (Ed.)., *Neonatology: Pathophysiology and management of the newborn* (3rd ed.) (pp. 985-1011). Philadelphia: J. B. Lippincott.

Exstrophy of the Bladder

King, L. (1980). Exstrophy of the bladder and epispadius. In J. Raffensperger (Ed.)., *Pediatric surgery* (pp. 7531-768). New York:Appleton-Century-Crofts.

Moore, K. (1982). *The developing human: Clinically oriented embryology* (pp. 269-270). Philadelphia: W.B. Saunders.

Prune-Belly Syndrome

Griggs, C. (1982). What is prune-belly syndrome? *Maternal-Child Nursing Journal, 7,* 253-257.
Short, K., Groft, D., & Cook, L. (1985). The concomitant presence of gastroschisis and prune-belly syndrome in a twin. *Journal of Pediatric Surgery, 20,* 186-187.

Inguinal Hernia

Rescorla, F., & Grosfeld, J. (1984). Inguinal hernia repair in the perinatal period and early infancy: Clinical considerations. *Journal of Pediatric Surgery, 19,* 832-836.

Undescended Testes

Moore, K. (1982). *The developing human* (pp. 271-294). Philadelphia: W. B. Saunders.

Torsion of the Testis

Rescorla, F., & Grosfeld, J. (1984). Inguinal hernia repair in the perinatal period and early infancy: Clinical considerations. *Journal of Pediatric Surgery, 19,* 832-836.
Wright, J. E. (1986). Impalpable testes: A review of 100 boys. *Journal of Pediatric Surgery, 21,* 151-153.

BIBLIOGRAPHY

Glick, P., Harrison, M., Noall, R., & Villa, R. (1983). Correction of congenital hydronephrosis in utero. III. Early mid-trimester ureteral obstruction produces renal dysplasia. *Journal of Pediatric Surgery, 18,* 681-683.
Griggs, C. (1982). What is prune-belly syndrome? *Maternal-Child Nursing Journal, 7,* 253-257.
Harrison, M., Ross, N., Noall, R., & de Lorimier, A. (1983). Correction of congenital hydronephrosis in utero. I. The model: Fetal urethral obstruction produces hydronephrosis and pulmonary hypoplasia in fetal lambs. *Journal of Pediatric Surgery, 18,* 247-256.
Howell, C., Caldamone, A., Snyder, H., Ziegler, M., & Duckett, J. (1983). Optimal management of cloacal exstrophy. *Journal of Pediatric Surgery, 18,* 365-369.

Inturrisi, M., Perry, S., & May, K. (1985). Fetal surgery for congenital hydronephrosis. *Journal of Obstetric, Gynecologic, and Neonatal Nursing, 14*, 271-276.

James, J. (1972). *Renal disease in childhood.* St. Louis: C. V. Mosby.

King, L. (1980). Exstrophy of the bladder and epispadius. In J. Raffensperger (Ed.)., *Pediatric Surgery* (pp. 753-768). New York:Appleton-Century-Crofts.

Murphy, P., Holder, T., Ashcraft, K., Sharp, R., Goodwin, C., & Amoury, R. (1984). Ureteropelvic junction obstruction in the newborn. *Journal of Pediatric Surgery,19*, 642-648.

O'Donnell, B. (1984). The lessons of forty bladder exstrophies in twenty years. *Journal of Pediatric Surgery, 19*, 547-549.

Rescorla, F., & Grosfeld, J. (1984). Inguinal hernia repair in the perinatal period and early infancy: Clinical considerations. *Journal of Pediatric Surgery, 19*, 832-836.

Schwoebel, M., Sacher, P., Bucher, H., Hirsig, J., & Stauffer, U. (1984). Prenatal diagnosis improves the prognosis of children with obstructive uropathies. *Journal of Pediatric Surgery, 19*, 187-190.

Short, K., Groft, D., & Cook, L. (1985). The concomitant presence of gastroschisis and prune belly syndrome in a twin. *Journal of Pediatric Surgery, 20*, 186-187.

Tank, E., & McCoy, G. (1983). Limited surgical intervention in prune belly syndrome. *Journal of Pediatric Surgery, 18*, 686-691.

Vestal, K., & McKenzie, C. (1983). *High risk perinatal nursing.* Philadelphia: W. B. Saunders.

Chapter 7

Alterations in the Neurological System

Ann Brueggemeyer   *Carole Kenner*

The infant born with neurological defects is at risk for long-term problems. Neural-tube defects constitute the majority of these defects. During the early first trimester, neural-tube closure should be complete. An interference with this closure prevents the normal development of an intact nervous system. Manifestations of these defects vary from mild to severe. Each defect has its own variation in severity. Long-term prognosis often cannot be determined until after surgery is performed. The infant may present with more severe problems after surgery.

Assessment is a very important aspect in the care of these infants. Attention must be paid to small changes that occur. Symptoms may be subtle. Infection is a major concern with these infants. Meningitis is more prevalent in infants with neural-tube defects than in infants with any other kind of defect. Postoperatively, open wounds provide direct access to invading organisms. Effects from meningitis complicate the already neurologically unstable infant.

DIAGNOSIS

Amniocentesis may be performed in anticipation of neural-tube defects in the infant. Elevated levels of alpha-fetal protein are present with these defects. Although not diagnostic of a specific defect, these increased levels may guide the physician in performing more fetal testing. Prenatal ultrasound can also detect some of the lesions. An enlarged skull may indicate hydrocephalus, which may be a sign of intracranial blockage or may be in conjunction with other neural-tube defects.

In most cases, the defect is detected at the time of birth. In the case of mild hydrocephalus, head enlargement may not be greater than normal for several days or weeks. The birth of an infant with neurological problems can be devastating. The defect may be quite obvious. What is not so obvious is the long-term medical and surgical problems that face the infant and family. Much support must be given to the parents in order for them to cope with this situation.

TRANSPORT

The nursing goal for transport is to assess neurological baseline data and prevent further physical trauma and an increase in intracranial pressure.

1. See Appendix A.

2. Decrease potential for injury or pressure to the defect:
   a. Do not place the infant on defect.
   b. Cover draining or open defect with sterile nonadhering dressings (i.e., Telfa).
   c. Support defect when moving or turning infant.

3. Monitor neurological status:
   a. Record routine vital signs every 15 minutes until stable.
   b. Record pupil size and pupil response.
   c. Record level of consciousness and signs of increased intracranial pressure:
      i. Behavior or activity level
      ii. Symptoms of increased intracranial pressure include high-pitched cry, lethargy, irritability, sunset or bulging eyes, and changes in vital signs
   d. Record motor function:
      i. Movement of all four extremities
      ii. Presence of anal wink, indicating neurological function of anal muscle
   e. Measure and record head circumference for baseline data.
   f. Assess fontanelles for fullness and firmness.

4. Monitor infant's intake and output, as lack of innervation may cause retention and distention.

5. Prevent skin breakdown by using sheepskin or other protective materials.

6. Maintain adequate nutrition and fluid and electrolyte balance. See Fluid Requirements and General Nutritional Considerations (pp. 263-290) in Chapter 9 for specific guidelines.

7. Parent care: See Chapter 3 for general guidelines.

PREOPERATIVE STABILIZATION

Nursing goal for stabilization is to assess neurological baseline data and prevent further physical trauma and an increase in intracranial pressure.

1. See Appendix B for admission setup.

2. See Transport above for general care.

3. Provide support to parents:
   a. Verify informed consent for surgery.
   b. Prepare parents for potential outcomes after surgery. Surgical intervention for neurological defects often requires the removal of nerve tissue. Normal motor function prior to surgery may not be intact after surgery. If brain tissue must be sacrificed, the infant's mental capacity may be greatly altered.

4. Assist with diagnostic tests, which may include radiographs, computed tomographic (CT) scan, and ultrasonogram.

5. Maintain neutral thermal environment as infant may be incapable of temperature stabilization if the neural temperature control mechanism is affected.

6. Maintain nutrition and fluid and electrolyte balance. See Chapter 9 for specific guidelines.

POSTOPERATIVE STABILIZATION

1. Monitor neurological status:
   a. Record routine vital signs every 15 minutes four times, every 30 minutes four times, and every hour until stable; check routine vital signs every 2-4 hours.
   b. Record pupil size and pupil response.
   c. Record level of consciousness and signs of increased intracranial pressure.
      i. Behavior or activity level
      ii. Symptoms of increased intracranial pressure to include high-pitched cry, lethargy, irritability, sunset or bulging eyes, and change in vital signs
   d. Record motor function:
      i. Movement of all four extremities
      ii. Presence of anal wink, indicating neurological function of anal muscle
   e. Measure and record head circumference daily. An increase >1cm per week may indicate hydrocephalus. Rapid growth within the first few days after surgery may require early intervention.
   f. Assess fontanelles for fullness and firmness. An increase may indicate an increase in intracranial pressure. A rapid decrease may lead to internal trauma due to shifting of brain tissue within the cranium.

2. Monitor intake and output:
   a. Report output < 1cc/kg/h. Lack of urine output or small voids may indicate a neurogenic bladder. Renal ultrasound and straight catheterization procedures after voids may indicate the need for regular bladder catheterizations. The Credé method is sometimes used but may lead to reflux and kidney damage.
   b. Report output that is significantly greater than intake. The syndrome of inappropriate antidiuretic hormone (SIADH) can occur when cranial surgery

is performed or infection is present. Large amounts of fluids are excreted causing a major disturbance in fluid and electrolyte balance.

3. Prevent skin breakdown:
   a. Place sheepskin or other protective materials under infant.
   b. Maintain a clean and dry dressing over suture areas. When a back or buttock wound is present, an occlusive clear dressing should be used. To prevent contamination of wound, a plastic shield may be secured between the dressing and the anus. This shield may be cleaned or replaced with every cleaning. A diaper should not be used until skin edges have completely healed to prevent wound contamination.

4. Provide adequate nutrition and fluid and electrolyte balance. See Fluid Requirements and General Nutritional Considerations (pp. 263-290) in Chapter 9 for specific guidelines. Oral fluids may be administered as soon as the infant recovers from surgery unless otherwise indicated.

5. Assessment and prevention of serious infection:
   a. Prevent contamination of wound sites.
   b. Observe for and report any signs of infection.

6. Observe for and report any signs of seizure activity.

PARENT CARE

The birth of an infant with a neural-tube defect can be a great burden to the parents. The defect can produce physical changes that make the infant look very different from the expected normal newborn. Even after correction, the infant may not appear normal.

The child may face a lifetime of frequent hospitalizations. Revisions of shunts and orthopedic procedures may seem endless. Along with support from the health care team, support services should be offered to the parents. Emotional as well as financial support will help to relieve some of their burden. The family should be encouraged to be involved in the care of their infant from the very beginning. Teaching begins from the time of diagnosis. Parents will need to be aware of the symptoms of infection, increased intracranial pressure, and any other complication that may arise in relation to the diagnosis. Follow-up care should be arranged prior to discharge. The nurse should make arrangements to coordinate the various health care providers that are necessary to give comprehensive care to this infant.

Meningomyelocele
Carole Kenner

DESCRIPTION

Meningomyelocele is a defect of the spinal cord that involves herniation of the meninges and the cord itself. This defect may or may not be covered with a membrane. While the meningomyelocele can occur anywhere along the spinal cord, the usual location is the lumbar or sacral region. The location of the defect determines the degree of neurological impairment.

ETIOLOGY AND EMBRYOLOGY

The commonly accepted theory of the cause of meningomyelocele is the failure of the neural tube to close during fetal development. Closure occurs cephalocaudal, often leaving the most distal portions open. It is also believed that rupture may occur after the tube has formed. Although variations occur, meningomyelocele is the most common neural tube defect.

INCIDENCE

The rate of occurrence fluctuates from 1 to 4 of every 1000 births.

SYMPTOMS

1. A visible defect in the vertebral column that may or may not be leaking cerebrospinal fluid (CSF).

2. Depending on the size and location of the defect, there may be no movement of the lower extremities.

3. There may be urinary retention due to impaired neurological impulses to the bladder.

4. No response to painful stimuli in the lower extremities is possible.

5. No anal wink; however, this along with decreased response to pain may be unreliable signs of the defect.

6. Dislocation of the hips.

7. Deformities of the knee—flexion or extension.

8. Deformities of the feet such as inward or outward rotation.

9. Abnormally large head circumference, as hydrocephalus often accompanies this defect.

DIAGNOSIS

The diagnosis is usually made by visual inspection of the infant's spine. The extent of the neurological deficiency is determined by physical and neurological exams as described above in Signs and Symptoms.

TRANSPORT

The nursing goal in transport and stabilization is to prevent trauma to the exposed sac and to preserve neural integrity.

1. Maintain tissue integrity:
   a. Keep infant in prone position to decrease the chance of pressure on the spinal area.
   b. If CSF is leaking from the defect or if the meningomyelocele is open, place sterile gauze soaked in warm saline solution to the area to keep it moist. If according to institutional policy, place the infant in plastic baby bag.
   c. If the defect is not open, place sterile dressing over the site.
   d. If the head is enlarged, place infant in the head-down position with the feet raised about 20° to decrease pressure on the defect. Caution: this position can increase intracranial pressure.

2. Preserve nerve function.
   a. Keep infant's lower extremities and hips in a neutral position with a small towel roll under the hips. This position decreases tension on the hips and decreases pressure on exposed nerves.
   b. Observe infant's lower extremities during the transport for any cyanosis or mottling. If these changes occur, infant's position should be changed. Remember that this infant may be unable to move the lower extremities.

3. See Appendix A for general transport guidelines.

PREOPERATIVE STABILIZATION

1. See Appendix B and Transport (p. 220) and Preoperative Stabilization (p. 220) at the beginning of this chapter for general guidelines.

2. Assist with head ultrasound and spinal radiographs to be taken in prone position to prevent trauma to back.

3. Assess vital signs for baseline measurements; include temperature, heart rate, respiratory rate and effort, and BP.

4. Assess infant: include a thorough neurological exam; examination of the head and fontanelles, size and quality; observation for movement or hypotonia of extremities; observation and palpation of bladder for urinary retention; and observation for knee, foot, or hip deformities. All physical exams should be carried out with the infant prone or on side. Do not lay the infant on defect. If resuscitation is necessary, care must be taken to prevent trauma if infant must be laid on the back. The use of towel rolls on either side of the defect or a doughnut-shaped cloth ring placed around the defect may help to take pressure off the defect and prevent trauma.

5. Maintain tissue integrity:

   a. Place sterile gauze over defect if a membrane covers the defect.

   b. Place sterile gauze soaked in warm saline solution over an open defect to prevent contamination or drying of the wound.

   c. If the infant is to be fed orally, the infant must remain prone with head turned to side. To burp the infant, rub or pat between scapula.

6. Preserve neurological function:

   a. Place towel roll under hips.

   b. Place infant's extremities and hips in a neutral position to prevent contractures and to decrease tension on the sac.

   c. Place infant in head-down position if hydrocephalus is present but only if so ordered. Decreasing pressure on the defect may increase intracranial pressure.

   d. Observe extremities for mottling or cyanosis. Check capillary refill of feet. If any cyanosis, mottling, or sluggish capillary refill is present, change the infant's position.

7. Prevent infection from fecal contamination of wound. Tape a small sheet of plastic flush to skin between wound and anus. This sheet should not be taped over defect or dressing.

8. Preserve urinary elimination.

   a. If urinary retention is present, place indwelling urinary catheter to closed gravity system. An alternative to this is to use the Credé method using gentle rolling pressure from the umbilicus to pubic area. This should be performed every 2-4 hours. This method may cause reflux leading to renal damage and may not be recommended.

   b. Record intake and output every 8 hours.

   c. Change diaper (which is under the infant but not fastened over defect) frequently as infant in prone position is very susceptible to diaper rash and excoriation.

SURGERY

The surgery may be performed only hours after birth; or if the defect is not open and draining, surgery may be postponed for several days. The surgery involves removing the herniated tissue and then covering the defect with surrounding skin from a local or rotated flap.

POSTOPERATIVE STABILIZATION

Nursing goals are to prevent contamination and trauma to wound site. Observation for and prevention of complications are secondary goals.

1. Prevention of trauma to site:

a. Keep infant in prone position.

b. Observe for swelling or collection of fluid pocket near suture line. If present, report it to the surgeon. Pressure on the suture line may occur from leaking spinal fluid or hematomas.

c. Maintain infant's lower extremities in neutral position with roll under hips. Flexion or hyperextension may place pressure on defect leading to trauma before healing has occurred.

d. Prone position is maintained even when holding the infant, for 10-14 days until suture line is healed.

2. Prevention of infection:
   a. Keep sterile dressing over suture line.
   b. Observe for drainage from suture line, including dampened dressing.
   c. Observe for signs of infection: irritability, unstable temperature, and increased respiratory or heart rate.
   d. Keep plastic protector in place to prevent fecal contamination of dressing.

3. Observation and maintenance of neurological function:
   a. Observe for movement, hypotonia, cyanosis, decreased capillary refill, or mottling in lower extremities.
   b. Check femoral, popliteal, and pedal pulses every 2 hours.
   c. Gently check range of joint motion to the extremities every 2-4 hours. Do not place tension on suture line.
   d. Measure and record head circumference every day. Once leaking sacs are closed, head circumference may increase rapidly due to a disruption of flow of circulating CSF. Shunting to treat hydrocephalus may need to be performed within the first few days after meningomyelocele closure to prevent increased intracranial pressure.

4. Maintain urinary elimination.
   a. Observe for urinary retention. Indwelling or intermittent catheterization or Credé method may be used. The use of the Credé method may not be recommended as it must be perfomed while infant is supine.
   b. Maintain accurate intake and output records.

5. Maintain nutrition and fluid and electrolyte balance. See Parenteral Nutrition: Peripheral and Total Parenteral (pp. 280-285) in Chapter 9 for specific guidelines. Oral fluids may be started as soon as infant recovers from anesthesia. Feedings are given in prone position as they are preoperatively.

6. Parent care; see Chapter 3 for general guidelines:
   a. Provide support to parents as their infant may require long and frequent hospitalizations for shunt revisions and orthopedic surgery.
   b. Prepare parents for further surgery if hydrocephalus is present.
   c. Utilize multidisciplinary approach for the variety of problems that will arise. Provide referrals to social service, orthopedist, urologist, and occupational and physical therapists if appropriate.
   d. Begin early teaching parents home management of the infant, to include:

   i. Catheterization or Credé method if appropriate. See Intermittent Bladder Catheterization (pp. 262-263.) in Chapter 12 for guidelines.
  ii. Cast or splint care if appropriate for correction of orthopedic problems.
 iii. Signs of increased intracranial pressure.

Hydrocephalus
Carole Kenner

DESCRIPTION AND PATHOPHYSIOLOGY

Hydrocephalus is an abnormal or excessive enlargement of the cranium. The enlargement results from an obstruction, either partial or complete, in the pathway of the CSF. The hydrocephalus may be communicating where the obstruction occurs, usually in the subarachnoid space, or noncommunicating where the obstruction is usually found in the aqueduct of Sylvius.

ETIOLOGY AND EMBRYOLOGY

This cranial enlargement may be either congenital or acquired. The congenital type is largely attributable to cysts, masses, stenosis, atresia, Arnold-Chiari malformation (often associated with meningomyelocele), or encephalocele. It can occur at any point in embryological development, causing constriction to the flow of CSF. The acquired hydrocephalus may result from masses, subarachnoid hemorrhages, inflammation from infections, meningeal hemorrhages, or tumors. In the perinatal period, hydrocephalus can also occur secondary to trauma, infection, or intracranial bleeding.

INCIDENCE

Hydrocephalus occurs in almost 2 of every 1000 births.

SYMPTOMS

1. Increasing head circumference above acceptable level for gestational age.

2. Bulging fontanelles.

3. Cracking sound elicited when forehead is tapped with finger indicating the ventricle is dilated.

4. Sunset eyes.

5. Irritability or lethargy, depending upon severity of intracranial pressure.

6. Vomiting with feedings, or anorexia.

7. Transillumination of skull.

8. Unilateral bulging of skull.

9. Symmetrical enlargement of skull.

10. Size of fontanelle above acceptable level for gestational age.

DIAGNOSIS

1. Visual inspection of cranium.

2. Head circumference increasing in size at abnormal rate or above acceptable level for gestational age.

3. Physical examination with positive findings for increased intracranial pressure.

4. Transillumination of the skull.

5. Cranial ultrasonogram or cranial CT scan.

6. Anteroposterior (AP) and lateral skull radiographs.

7. Ventriculogram may be done if necessary but is not routinely performed.

8. Pneumoencephalogram may be done but may be inadvisable if intracranial pressure is severely elevated.

9. Cerebral angiography may be done but is not routinely performed.

TRANSPORT

Nursing goals during transport include maintenance of thermoregulation and prevention of occlusion of airway secondary to head positioning.

1. Maintain position of comfort for infant:
   a. Support head well when lifting if head size is excessive.
   b. Position infant on side or prone so that head does not fall forward, potentially cutting off airway.

2. Maintain thermoregulation. Cover head if possible as infant's heat loss through a large body surface can be enormous.

3. See Appendix A.

PREOPERATIVE STABILIZATION

1. See Appendix B for admission setup.

2. Assessment for neurological function to include the following:
   a. Observe quantity and quality of fontanelles.
   b. Palpate fontanelles to evaluate fullness and firmness.
   c. Percuss for cracking sound by tapping infant's forehead with finger.
   d. Auscultate fontanelles and temporal arteries for bruit or venous hum.
   e. Observe for anorexia, vomiting, irritability, sunset eyes, hypotonia, or lethargy.
   f. Observe for symmetrical or asymmetrical enlargement of cranium.
   g. Observe for high-pitched cry.
   h. Assess for the presence of any other congenital anomalies such as meningomyelocele.
   i. Measure head circumference for baseline and continue to measure daily.

3. Maintain airway:
   a. Position infant on side or prone, so that head may not fall forward potentially cutting off airway.
   b. Support infant's head and neck when lifting or moving infant.

4. Maintain skin integrity:
   a. If head is excessively large, place sheepskin or other protection under head to decrease occurrence of pressure areas.
   b. Turn and reposition infant at least every 2 hours.

5. Maintain thermoregulation. Cover newborn's head if possible to decrease heat loss.

6. Maintain nutrition and fluid and electrolyte balance. See Fluids, General Nutritional Considerations in the Neonate, and Protein Caloric Malnutrition (pp. 263-280) in Chapter 9 for specific guidelines.
   a. Feedings may be given by nipple or gavage.
   b. Since hydrocephalus is associated with meningomyelocele, feed in prone position.

SURGERY

The surgery involves placement of a shunt in one of two ways: ventriculoatrial or ventriculoperitoneal. These shunts contain valves that regulate the flow of CSF. The shunt drains the spinal fluid from the dilated ventricle into the atrium or peritioneal cavity where it then is absorbed and removed as are other body fluids. The shunt, when placed in an infant, may require multiple revisions as the child grows.

A temporary shunt may be used and is drained externally into a sterile closed system container. Care must be taken not to disturb the placement of this container since gravity, not a valve, regulates the flow of CSF. An external drain may be used when infection (of the peritoneum or heart) or overwhelming sepsis is present in either the ventricle or the drain site.

If the presence of a cyst, tumor, or mass is known, surgical removal of this obstruction is performed. In these cases, a shunt may not be necessary.

POSTOPERATIVE STABILIZATION

Major nursing goals are to prevent infection and prevent complications from shifts in CSF.

1. Maintain proper positioning of infant:
    a. Keep infant in flat position off the shunt site unless otherwise ordered.
    b. After scalp dressing is removed and infant is to be turned on shunt site, place a cloth or foam ring or "doughnut" under shunt site to decrease pressure on the area.
    c. Position head with slight support to maintain patent airway if head size is excessively large.

2. Prevent infection:
    a. Observe head and abdominal and chest dressing over suture lines for moisture or drainage. Leakage of CSF could lead to serious infection.
    b. Observe infant for signs of infected shunt such as hyperirritability, lethargy, or change in vital signs.

3. Assess neurological function:
    a. Measure head circumference daily to observe for dramatic shifts of fluid.
    b. Observe and record characteristics of fontanelles. Report any changes since fluid may drain too quickly and cause shifting of brain tissue leading to permanent tissue damage. If fontanelles remain full, shunt may not be functioning.
    c. Observe for signs of an obstructed shunt such as vomiting, anorexia, increasing head circumference, high-pitched cry, or any symptom that the infant may have exhibited before surgery.
    d. Maintain function of external drain if used. Drainage container must be secured in a fixed position at the position of the infant's head. If the container is elevated, CSF will not readily drain causing an increase in intracranial fluid. If the level of the container is lowered, excessive drainage may occur causing a shift in cerebral contents. If a dramatic shift occurs, brain trauma and swelling may occur causing permanent damage. Accurate measurement of fluid must be maintained. In some instances, fluid replacement therapy may be instituted to prevent electrolyte and fluid imbalance.

4. Maintain nutrition and fluid and electrolyte balance. See Chapter 9 for specific guidelines. Oral feedings may be begun as early as 24 hours postoperatively,

once infant is awake and alert. If an external drain is in place, the infant cannot be moved for feedings since a change in position would alter the gravity flow of CSF and could lead to serious consequences.

5. Begin early teaching the parents how to care for the baby at home:
   a. Teach parents symptoms of shunt infection and obstruction as these may occur once the infant is at home.
   b. Instruct parents on the need for frequent checkups and the need for shunt revisions, usually beginning when the child is between 1 and 3 years old.
   c. See Chapter 3 for general guidelines.

Teratoma
Ann Brueggemeyer   Carole Kenner

DESCRIPTION

A teratoma is a tumor or mass that may be cystic or solid. A teratoma may occur anywhere in the body; however, it is more frequently found in the sacrococcygeal area. The teratoma sometimes contains calcium that can be seen on radiographs. Rarely are these neoplasms malignant. The sacrococcygeal tumors can be totally external or partially external with the remainder being intrapelvic or retroperitoneal.

ETIOLOGY AND EMBRYOLOGY

During the first trimester of development the primitive streak, which is a thickened portion of the ectoderm, generally forms the mesenchyme. In so doing, the primitive streak gradually disappears. Failure to disappear, remaining a part of the ectoderm, may eventually produce a tumor, mass, or teratoma (Moore, 1982).

INCIDENCE

Teratoma occurs in 1 of every 40,000 newborns and is generally more common in female than male newborns (Arceci & Weinstein, 1987).

DIAGNOSIS

1. Visual inspection of the sacral and coccygeal area.
2. Spinal radiographs to demonstrate the presence of any calcifications and to

provide a clear picture of the spinal column. (Presence of teeth or bones may be shown on radiographs, signs of the theory that teratoma results from incomplete twinning.)

3. Complete physical examination to look for any other congenital anomalies such as imperforate anus, cardiac defects, meningomyelocele, or spina bifida.

TRANSPORT

The nursing goal is to prevent trauma to the defect site.

1. Prevention of trauma: Keep infant prone to protect from pressure on the teratoma, which might result in trauma or hemorrhage. Occasionally the teratoma actually extends in such a manner to bulge the perineum and necessitate positioning of the infant on the side.

2. See Appendix A for general guidelines.

PREOPERATIVE STABILIZATION

1. See Appendix B for general admission guidelines.

2. Assist with spinal, AP, and lateral abdominal radiographs. An IV pyleogram may be done to identify any urinary problems that may result if part of the teratoma is retroperitoneal or intrapelvic.

3. Assess the infant to include:
   a. Observation of appearance of mass.
   b. Palpation of mass, if closed, to determine if cystic or solid.
   c. Palpation of abdomen for any masses.
   d. Palpation of kidneys, as hydronephrosis sometimes accompanies a teratoma (sacrococcygeal).
   e. Observation for urinary retention. Uropathy sometimes occurs in conjunction with a teratoma.
   f. Observation of tumor for any sign of hemorrhage or rupture.
   g. Observation for any other congenital anomalies such as meningomyelocele, spina bifida, or imperforate anus.
   h. Evaluation for any presence of heart murmur as cardiac defects may be associated with teratomas.

4. Maintain nutrition and fluid and electrolyte balance. See Chapter 9 for specific guidelines. Antibiotics may be given if the teratoma is ruptured.

5. Maintain skin integrity: place sheepskin under the infant's knees to keep skin breakdown to a minimum.

6. Parent care: see Chapter 3 for general guidelines.

SURGERY

The complete excision of the teratoma is accomplished by a transverse incision in the sacral area and extending across the buttocks. An incision is also made from the anus to the coccygeal area. The rectum may be packed during the surgery. The coccyx also may be removed during the surgery as this may be the point of origin of the tumor and serve as a site for recurrence of the tumor. Drains may be placed in either side of the incision.

POSTOPERATIVE STABILIZATION

Nursing goals focus on preservation of skin integrity and prevention of infection.

1. Maintain skin and tissue integrity:
    a. Keep infant in prone position.
    b. Observe dressing for drainage.
    c. Observe and record drainage from incisional drains.
    d. Loosely restrain lower extremities to keep pressure from suture line.
    e. Keep sheepskin under infant's knees to prevent skin breakdown.
    f. Feed infant in bed in a position to prevent aspiration, until suture line is well healed.
    g. If infant is held by parents prior to complete closure of the suture line, maintain a position that minimizes pressure to the site.

2. Prevent infection:
    a. Observe suture line for swelling, redness, and drainage.
    b. Observe quantity and quality of drainage.

3. Maintain normal nutrition and fluid and electrolyte balance. See Fluid Requirements and General Nutritional Considerations (pp. 263-290) in Chapter 9 for specific guidelines.

4. Assess neurological function:
    a. Measure intake and output every 8 hours; include diaper weights for the first 2-3 days postoperatively to assess for normal renal functioning.
    b. Observe movement of lower extremities.
    c. Observe color of lower extremities, especially for mottling, cyanosis, or poor capillary refill; if any of these signs are present notify the physician.
    d. Observe for urinary retention; if present , notify the physician.

5. Begin early to teach parents how to care for the newborn:
    a. Special positioning of the infant
    b. Suture line care:
        i. Keep area clean and dry.
        ii. Change dressing frequently with diaper changes.

Encephalocele
Ann Brueggemeyer

DESCRIPTION

Encephalocele is the protrusion of meninges and brain tissue through the cranium. It can occur anywhere along the cranial wall but usually is a midline defect that occurs through a suture line. Defects commonly occur in the occipital region. Other areas include the frontal ethmoid bone region and basal regions (Reigel, 1982).

ETIOLOGY AND EMBRYOLOGY

Encephaloceles occur as a failure of the closure of the neural tube in the middle of the first trimester. This failure to close may be a result of teratogens present during this time. In some instances, encephaloceles are thought to occur as a rupture of the closed neural tube (Reigel, 1982).

The extent of the damage to the infant cannot be determined by size alone. Large defects do not necessarily cause more permanent problems than small lesions. The extent of permanent disability is dependent on the amount and type of neural tissue that is enclosed within the defect and how much of it must be sacrificed during surgery. Encephaloceles may occur in conjunction with other neural tube and systemic defects.

INCIDENCE

Encephalocele may occur as commonly as in 1 of every 2000 live births.

SYMPTOMS

1. Protrusion of meninges through cranial vault:
   a. May occur along suture line or through central skull area
   b. May be covered with skin or membrane

2. May be associated with hydrocephalus.

3. Neurological effects may be observed, including paralysis or seizure activity.

DIAGNOSIS

1. Ultrasonography may sometimes identify defect but is not conclusive.

2. Amniocentesis may show elevated alpha-fetal protein levels, suggestive of neural-tube defects but not directly identifying an encephalocele.

3. Visible defect upon physical examination.

4. Radiographs, ultrasonography, and CT scans show structural defects and contents of the sac.

TRANSPORT

Nursing goals during transport include prevention of trauma to the defect and maintenance of thermoregulation.

1. See Appendix A for general guidelines.

2. Prevent trauma to site:
   a. Do not lay the infant on defect.
   b. Position infant to maintain patent airway.

3. Prevent infection at site. If leakage of CSF is apparent, cover defect with sterile dressing.

PREOPERATIVE STABILIZATION

Nursing goals are to prevent infection and to preserve maximum amount of neurological function.

1. Assess infant to include neurological status.

2. Maintain tissue integrity. Do not lay infant on defect.

3. Prevent infection at site:
   a. If leakage of CSF is present, cover defect.
   b. Antibiotics may be ordered to prevent infection. See Antibiotics in Chapter 9 for specific guidelines.

4. Maintain nutrition and fluid and electrolyte balance. See Fluid Requirements and General Nutritional Considerations (pp. 263-290) in Chapter 9 for specific guidelines.

5. Provide parent support:
   a. Because prognosis may not be positive, make sure parents understand the implications of surgery. Removal of defect may require removal of an extensive amount of brain tissue.
   b. Verify informed surgical consent.

SURGERY

Surgery is performed to close the cranial defect. In doing so, the tissue that is external to the cranium must be removed. Rarely is it possible to place neural tissue back into the cranial vault. The tissue that is removed determines the prognosis of the infant after surgery. Although the infant may have appeared healthy before surgery, the infant may be returned to the unit with multiple neurological problems. Paralysis, mental retardation, and inability to support life unassisted may occur. Surgical closure of the defect may not correct facial deformities. If left untreated, the encephalocele may enlarge. Risk of infection may also increase.

POSTOPERATIVE STABILIZATION

1. Monitor neurological status:
   a. Assess vital signs frequently: every 15 minutes four times, every 30 minutes four times, every hour until stable, and then every 2 hours.
   b. Record pupil size and response.
   c. Record level of consciousness.
   d. Record motor function in all extremities.
   e. Record accurate intake and output:
      i. Report output <1 cc/kg/h.
      ii. Report output that greatly exceeds intake, suggestive of syndrome of inappropriate secretion of ADH.

2. Support respiratory status as needed if cerebral function is lost or damaged.
   a. Provide ventilatory support to infant who has lost ability to breathe independently. This may be temporary or long-term support.
   b. Suction airway frequently to remove buildup of secretions. Infant may not be able to cough or clear the throat.

3. Prevent trauma and infection at incision site.
   a. Observe dressing for drainage or leakage of CSF.
   b. Do not lay infant on suture site.
   c. Maintain sterile dressing, as infection may cause serious neurological consequences.
   d. Turn or reposition infant every 2 hours to prevent pressure areas or skin breakdown.

4. Maintain fluid and electrolyte balance. See Fluid Requirements and General Nutritional Considerations (pp. 263-290) in Chapter 9 for specific guidelines.

5. Provide parent support.
   a. Prepare parents for potential consequences of surgery. Infant may be seriously impaired after defect is repaired.
   b. Provide early instructions on how to care for the infant at home, in line with infant's condition. Long-term institutional care may be required if extensive neurological function is lost. Parents may require assistance in identifying local, long-term infant placement.
   c. See Chapter 3 for general guidelines.

REFERENCES

Teratoma

Arceci, R. J. & Weinstein, H. J. (1987). Neoplasia in the neonate and young infant. In G. B. Avery (Ed.), *Neonatology: Pathophysiology and management of the newborn* (3rd ed.) (pp. 1012-1032). Philadelphia: J. B. Lippincott.
Moore, K. L. (1982). *The developing human: Clinically oriented embryology* (2nd ed.) (pp. 35-42). Philadelphia: W. B. Saunders.

Encephalocele

Reigel, D. (1982). Encephalocele. In R. McLaurin (Ed.), *Pediatric neurosurgery: Surgery of the developing nervous system* (pp. 49-58). Orlando, FL: Grune & Stratton.

BIBLIOGRAPHY

Chervenak, F., Isaacson, G., Mahoney, M., Burkowitz, R., Tortora, M., & Hobbins, J. C. (1984). Diagnosis and management of fetal cephalocele. *Obstetrics and Gynecology, 64,* 86-90.
Cotton, J. (1984). A comprehensive nursing approach to the neonate with myelomeningocele. *Neonatal Network, 2,* 7-15.
Glick, P. L., Harrison, M. R., Halks-Miller, M., Adzick, N. S., Nakayama, D. K., Anderson, J. H., Nyland, R. G., Villa, R., & Edwards, M. S. B. (1984). Correction of congenital hydrocephalus in utero: Efficacy of in utero shunting. *Journal of Pediatric Surgery, 19,* 870-881.
Hausman, K. (1983). Neurological crises. In K. Vestal & C. McKenzie (Eds.), *High risk perinatal nursing* (pp. 399-428). Philadelphia, W. B. Saunders.
Reigel, D. (1982). Encephalocele. In R. McLaurin (Ed.), *Pediatric neurosurgery: Surgery of the developing nervous system* (pp. 49-58). Orlando, FL: Grune & Stratton.

Chapter 8

Alterations in the Circulatory System

Ann Brueggemeyer   *Carole Kenner*

The infant with congenital or acquired heart disease is one of the most difficult and challenging infants in relation to nursing care. The infant will require a high degree of assessment skills and will challenge the most experienced nurse. Sophisticated equipment is often required during the surgical procedures and in the early postoperative stabilization period. It is highly recommended that only those medical centers prepared to provide the type of care necessary for this infant attempt to perform the delicate procedures.

INCIDENCE

The congenital heart diseases are found in almost 10 of every 1000 births. Premature newborns have a somewhat higher incidence. Other anomalies are found in infants with congenital heart disease, with an incidence of 25-45 percent (Noonan, 1978; Hazinski, 1983). This association with other defects and problems compromises the care of these infants greatly.

ETIOLOGY

Because fetal heart development occurs prior to the eighth week of gestation, congenital heart disease is often linked with teratogens. The most commonly associated causative agents include maternal rubella in the first trimester, maternal diabetes mellitus, maternal drug ingestion, and fetal alcohol syndrome.

Neonatal Surgery: A Nursing Perspective
ISBN 0-8089-1893-1

Genetic syndromes, especially Down's syndrome, have a high rate of concurrent cardiac anomalies. Although these congenital anomalies can sometimes be identified with causative agents, most cardiac anomalies cannot be linked to a specific cause. It is most important that nurses help parents realize that they are not at fault for these defects.

TRANSPORT

Nursing goals focus on maintenance of oxygenation and acid-base balance.

1. See Appendix A for basic transport guidelines.
2. Maintain adequate respiratory support:
   a. Provide supplemental oxygen via oxygen hood if needed. It must be remembered that cyanotic lesions may not respond to the use of oxygen. If ductal-dependent lesions are present the use of oxygen may be contraindicated, as it may encourage the closure of the ductus arteriosus.
   b. Provide ventilatory assistance if required, as indicated by infant's condition or blood gas analysis. Intubation should be performed before transport as this is a difficult procedure to attempt in transit. See Chapter 10 for specific ventilatory guidelines.
3. Maintain fluid and electrolyte balance. See Chapter 9 for specific guidelines. Observe for hypoglycemia and hypocalcemia and provide replacement fluids.
4. Maintain cardiac output. Provide therapeutic medications as required to improve perfusion and cardiac output or to maintain patent ductus. For ductal-dependent lesions, the use of prostaglandin E_1 (PGE_1) may be indicated to maintain optimal perfusion. Prostaglandin E_1 is a vasodilator that delays the closure of the ductus arteriosus. A patent ductus arteriosus will allow for improved peripheral oxygenation due to shunting. Prostaglandin E_1 may also improve systemic BP and improve renal perfusion. Hypotension is rarely a problem since PGE_1 is deactivated in the lungs. Apnea is a common side effect and the infant must be monitored constantly (Lynch, 1986).

PREOPERATIVE STABILIZATION

1. See Appendix B for general guidelines.
2. Assess infant to include the following:
   a. Auscultate chest to include breath sounds and heart sounds.
   b. Observe for and record presence of other congenital anomalies.
   c. Peripheral perfusion:
      i. Note color, warmth, and capillary refill of extremities.
      ii. Palpate for position of liver.
      iii. Note presence of edema.

iv. Record urine output every hour; report an output <1 cc/kg/h.

d. Perform neurological exam to determine effects of hypoxia.

3. Assist with diagnostic tests to include chest radiograph, echocardiogram, ultrasonogram, and angiogram.

4. Maintain neutral thermal environment, maintaining an axillary temperature of 36°-37°C and skin temperature of 35°-36°C.

5. Maintain fluid and electrolyte balance. See Chapter 9 for specific guidelines. Careful administration of fluids is most important. Care must be taken to maintain adequate levels of glucose and minerals without placing a fluid overload on the heart. An air embolus can be especially dangerous to the infant with congenital heart disease because of the increased risk of stroke due to the shunting of blood.

6. Feedings may be withheld to prevent aspiration due to tachypnea or necrotizing enterocolitis due to hypoxia.

SURGERY

The type of surgery performed is based on the type of defect present and the infant's current condition. In many cases, several defects may be present. Palliative surgery is often performed until the infant stabilizes and grows. Postoperative concerns focus on the type of defect present and the type of surgery performed.

Infants who have been placed on bypass pump oxygenation have specific postoperative concerns. The risk of infection and leakage at the site of the insertion catheters is high. Since large amounts of anticoagulants are used to prevent clotting, bleeding may be a significant problem. As in any thoracic surgery, there may be problems with atelectasis, pneumothorax, chylothorax, or phrenic nerve paralysis. The risk of cerebral vascular accidents is high due to air emboli or clot formation. Acidosis may be a problem as the infant tries to compensate for the dramatic changes that have occurred during surgery. Cardiac output may be compromised and may be further altered due to arrhythmias.

POSTOPERATIVE STABILIZATION

1. Provide respiratory support:
   a. Ventilatory support may be needed for several days after surgery. See Chapter 10 for specific ventilatory care.
   b. Frequent assessment of blood gases should be performed to provide for appropriate ventilation. Arterial samples and/or transcutaneous monitoring should be utilized. It may be necessary to obtain both preductal and postductal samples.
   c. Palliative procedures for cyanotic lesions may not provide sufficient

peripheral oxygenation to allow infant to look pink. Parents should be aware of this prior to surgery. Ventilator settings should not be managed according to arterial blood gas samples without taking into consideration whether the surgery was palliative or corrective. Palliative surgery may improve perfusion and shunting but may not improve oxygenation. Altering the amount of inspired oxygen may not affect the pO_2.

2. Monitor vital signs:
   a. Vital signs should be monitored frequently for several days; apical pulse, respiration rate and effort, temperature, and BP should be recorded every 15 minutes four times, every 30 minutes four times, and every hour for first few days. Any changes should be reported immediately.
   b. Electronic monitoring devices should be used at all times for heart rate, respiratory rate, and BP.
   c. Urine output should be monitored hourly. Report any output <1 cc/kg/h.
      i. Obtain specific gravity value every 2-4 hours to assess for adequate hydration.
      ii. Perform urine dipstick test every 2-4 hours.
   d. Frequently monitor blood tests, including electrolyte, CBC, glucose, calcium, blood urea nitrogen (BUN), and creatinine levels.

3. Observe for alterations in cardiac output:
   a. Changes in vital signs
   b. Increase in drainage from chest tubes or drains
   c. Drainage noted on dressings
   d. Decrease in breath sounds or chest expansion
   e. Alterations in hemoglobin and hematocrit levels

4. Maintain fluid and electrolyte balance. See Chapter 9 for specific guidelines.
   a. Provide maintenance fluids.
   b. Maintain constant infusion of medications required for BP or perfusion. Such medications include epinephrine, dopamine, hydrochloride, levarterenol bitartrate, and phentolamine.
   c. Irrigate arterial lines with heparinized saline solution per hospital protocol. Air must not be allowed to enter any lines since shunting of blood may lead to cerebral emboli.

5. Maintain patency of chest tubes:
   a. Connect chest tubes to drainage container, may be connected to gravity drainage or suction as determined by the surgeon.
   b. Measure and record output every 2-4 hours.
   c. Milk or strip tubes according to hospital protocol every 2 hours.
   d. Observe for patency of system by consistent flow of bubbles in underwater seal container.

6. Maintain nasogastric decompression:
   a. Keep size 8 F indwelling tube in place and at low–intermittent suction.
   b. Irrigate nasogastric tube every 2 hours with 2 cc of saline solution or air.

   c. Check gastric aspirate for occult blood; antacids may be given.

   d. Record and discard aspirate. Unless output is large, replacement fluids may not be given. Electrolyte balance should be maintained through maintenance fluids to not increase the work load of the heart.

7. Provide parent support.

   a. Provide parents with accurate information about the infant's condition to prevent misconceptions.

   b. When the infant is stable, begin early teaching the parents how to care for the infant at home:

      i. Infant should be given small, frequent feedings without tiring the infant.

      ii. Infant will have slow or delayed growth.

      iii. Infant will have specific rest needs.

      iv. Infant should be protected from infections. Infants with congenital cardiac defects are more susceptible to bacterial endocarditis. These patients may be placed on prophylactic antibiotics for surgical procedures or during high-infection seasons during the school years.

      v. Parents should be informed about medications, including types, amounts, actions, and side effects.

      vi. The infant will need continued follow-up medical care.

      vii. The parents may need to be able to treat cyanotic spells if applicable.

Acyanotic Heart Disease

Ann Brueggemeyer

DESCRIPTION

Acyanotic heart disease is so named because it does not itself induce cyanosis in the newborn. Acyanotic lesions are those that produce a left-to-right shunting of blood in the heart. As long as the pressures within the left side of the heart remain higher than in the right side of the heart, left-to-right directional shunting will take place. When more than one lesion occurs or when the lesion is so large that right-to-left shunting occurs, then cyanosis will occur. Obstruction to pulmonary circulation will also lead to hypoxia and cyanosis.

Coarctation of the aorta occurs as a narrowing of the aorta, usually along the aortic arch at the point of the ductus arteriosus. This narrowing causes a constriction of blood flow through the lesion with an increase in BP proximal to the lesion. In a preductal lesion (the lesion occurs proximal to the ductus arteriosus), BP in the lower extremities may be similar to that in the upper extremities. The distal portion of the aorta is perfused by blood from the right ventricle through the patent ductus arteriosus. Cyanosis is present in the lower portions of the body due to this defect. The upper body, however, is perfused with oxygenated blood from the left ventricle through the aortic arch. In the postductal lesion (occurring distal to the ductus arteriosus), the supply of blood to the lower portions of the body occurs from the amount of blood able to pass through the coarctation and from collateral circulation. In this lesion, there is a dramatic difference between the BP readings of the upper and lower extremities.

Atrial septal defect is an opening between the left and right atria through the septal wall. Often this lesion occurs as the failure of the foramen ovale to close. Blood flow is directed from the left atrium to the right atrium.

Ventricular septal defect is a defect that occurs as single or multiple openings between the left and right ventricular septum. Blood is usually shunted from left to right as the force of pressure is greater in the left. When multiple lesions or a single but large lesion occurs, blood can often mix between the two ventricles, producing cyanosis.

The term "acyanotic" can be misleading, however, since cyanosis can occur as a result of heart failure or pulmonary edema. Because these lesions produce an increase in blood flow to the right ventricle, there is an increase in the amount of blood being circulated to the lungs. Increased pulmonary circulation can lead to pulmonary edema and heart failure. In the newborn, cyanosis may be one of the first signs of problems even in the infant with an acyanotic lesion.

SYMPTOMS

1. Murmur may or may not be heard on auscultation.

2. Enlarged heart shown on radiograph.

3. Peripheral BP significantly greater in the upper extremities than in the lower if the lesion is postductal coarctation. Peripheral pulses may be bounding if defect is high output, or decreased if high cardiac output is low.

4. Congestive heart failure:
   a. Duskiness or cyanosis
   b. Respiratory distress
   c. Feeding intolerance
   d. Ventricular hypertrophy as indicated by electrocardiogram
   e. Decreased urine output

5. Cyanosis:
   a. If the lesion is preductal coarctation, cyanosis may be seen in the lower portions of the body, especially in the legs.
   b. Overall cyanosis will occur if the defect is severe enough to cause early congestive heart failure.

DIAGNOSIS

1. Presence of murmur.

2. Enlarged heart shown on radiograph.

3. Cardiac studies:
   a. Electrocardiogram: in isolation, electrocardiogram may not be helpful in the newborn period.
   b. Echocardiogram.
   c. Cardiac catheterization with angiogram.

4. Blood pressure readings from all four extremities.

TRANSPORT

Nursing goal of transport is to maintain thermoregulation and provide optimum oxygenation.

1. See Appendix A for general guidelines.

2. Maintain cardiac output.
   a. Maintain fluid and electrolyte balance. See Chapter 9 for specific guidelines.
   b. Infusion of PGE_1 if ductal-dependent lesion is present.

3. Provide respiratory support:
   a. Provide supplemental oxygen to maintain oxygenation if the lesion is not ductal dependent.
   b. Avoid the use of excessive oxygen therapy if the lesion is ductal dependent. Oxygen is believed to be partly responsible for the mechanism that closes the ductus arteriosus. The use of oxygen in the infant with acyanotic heart disease may be diagnostic or palliative treatment for the underlying defect.

PREOPERATIVE STABILIZATION

The nursing goal is centered on the maintenance of cardiac output and maximization of oxygenation.

1. See Appendix B for general guidelines.

2. Maintain fluid and electrolyte balance: see Chapter 9 for specific guidelines.
   a. Normal fluid and electrolyte balance
   b. Prostaglandin E_1 infusion for ductal-dependent lesion

3. Provide respiratory support:
   a. Provide oxygen as needed through an oxygen hood to keep infant optimally oxygenated, unless the lesion is ductal dependent.
   b. Assist ventilation as needed for adequate gas exchange.

4. Monitor vital signs: temperature, pulse, respiratory rate and effort, and BP at least every 2 hours.

5. Assist with cardiac studies:
   a. Chest radiograph
   b. Electrocardiogram and echocardiogram
   c. Cardiac catheterization with angiogram

6. Assess and record peripheral perfusion:
   a. Check peripheral BP and record at least every 2 hours.
   b. Measure and record urine output every 2 hours.

SURGERY

Unless surgery is needed immediately to correct congestive heart failure untreatable with drugs, the procedure is delayed until the child is older. Surgery is required in the neonatal period when the lesion is severe or when heart failure cannot be controlled with medications. The surgical procedure that is often performed for coarctation is a patch graft to the area of stenosis. A prosthetic patch or a grafting of the left subclavian artery may be used. When the subclavian is used, the distal portion of the artery is tied off. Collateral circulation builds to replace the loss of the artery. Care should be taken to avoid venopuncture or trauma to the left arm until collateral circulation has taken place. No long-term side effects are expected from using this surgical approach. Patch grafts are also used for atrial and ventricular septal defects when the child is older. It is generally accepted that the majority of these two lesions will close on their own by 1 year of age. Palliative surgery in the newborn period involves the application of a band around the pulmonary artery to limit the blood flow to the lungs.

POSTOPERATIVE STABILIZATION

1. Monitor and record vital signs including temperature, pulse, respiratory rate and effort, and BP every 15 minutes four times, every 30 minutes four times, every hour four times, and every 2 hours until stable.

2. Assess and record peripheral perfusion:
   a. Record color, warmth, and capillary refill in all four extremities.
   b. Assess and record peripheral edema.
   c. Measure and record urinary output at least every 4 hours. Report output <1 cc/kg/h.

3. Maintain fluid and electrolyte balance. See Chapter 9 for specific guidelines.
   a. Maintain fluid and electrolyte balance.
   b. Maintain patency of arterial and pressure lines.

4. Provide respiratory support as needed:
   a. Provide oxygen per oxygen hood to provide optimal oxygenation.
   b. Provide assisted ventilation as needed for adequate aeration.

    c. Provide nasotracheal or nasopharyngeal suctioning to provide patent airway.

5. See Postoperative Stabilization (p. 240) in the introduction to this chapter for more specific information.

Patent Ductus Arteriosus
Ann Brueggemeyer

DESCRIPTION AND EMBRYOLOGY

Patent ductus arteriosus is the failure of the ductus arteriosus to close at birth. The ductus connects the aorta with the pulmonary artery supplying oxygenated blood to the body in utero. In utero, the blood is shunted through the ductus from the pulmonary artery to the aorta, bypassing the lungs. After birth, the shunting of blood reverses, due to the shift in pressures within the heart and the change in vascular resistance in the lungs. Within a few hours, the ductus functionally closes. After several days, the shunt should permanently close. Failure to close can occur secondary to prematurity, concomitant cardiac anomalies, and perinatal stress.

ETIOLOGY

Patent ductus arteriosus often occurs in association with prematurity and congenital heart disease. Although the exact causative mechanism is not known, the closure may be related to the change in arterial pressure and oxygenation that occurs at the time of birth. Normally, complete closure does not take place for several days.

INCIDENCE

The abnormality occurs in approximately 12 percent of all cardiac anomalies.

SYMPTOMS

1. Murmur: often loud and harsh
2. Congestive heart failure:
    a. Cyanosis or dusky spells

b. Increased respiratory rate and effort
c. Increased heart rate
d. Poor tolerance of feedings
e. Failure to grow, yet an increase in body weight due to retention of fluids
f. Decreased peripheral perfusion
g. Increase in $paCO_2$
h. Increased ventilatory support needs
i. Bounding peripheral pulses
j. Wide pulse pressure

DIAGNOSIS

1. Presence of loud murmur heard on auscultation

2. Enlarged heart shown on radiograph

3. Cardiac studies:
   a. Electrocardiogram
   b. Echocardiogram
   c. Cardiac catheterization with angiogram

TRANSPORT

Nursing goal during transport is to maintain cardiac output.

1. See Appendix A for general guidelines.

2. Decrease workload of the heart:
   a. Maintain fluid and electrolyte balance and provide glucose infusion to prevent hypoglycemia.
   b. Provide oxygen via oxygen hood to optimize oxygenation.
   c. Maintain neutral thermal environment.

PREOPERATIVE STABILIZATION

1. See Appendix B for general guidelines.

2. Provide respiratory support as needed:
   a. Oxygen via oxygen hood to maximize oxygenation.
   b. Assisted ventilation as needed. See Chapter 10 for specific guidelines.

3. Maintain nutritional support. See Chapter 9 for specific guidelines.
   a. Oral or gavage feedings may continue as long as they do not stress the infant.

b. Maintain IV access to provide fluid and electrolytes if oral feedings are contraindicated.

4. Provide adequate rest for the infant. Handle infant only when necessary.

SURGERY

Surgical intervention is not always necessary. In some infants, the ductus will close on its own when pulmonary or oxygenation problems are corrected. In some infants, drug therapy is successful in treating and closing the defect. The use of indomethacin can be effective in closing the patent ductus in some selected infants. Indomethacin blocks prostaglandin's effects on the vessel, which then allows the ductus to close on its own.

Ligation of the ductus is a relatively simple cardiac procedure, often performed in the neonatal unit. Cardiopulmonary bypass is not needed.

POSTOPERATIVE STABILIZATION

1. Closely monitor vital signs: apical pulse, respiration rate and effort, temperature, and BP should be recorded every 15 minutes four times, every 30 minutes four times, every hour four times, and then every 2 hours until stable.

2. Monitor and record perfusion:
   a. Observe and record peripheral pulses and capillary refill.
   b. Record and report urine output at least every 4 hours. Urine output of <1 cc/kg/h should be reported immediately.

3. Maintain fluid and elecrolyte balance. See Chapter 9 for specific guidelines. Fluid volumes must be monitored and calculated closely to avoid overhydration and stress on the heart.

4. Maintain respiratory support:
   a. Provide oxygen as needed through an oxygen hood to optimize oxygenation.
   b. Assist ventilation as needed to decrease respiratory effort and to provide adequate ventilation.
   c. Observe for respiratory distress and report.
      i. Assess breath sounds with vital signs and be alert for signs of pneumothorax or hemothorax.
      ii. Provide nasopharyngeal and oropharyngeal suctioning as needed to keep airway clear.

5. Maintain skin integrity:
   a. Keep suture site clean and dry.
   b. Record and report any signs of redness, puffiness, or exudate.
   c. Turn and reposition infant at least every 2 hours.

6. Provide support for parents:
   a. Begin early teaching them how to care for the newborn at home. See Post-operative Stabilization (p. 241) at the beginning of this chapter for specific guidelines.
   b. See Chapter 3 for general guidelines.

Cyanotic Heart Disease
Ann Brueggemeyer

DESCRIPTION, PATHOPHYSIOLOGY, AND EMBRYOLOGY

Cyanotic heart disease occurs from a defect that does not allow adequate oxygenation of tissues. Cyanosis results from the shunting of blood from right to left or a major mixing of blood prior to transport through the body. There are several defects in a variety of combinations or severity that also yield cyanosis. Respiratory complications can also produce cyanosis in an infant with acyanotic heart disease. The major cyanotic lesions include tetralogy of Fallot, transposition of the great vessels, tricuspid atresia, truncus arteriosus, and total anomalous pulmonary venous return.

Tetralogy of Fallot is the most common of the cyanotic heart defects. It includes four defects: a ventricular septal defect, pulmonary stenosis, overriding aorta, and right ventricular hypertrophy. Blood flow is diverted from the lungs requiring the patency of the ductus arteriosus to maintain pefusion to the lung tissue.

Transposition of the great vessels occurs when the heart is developing from a curved tube. The main vessels fail to twist, causing the aorta to arise from the right ventricle and the pulmonary artery to arise from the left ventricle. In this defect, the circulation is divided into two separate systems. If the infant is to survive, mixing of oxygenated and unoxygenated blood must occur. A patent foramen ovale or ductus arteriosus must be present.

Tricuspid atresia is the failure of the growing heart to develop a valve between the right atrium and ventricle. This defect is often found in association with other cardiac defects. Because blood is not reaching the right ventricle, lung perfusion must be maintained through a ventricular septal defect or patent ductus arteriosus.

Truncus arteriosus occurs when the main vessels fail to separate into two distinctive tubular structures. In conjunction with this the ventricular septum fails to close, providing a mixture of oxygenated and unoxygenated blood to flow to the systemic and pulmonary circulation.

Total anomalous pulmonary venous return results when the pulmonary venous blood returns to the right atrium either directly or systemically. In order for the infant to survive, an atrial septal defect must be present.

The administration of oxygen does not improve the color or oxygenation of these infants. In some cases, maintaining a patent ductus arteriosus is necessary to provide oxygenation to the tissues. Although the exact mechanism is not understood, it is believed that an increase in paO_2 is part of the mechanism that closes the ductus. Complicating the already seriously ill infant are the adverse effects on other bodily functions. The infant with cyanotic heart disease is prone to acidosis, hypoxia, dehydration, poor peripheral perfusion, hypoglycemia, and hypocalcemia.

SYMPTOMS

1. Cyanosis that is not relieved with the administration of oxygen

2. Tachypnea, especially with feedings

3. Poor peripheral perfusion and low BP

4. Hemoconcentration and dehydration

5. Presence of a murmur on auscultation

6. Metabolic disturbances:
   a. Hypoglycemia
   b. Hypocalcemia
   c. Temperature regulation

7. Congestive heart failure

DIAGNOSIS

1. Presence of murmur

2. Enlarged heart shown on radiograph

3. Cardiac studies:
   a. Electrocardiogram
   b. Echocardiogram
   c. Cardiac catheterization with angiography

4. Hyperoxygenation test:
   a. Administration of high concentrations of oxygen
   b. Frequent analysis of arterial paO_2
   This test is controversial in its application. In an infant with cyanotic heart disease, peripheral blood oxygen levels are not expected to rise with the administration of high concentrations of oxygen. This test may be misleading in that a rise in paO_2 levels may not reflect accurate cardiac conditions but may reflect underlying respiratory disease in an infant with a cyanotic lesion.

TRANSPORT

The nursing goal during transport is to maintain thermoregulation and prevent increase in hypoxia.

1. See Appendix A for general guidelines.
2. See the beginning of this chapter (p. 240) for specific guidelines.

PREOPERATIVE STABILIZATION

The nursing goal in the preoperative period is to decrease the workload of the newborn's heart, maintain optimal perfusion, and prevent infection.

1. Assess vital signs to include heart rate, respiratory rate and effort, and BP.
2. Assess peripheral perfusion:
   a. Check color, warmth, and capillary refill of all extremities.
   b. Record urine output every hour. Output may be lower than normal limits.
   c. Provide medications to assist in providing optimal perfusion. The type and concentration of medication will be determined by the type of lesion and the condition of the infant. Such medications may include prostaglandin E_1 or other drugs to improve cardiac output or peripheral perfusion.
3. Maintain metabolic stabilization:
   a. Provide adequate glucose infusion for maintenance of normal blood glucose levels.
   b. Correct acidosis through ventilator changes or chemical buffers.

SURGERY

The type of surgery performed will depend on the type of lesion and the preference of the surgeon. In the newborn period, corrective surgery is not usually performed. Palliative surgery is performed until the infant grows and stabilizes. Such procedures involve opening atrial shunts through the use of balloon septotomy or the surgical creation of an atrial septal defect. Some palliative procedures include the creation of an artificial or vessel-to-vessel graft. The specific procedures are not discussed here.

POSTOPERATIVE STABILIZATION

1. Assess baseline measurements. Monitor and record vital signs including temperature, pulse, respiratory rate and effort, and BP every 15 minutes four times, every 30 minutes four times, every hour four times, and every 2 hours until stable.
2. Assess and record peripheral perfusion:
   a. Record color, warmth, and capillary refill in all four extremities.
   b. Assess and record peripheral edema.
   c. Measure and record urinary output at least every 4 hours. Report output <1 cc/kg/h. It is not unusual for infants with cyanotic heart disease to have urine output below set standards.

3. Maintain fluid and electrolyte balance. See Chapter 9 for specific guidelines.
   a. Provide maintenance and replacement fluids as needed.
   b. Maintain patency of arterial and pressure lines. Irrigate lines carefully to prevent air from entering system. Infants with shunts risk developing cerebral air emboli when air is introduced into central lines.

4. Provide respiratory support as needed:
   a. Provide oxygen to maintain optimum tissue oxygenation. Oxygen administration may be palliative as infants with uncorrected cyanotic defects will not achieve normal arterial oxygen levels.
   b. Provide assisted ventilation as needed for adequate aeration.
   c. Provide nasotracheal or nasopharyngeal suctioning for a patent airway.

5. See the beginning of this chapter for general considerations.

6. Provide parent support:
   a. Provide cardiac teaching:
      i. Anatomy and physiology of the cardiac defect
      ii. Implications for growth and development
      iii. Medications, use and side effects:
         a) Diuretics
         b) Digoxin
      iv. Symptoms of congestive heart failure
   b. Describe the long-term follow up care:
      i. Frequent visits to the physician
      ii. Revision of palliative surgery
      iii. Corrective surgery

Persistent Pulmonary Hypertension
Carole Kenner

DESCRIPTION

Persistent pulmonary hypertension is often referred to as persistent fetal circulation. It occurs when the pulmonary vascular resistance remains high following birth, thus impeding blood flow into the pulmonary system. The fetal shunts continue to function, especially the ductus arteriosus and often the foramen ovale.

ETIOLOGY AND PATHOPHYSIOLOGY

In the fetus, the placenta serves a low circuit of resistance. Thus blood flows from the placenta, through the umbilical vein, and into the ductus venosus. The ductus venosus bypasses the portal circulation. Blood then travels through the ductus to the inferior vena cava and into the right atrium. It is then shunted through the foramen to the left atrium. Blood also enters the right atrium from the superior vena cava. This blood then goes into the right ventricle and into the pulmonary artery. Blood flow into the pulmonary system is impeded due to the high pulmonary resistance present. It must be remembered that the fetal lungs are fluid filled and offer great resistance to blood flow. Thus blood is shunted across the patent ductus arteriosus and into the descending aorta, and finally into the umbilical arteries back to the placenta for oxygenation.

In the newborn, circulatory pathways change. The ductus venosus is rendered useless after the cord is clamped. Once the first breath is taken and the lungs expand, fetal lung fluid is expelled or absorbed. Thus the pulmonary vascular resistance is decreased. With the loss of the low resistance circuit in the form of the placenta, the systemic resistance rises. Pressures in the heart then change. The pressures in the right atrium and ventricle are lower than the left atrium and left ventricle. This facilitates movement of the blood into the pulmonary circuit. It also creates a pressure gradient between the two atria, thus putting pressure on the foramen ovale and functionally closing the flap. The ductus arteriosus closes as a result of the rise in aortic pressure and the decrease in pulmonary vascular resistance, thus reducing pulmonary artery pressure (Hazinski, 1983) . As more blood becomes oxygenated, the oxygen level rises. This high oxygen content may cause the ductus to close. There is also a theory that the ductus constricts to stop the back flow of blood from the aorta to the pulmonary artery (Edwards & Millay, 1981).

Sometimes this shift to newborn circulation does not occur. This failure to convert from fetal circulation may be due to a number of prenatal or postpartal complications. When the pulmonary vascular resistance fails to decrease, a pulmonary vasospasm occurs, raising the pulmonary vascular resistance even further. At this point the pulmonary vascular resistance may actually exceed the systemic resistance, thus resulting in a right-to-left shunting of blood across the ductus arteriosus and possibly the foramen ovale. Since blood is not entering the pulmonary circuit for oxygenation, the baby becomes hypoxemic and eventually acidotic. The low levels of oxygen and buildup of acid only further increase the pulmonary constriction and thus elevate the pulmonary resistance even more.

Another cause of persistent pulmonary hypertension relates to the fetus's development of smooth vascular muscle. As the fetus matures, smooth vascular muscle develops. When too much smooth vascular muscle develops, the pulmonary resistance is further raised and pulmonary hypertension occurs in extrauterine life. Since this smooth-muscle development occurs late in gestation, it is not surprising that persistent pulmonary hypertension is more often associated with an infant older than 37 weeks' gestation.

Thus any event that precipitates fetal or extrauterine hypoxia can result in persistent pulmonary hypertension. Prognosis is dependent on early recognition and treatment. It is, however, a guarded prognosis.

INCIDENCE

Persistent pulmonary hypertension occurs in approximately 1 of every 1500 births (Edwards & Millay, 1981), with the majority being full-term or postmature infants. It is more common in male than female newborns.

RISK FACTORS

1. Persistent or chronic hypoxemia in utero or during the intrapartal period

2. Fetal hypertension

3. Premature closure or constriction of ductus arteriosus, often secondary to maternal intake of salicylic acid, indomethacin, or other drugs (Merenstein & Gardner, 1985)

4. Postnatally:
   a. Hypoxemia
   b. Meconium aspiration
   c. Acidosis
   d. Polycythemia
   e. Cold stress
   f. Pulmonary dysfunction
   g. Asphyxia
   h. Cardiac dysfunction
   i. Hypoglycemia
   j. Pneumonia
   k. Transient tachypnea

5. Surgical problem: diaphragmatic hernia

SYMPTOMS

1. Tachypnea.

2. Cyanosis.

3. Chest retractions, usually deep; may be accompanied by grunting.

4. Paleness.

5. Poor capillary refill.

6. Poor peripheral perfusion.

7. Decreased pulmonary vascularity shown on radiograph.

8. Cardiomegaly may or may not be present.

9. Higher right radial paO_2 compared to a sample drawn from the umbilical arterial line, suggesting a shunting of blood at the level of the ductus.

10. Murmur associated with tricuspid insufficiency.

DIAGNOSIS

1. Preductal arterial blood sample from the right radial artery, for example, with a higher arterial oxygen level than a blood sample obtained postductally from a

site such as the umbilical artery. A paO_2 difference of 15 mm Hg is usually indicative of persistent pulmonary hypertension (Lynch,1986). Placement of two transcutaneous monitor probes should yield the same results. Preductal site includes left arm and shoulder. Postductal site is usually considered below the umbilicus.

2. Chest radiograph demonstrating slight or moderate cardiomegaly, with decreased or normal pulmonary vascularity. The lungs may be hyperexpanded and pushing on the diaphragm so as to give it a flattened appearance.

3. Results of electrocardiogram are either within normal limits or demonstrate right ventricular hypertrophy and myocardial ischemia; nonspecific ST and T wave changes may also be noted.

4. Echocardiogram demonstrates no cardiac lesions but increased pulmonary artery pressure and increased pulmonary vascular resistance. Left ventricular dysfunction can be confirmed by measuring the right ventricular and left ventricular ejection period; the right ventricular ejection period is increased as is the left ventricular ejection period.

5. A hyperoxia-hyperventilation test may be performed although it may not differentiate the diagnosis from congenital heart defects. The test is performed by first identifying arterial blood gas values. Manual ventilation with 100 percent oxygen is provided at a rate of at least 100 breaths per minute. If the PaO_2 rises from 50 to at least 100 mm Hg, then pulmonary hypertension probably exists (Lynch,1986).

TRANSPORT

Nursing goals prior to and during transport are to maintain adequate aeration and oxygenation.

1. See Appendix A for general guidelines.

2. Early transport and intervention to maintain adequate ventilation is essential for survival of these infants.

3. Support of the respiratory status often requires early intubation with high ventilation rates and pressures.

4. Provide a neutral thermal environment to decrease the chance of cold stress, further compromising oxygenation.

ADMISSION EQUIPMENT

1. See Appendix B for general guidelines.

2. A radiant warmer is usually the bed of choice for easy access.

3. Syringe pumps or microdrip infusion pumps should be available for medication infusions.

4. Blood pressure transducer.

5. Extracorporeal membrane oxygenation (ECMO) setup if transporting infant to an ECMO center (See Chapter 10).

6. Transcutaneous oxygen monitor.

7. Emergency drugs.

8. Intubation equipment.

9. Blood gas supplies.

10. Umbilical-artery catheter and tray for placement.

11. Medications for treatment of persistent fetal circulation such as dimethyl tubocurarine, pancuronium bromide, tolazoline hydrochloride, and dopamine.

12. Ventilator capable of delivering high ventilation rates and pressures.

13. Chest tubes, sizes 12 and 14 Malecot catheters, and chest tube setup, either self-contained or bottles and suction apparatus.

14. Chest-tube tray for insertion of chest tubes.

NURSING CONSIDERATIONS

The treatment of persistent pulmonary hypertension is to correct the acidosis and hypoxemia, thus reducing pulmonary vascular resistance and converting the infant to normal postnatal circulation.

1. Monitor vital signs including temperature and BP at least hourly.

2. Assess infant for signs of increasing respiratory distress:
    a. Grunting and nasal flaring
    b. Increasing chest retractions
    c. Increasing cyanosis
    d. Tachypnea
    e. Activity intolerance with resulting cyanosis

3. Place infant in a radiant warmer with skin probe to measure skin temperature; a neutral thermal environment is crucial to prevent hypothermia and increased acidosis.

4. Monitor serum electrolyte and glucose levels every 2-4 hours or more often if unstable.

5. Obtain a dextrostick only if absolutely necessary as this is an invasive and disturbing procedure.

6. Check CBC for the presence of polycythemia.

7. Place a transcutaneous oxygen monitor both preductally and postductally to obtain continuous readings. Nursing care adjustments may be made according to noted changes in the readings. If transcutaneous oxygen levels decrease during routine care, such as diaper changes, turning, and oral care, these procedures should be kept to a minimum. Oxygen level decreases may indicate the need for suctioning or changes in ventilation rate or pressure. When high ventilation rates and pressures are being utilized, pneumothorax should be ruled out when oxygen levels decline rapidly.

8. Assess for signs of poor peripherial perfusion such as decreasing BP, decreasing or poor capillary refill, and increasing peripheral cyanosis.

9. Assist with intubation; the infant is usually intubated immediately once persistent pulmonary hypertension is suspected.
   a. Place infant on 100–percent oxygen and administer peak inspiratory pressures usually between 30-40 and at rates of 60-100 to hyperventilate the infant; hyperventilation places the infant in an alkalotic state with a resulting pH ≥ 7.45.
   b. Monitor arterial blood gases after any ventilator changes.
   c. Manually bag breath the infant if arterial oxygen levels are not rising with mechanical ventilation; arterial carbon dioxide levels should be kept from 25 to 30 mm Hg. Arterial oxygen levels may be kept around 100 mm Hg.

10. Monitor intake and output every 4 hours.
    a. Check urine-specific gravity every 2–4 hours.
    b. Test urine with a dipstick every 2–4 hours.

11. Administer IV fluids to maintain fluid and electrolyte balance; the physician may wish to restrict the infant's fluids. See Chapter 9 for specific guidelines.

12. Assess infant for signs of dehydration or overhydration:
    a. Alterations in vital signs from baseline measurements
    b. Presence of a cardiac murmur
    c. Bounding femoral pulses
    d. Fluctuation in BP
    e. Alterations in serum electrolyte levels
    f. Sunken fontanelles or eyeballs if dehydrated; bulging fontanelles if overhydrated
    g. Taut shiny skin or poor skin turgor
    h. Presence of rales
    i. Presence of edema or ascites
    j. Descended liver edge

13. Weigh infant daily if procedure can be tolerated by infant.

14. Give rest periods between care-giving activities and be an advocate for the infant. The baby cannot tolerate disturbances yet health professionals from many disciplines will be working on providing care. It is the nurse who can monitor these disturbances and coordinate the team. Nurses and physicians, con-

cerned about the infant, may be tempted to check or handle the infant frequently. If manual ventilation is being used, the number of persons being involved with this procedure should be limited to maintain consistency.

15. Minimal handling of the newborn is essential.

16. Obtain a chest radiograph for visualization of lung fields and cardiac borders.

17. Assist in diagnostic tests such as an electrocardiogram or echocardiogram.

18. Assess breath sounds frequently for signs of decreased breath sounds indicative of a pneumothorax (a common occurrence with high pressure and rate ventilation).

19. If dimethyl tubocurarine (0.5 mg/kg IV push every 2-3 hours as needed) or pancuronium bromide (0.04-0.10 mg/kg IV as needed) is given to "paralyze" the infant, the nurse must observe the infant closely.
   a. Observe for skin flush (due to histamine release).
   b. Observe for tachycardia.
   c. Check BP frequently, at least every 30 minutes, as hypotension often results.
   d. Check mechanical ventilation equipment frequently, as the infant is dependent on ventilatory assistance.
   e. One-to-one nursing care is imperative.
   f. Frequent suctioning of oral secretions may be necessary.
   g. Performing Credé maneuver of bladder may be necessary as urinary retention is common.
   h. Artificial tears may be needed as blink reflex is absent.
   i. Provide frequent mouth care at least every 2-4 hours.

20. The newborn may be given tolazoline hydrochloride, a vasodilator, 1-2 mg/kg IV in dextrose 5 percent or dextrose 10 percent for a period of 15 minutes and then placed on a maintenance of 1-2 mg/kg/h IV in dextrose 5 percent or 10 percent with electrolytes by infusion pump if the newborn is maintaining a partial pressure of arterial oxygen <60 mm Hg.
   a. Administer medication through an upper extremity vein or scalp vein so that medication is directed into the right ventricle.
   b. Place a nasogastric tube and administer an antacid every 2-4 hours as needed, to prevent gastric irritation.
   c. Hematest all gastric apirate and perform guaiac tests on all stools.
   d. Check urine specific gravity every 4 hours.
   e. Measure intake and output every 4 hours.
   f. Continuously monitor BP via an arterial transducer.
   g. Monitor CBC and serum electrolyte levels including creatinine, BUN, SGOT, alkaline phosphatase, and calcium.

21. Administer dopamine (2 µg/kg/min per IV, continuous infusion per pump) for hypotension that often results following the start of tolazoline hydrochloride

therapy. Dosage is adjusted based on BP readings established by physician preference.

   a. Monitor BP continuously through the arterial transducer.

   b. Hypertension with a rise in diastolic pressure may result.

   c. The IV site should be watched carefully for signs of infiltration as dopamine causes tissue sloughing (phentolamine may be given to prevent sloughing if infiltration has occurred).

22. All of the drugs used in the treatment of persistent pulmonary hypertension are strong medications with many adverse side effects, especially when used simultaneously. The infant must be closely monitored via an electrocardiagram and respiratory monitor. This infant must also have an expert nurse to assess accurately subtle changes in the baby's condition.

23. Place the infant on ECMO if the infant meets the criteria for ECMO and the referral center is an ECMO center (See Chapter 10, Ventilatory Care[pp. 304-313], for the specifics of ECMO).

PARENT CARE

1. See Chapter 3 for specific guidelines.

2. Parents will need much support, especially since the infant is often full term and without obvious defects.

3. The aspect of minimal handling may be difficult for the parents as touching the infant is comforting to the parents.

4. Education of the parents about the equipment and the need for minimal stress in using it is essential.

5. If the baby is "paralyzed," prepare the parents for this, as the baby's appearance may be altered and motor response will not occur.

6. Prepare the parents for the baby's treatment and encourage them to express their feelings regarding baby's guarded prognosis.

7. Assess their support system (family and friends).

8. Encourage the parents to visit the baby and call the hospital regularly.

9. Answer any and all questions honestly and simply.

REFERENCES

Persistent Pulmonary Hypertension

Dazé, A. M. (1985). Respiratory development and disease in the newborn. In A. M. Dazé & J. W. Scanlon (Eds.), *Neonatal nursing* (pp. 112-161). Baltimore: University Park Press.

Edwards, N. S., & Millay, C. (1981). Persistent fetal circulation. In R. H. Perez (Ed.), *Protocols for perinatal nursing practice* (pp. 404-421). St. Louis: C. V. Mosby.

Hazinski, M. F. (1983). Congenital heart disease in the neonate: Part I: Epidemiology, cardiac development, and fetal circulation. *Neonatal Network, 1(4)*:29-42.

Lynch, T. M. (1986). Cardiovascular conditions in the newborn. In N. S. Streeter (Ed.), *High-risk neonatal care* (pp. 163-228). Rockville, MD: Aspen.

Merenstein, G. B. & Gardner, S. L. (1985). *Handbook of neonatal intensive care.* St. Louis: C. V. Mosby.

BIBLIOGRAPHY

Foster, S. (1982). Indomethacin: Pharmacologic closure of the ductus arteriosus. *Maternal Child Nursing, 7,* 171.

Greenwood, R. (1984). Cardiovascular malformation associated with extracardiac anomalies and malformation syndromes. *Clinical Pediatrics, 23,* 145-151.

Hazinski, M. F. (1983). Congenital heart disease in the neonate: Part V: Admission of the neonate with heart disease. *Neonatal Network, 2*(3), 7-19.

Hazinski, M. F. (1984). Congenital heart disease in the neonate: Part VI: Acyanotic defects producing increased pulmonary blood flow. Neonatal Network, 2(5), 12-25.

Hazinski, M. F. (1984). Congenital heart disease in the neonate: Part VII: Common congenital heart disease defects producing hypoxemia and cyanosis. *Neonatal Network, 2*(6), 36-51.

Malinowski, P., & Elixson, M. (1985). Transposition of the great arteries. *Critical Care Nurse, 5*(3), 35-48.

Noonan, J. (1978). Association of congenital heart disease with syndromes or other defects. *Pediatric Clinics of North America, 25,* 797-815.

Stachura, L. (1984). Care of the infant with ductus-dependent congenital heart disease receiving prostaglandin E_1. *Issues in Comprehensive Pediatric Nursing, 7,* 203-215.

Vestal, K., & McKenzie, C. (1983). *High risk perinatal nursing.* Philadelphia: W. B. Saunders.

Chapter 9

Fluids, Electrolytes, Nutrition, and Antibiotics

Pat Gorgone   *Susan Bondi Schilling*
Carole Kenner

The predictable growth and developmental patterns of the newborn can be severely altered when surgical intervention is necessary in the immediate newborn period. If adequate nutrition can be maintained during this period of time when the infant's health is compromised, optimal growth, good tissue repair, and fewer secondary complications can be achieved. One aspect of these neonatal surgical problems is that the infant is unable for multiple reasons to take in adequate oral nutrition. Total parenteral nutrition or parenteral nutrition in conjunction with some form of enteral intake is vital. This chapter reviews nutrition in the surgical neonate with a close look at total parenteral nutrition and fluid requirements. Antibiotic dosages, side effects, and considerations for the surgical neonate are included.

Fluid and Electrolyte Status:
Preoperative, Intraoperative, and Postoperative
Carole Kenner

DESCRIPTION

Fluid and electrolyte status for a sick newborn requires constant assessment and monitoring. A delicate balance is called for especially in the newborn undergoing the stress of surgery. Specific considerations exist for the preoperative, intraoperative, and postoperative periods. Before these considerations can be understood a review of kidney development is necessary.

Kidney development begins during the second month of the first trimester of pregnancy. Kidney function and production of fetal urine is established by the eighth week of gestation; however, development continues after birth. Even in the full-term newborn, the kidney remains immature. In the premature infant, this immaturity is accentuated. In utero, the placenta serves the function of eliminating fetal waste products. It also maintains the balance of fluid and electrolyte levels, so the fetus's kidney function is not critical (Page, Villee, & Villee, 1981).

Nephron formation begins at the end of the second month of gestation and continues until approximately the 34th week (Page et al.,1981). Nephrons multiply in number from the region of the medulla outward. Thus the more premature the infant the lower the glomerular filtration rate. A rate of <5 mL/min/1.73 mm^2 is not uncommon in the neonate of <27 weeks old. Rates rise to >20mL/min/1.73 mm^2 by the middle of the third trimester (José, Tina, Papadopoulou, & Calcagno, 1987). In the neonatal period, glomerular circumference is greater than that of the tubular circumference. Thus there is decreased filtration at the level of the glomeruli. This rate increases after birth even in the premature newborn. Continued growth of tubules is seen after birth, but they will not increase in number (Page et al., 1981). The neonatal concentrating capacity increases along with the glomerular filtration rate. Tubular excretion, reabsorption, and active transport of electrolytes increases as well (Johnson, Moore, & Jeffries, 1978).

KIDNEY FUNCTION

The kidney performs several critical functions in the neonate: (1) secretion; (2) reabsorption; and (3) excretion, all of which in turn regulate fluid and electrolyte balance, arterial BP, and levels of toxin in the body. These functions are all intimately tied to the formation of urine. This urine formation begins with renal blood flow. From the renal artery and into the afferent arteriole, plasma that is protein-free is acted upon by the glomeruli. Glomerular capillaries are permeable to small molecules or crystalloids, such as sodium, that are generally positively charged; however, colloids cannot be filtered within the glomerular apparatus. Colloids are a determinant in colloidal osmotic or oncotic pressure. If these colloids are reduced, as seen in alterations in the hepatic system, the oncotic pressure will be reduced. It is this pressure coupled with the opposing hydraulic pressure within the glomeruli that determines the net filtration pressure of the capillaries (Vander, 1985). This net filtration pressure varies as to the portion of the capillary being examined. Alterations in real blood flow will in turn alter the net filtration pressure. The reason for this is that the hydraulic pressure within the capillaries of the glomeruli are dependent upon renal arterial pressure. If renal arterial pressure decreases, the glomerular capillaries' increased resistance to blood flow into the capillaries will result in a lower hydraulic pressure at the level of the glomerular capillary, thus reducing the glomerular filtration rate (Vander, 1985). An obstruction in the urinary system will also reduce the glomerular filtration rate since hydraulic pressure within the capillary is dependent upon blood flow.

Albumin is an exception to the filtration rule, as it possesses a large molecular structure and does pass through the filtration system, finding its way, in small quantities, into the urine. Postively charged particles find passage easier as the glomerular capillaries are composed of polyanions (Vander, 1985). There through the glomerular capillaries plasma is either filtered into Bowman's capsule or leaves via the efferent arteriole and enters the renal vein. There it leads to the tubule where tubular secretion and finally either urinary excretion or absorption in the renal vein occur. Plasma that contains a high concentration of proteins that were impermeable to the filtration process possess a higher oncotic pressure, that is, they are more concentrated. Alteration in the permeability of the glomerular capillaries may result from inherent damage to the capillary, thus altering the pore size, or from a change in electrical charge within the membrane.

Tubular reabsorption, secretion, and excretion are closely tied together. These processes are concerned with maintenance of the internal homeostasis. This maintenance is dependent upon a flexible and dynamic reabsorption pattern that is responsive to other body systems. Tubular reabsorption occurs via transport and diffusion of substances across a semipermeable membrane in the direction of the lumen to the epithelial lining of the tubule (Vander, 1985). Much of the body's nutrients, electrolytes, and water is reabsorbed, thus achieving a balance for continued growth and normal physiological function.

Simple diffusion or passive transport involves the movement of substances down a gradient, from an area of higher to lower concentration, or according to polarization of the molecules, anions migrating towards cations. Active transport requires utilization of energy derived directly from adenosine 5′-triphosphate (ATP) since the net movement of substances is against a gradient (Wodniak & Szwed, 1986). Molecular structures may link together to carry one another across the membrane. Sodium first undergoes simple diffusion across the tubular membrane, then it is transported by this mechanism of active transport by the sodium pump (Wodniak & Szwed, 1986). Sodium filtration is dependent upon the glomerular filtration rate. Thus a higher glomerular filtration rate results in an increase in sodium reabsorption (Wodniak & Szwed, 1986). If the extracellar fluid volume increases, sodium reabsorption is decreased. Thus the regulation of fluids and electrolytes is highly complex. For sodium in turn influences other substances to move against their gradients yielding a net movement upward. Water follows the sodium ion across the membrane and into the capillary bed. This type of transport of a second substance is often referred to as secondary active transport (Vander, 1985). Simple facilitated diffusion is similar to active transport in that a carrier substance is used but the net movement is not against a gradient (Vander, 1985). Amino acids, water-soluble vitamins, albumin, and lactate are also transported in this fashion.

GLUCOSE

Glucose is an example of a secondary substance that is carried with sodium across the membrane by secondary active transport. Glucose is reabsorbed by the proximal tubules, thus only appearing in the urine when the renal threshold or maximal tubular transport capacity has been exceeded or the permeability of the filtering capillaries has been altered (Vander, 1985).

At birth the kidney suddenly is required to maintain a fluid and electrolyte balance that it has never maintained before. In the full-term, healthy newborn, brown fat stores are present and available to supply glucose for the energy that is expended in making the transition to extrauterine life. The infant may also develop hypoglycemia (<45 mg/dL) due to the utilization of glucose secondary to the cold stress from the cool external environment. Remember, too, that the body surface of a newborn is large, leading to greater energy expenditure to maintain a neutral thermal temperature in the sick or premature infant, and so the danger of hypoglycemia is even greater. Little or no fat stores may be present, or they may be depleted quickly. Added stress from a neonatal problem only increases the rapidity of this depletion of glucose. Therefore, monitoring glucose levels with a dextrostix is essential following birth and every 1-2 hours following birth until the infant is stable. Monitoring with a dextrostix may be necessary every 30 minutes if the infant has been greatly stressed, and already is hypoglycemic.

If allowed to continue, depletion of the glucose will lead to metabolic acidoisis since anaerobic metabolism will take over, increasing the lactic-acid levels in the infant. Unfortunately, the infant's kidney is less able to acidify urine; therefore, the acid is retained adding to the potentially dangerous problem of acidosis. This ensuing acidosis is not immediately treated with sodium bicarbonate in the premature newborn since this is a hypertonic solution and may lead to increased intracranial pressure and ultimately to intraventricular hemorrhage. Baumgart (1983) suggests that a glucose level of 45-90 mg/dL be maintained by giving 4-8 mg/kg/min of dextrose IV. Often in the first 24 hours of life no electrolytes are added to the solution because with the breakdown of the RBCs that normally occurs following birth, potassium is released raising the level of serum potassium. Sodium and chloride are found in many of the medications that infants receive.

FLUID BALANCE

The infant's fluid balance is affected by the cool extrauterine environment, the maturity of the infant, the stress level of the infant, as well as kidney function. When the newborn is placed under a radiant warmer in the delivery room, the wet skin and cool ambient temperatures cause insensible water loss accompanied by a loss of free sodium to occur. Normally, insensible water loss accounts for approximately 40-50 mL/kg/d (Filston & Izant, 1985).

While the temperature can be maintained under a radiant warmer, insensible water loss is not always easily controlled. In some institutions, clear plastic sheets are placed over infants under radiant warmers to decrease this type of fluid loss. Other institutions advocate the use of isolettes with warmed, humidified reservoirs to decrease this fluid loss. The infant in the isolette, however, radiates heat to the cool isolette walls, thus having to work to maintain a "normal" temperature.

Whatever the policy of the institution, fluid loss is an important consideration. If the baby also has a surgical problem such as gastroschisis, this loss may be greatly increased. A neutral thermal environment (see Thermoregulation in Chapter 2 for specific information) is essential to decrease insensible water loss.

Fluid maintenance varies greatly. Some physicians suggest that newborns need only 65 mL/kg/d of fluids; while others suggest that liberalization of fluids, up to 100 mL/kg/d is acceptable. Recommendations are usually for 60-80 mL/kg for the first 24 hours of life, then 120-160 mL/kg/d. The very small baby has greater insensible water losses and may need fluid maintenance at 180-200 mL/kg/d. The basis for fluid management is a urine output of at least1 mL/kg/h and a urine-specific gravity of 1.005-1.012. The goal is to maintain adequate hydration without fluid overload. Check your hospital protocol. These are only suggested guidelines and are based on newborns with adequate kidney function (Baumgart, 1983).

SODIUM, CHLORIDE, AND POTASSIUM

It should be remembered that extracellular fluid volume is greater in the premature infant and decreases as the fetus reaches maturity. A diuresis is normal in the newborn during the first 5-7 days of life; however, a newborn may not void until well after the first 24 hours of life. This diuresis also rids the body of excess sodium. Thus, if the baby is premature, sick, or stressed, and delay of this urine occurs, sodium may be retained.

Sodium is maintained at 2-3 mEq/kg/d (Baumgart, 1983; Filston & Izant, 1985). Potassium, an intracellular electrolyte, is maintained at 2 mEq/kg/d (Filston & Izant, 1985). Normal range for serum potassium is 4.5-6.7 mmol/L. If the infant has been stressed, or has suffered asphyxia, then hyponatremia (<133 mmol/L of serum) or hypocalcemia (<6 mg/dL of serum) may result. The hypocalcemia is especially characteristic of the premature infant, since calcium stores are obtained during the last few weeks of a normal gestational period.

INAPPROPRIATE SECRETION OF ANTIDIURETIC HORMONE

Antidiuretic hormone (ADH) is usually released in response to the presences of epinephrine and acetylcholine, stimulation of the osmoreceptors, and volume receptors. This hormone acts to preserve the fluid and electrolyte balance in the baby. Unfortunately in newborns who are premature or stressed, ADH may be released inappropriately. Fallon (1983) identified inappropriate secretion of ADH in other groups as well: infants with persistent pulmonary hypertension, congenital heart disease, or asphyxiation; infants requiring long-term ventilatory assistance, and those receiving (or with a history of receiving) certain medications such as diphenylhydantoin, calcium supplements, morphine sulfate, or other barbiturates.

ADH acts on the renal tubules to facilitate reabsorption of water, sodium urea in particular. If ADH acts inappropriately, the infant exhibits a low serum sodium level; increased excretion of sodium by the kidneys; high specific gravity of urine; serum potassium within normal limits; no signs of dehydration; urine output within normal limits; and normal renal, thyroid, and adrenal functions (Fallon, 1983). Treatment is aimed at restoring fluid and electrolyte balance. Fluid restriction and/or medications such as furosemide and mannitol are the usual modes of treatment (Fallon, 1983).

ANTIBIOTICS

Antibiotic therapy is often a mainstay of treatment for a surgical newborn. Kidney immaturity, however, places the infant at risk for nephrotoxicity due to antibiotic therapy. It must be remembered that many antibiotics are cleared through the kidney. Since kidney clearance is compromised due to kidney immaturity, the levels of antibiotics must be closely monitored. Also, attention must be given to urine output. If the infant's output is depressed, then antibiotics such as gentamicin may be held until urine output is stabilized. Medications should not just be given on a routine basis if urinary output is decreased. The physician should be notified and the medication should possibly be withheld.

MAINTENANCE OF FLUID AND ELECTROLYTES

Specific guidelines for maintenance of fluid and electrolytes are given in this chapter. The aim is to maintain the serum electrolyte levels in the normal ranges suggested: sodium, 133-146 mmol/L; chloride, 100-117 mmol/L; potassium, 4.6-6.7 mmol/L; calcium, 6.1-11.6 mg/dL (Avery, 1987); and glucose, 45 mg/dL (newborn), 80 mg/dL (1-2 days old) to 105 mg/dL (3 or more days old).

Fluids should be maintained so that urine output is 1 mL/kg/h. It must also be remembered that oral feedings can maintain this output; however, the gastrointestinal (GI) system is not colonized with bacteria until several feedings have been tolerated. Therefore, the nutrients and absorption rates are affected for several days following birth.

If gastric suction is being used, gastric losses of fluids and electrolytes, especially sodium, potassium, and chloride, must be replaced. Gastric losses consist mostly of sodium and chloride. The replacement therapy is aimed at replacing both of these electrolytes, usually with sodium given in greater amounts than necessary to ensure adequate chloride replacement. Some institutions use dextrose 5 percent and Ringer's lactate (Filston & Izant, 1985); others use dextrose 5 percent in N/2 saline solution with 10 mEq potassium chloride/L. The solution is given with 1 cc of fluid replacement for every 1 cc of fluid lost, given over a period of 4-8 hours. This amount is in addition to the maintenance fluids. The potassium is given to ensure adequate intracellular potassium in the presence of hyponatremia; potassium, an intracelluar product, will shift to the intravascular spaces. Thus a potassium serum electrolyte level reflecting within normal range may be a false indication of total body potassium.

SYMPTOMS

1. Alterations in urinary output < 1 mL/kg/h or > 5 mL/kg/h.

2. No urine output for the first 24-48 hours of life.

3. Edema.

4. Alterations in vital signs from baseline measurements.

5. Presence of a cardiac murmur.

6. Bounding femoral pulses.

7. Weight changes that exceed 30 g in 24 hours.

8. Fluctuation in BP.

9. Alterations in serum electrolyte levels.

10. Sunken fontanelles or eyeballs.

11. Taunt shiny skin or poor skin turgor.

12. Presence of rales.

13. Descended liver edge.

PREOPERATIVE STABILIZATION

The preoperative goal is to maintain fluid and electrolyte balance or to restore balance if an alteration is present.

1. Assess for subtle symptoms of fluid and electrolyte imbalance (see Symptoms above).

2. Monitor vital signs every 2-4 hours, including BP.

3. Assess breath sounds for presence of rales.

4. Palpate liver for potential hepatomegaly.

5. Monitor serum electrolyte levels every 8 hours, more often if altered.

6. Check dextrostix every 1-2 hours after birth, especially if the level alters, for at least the first 24 hours.

7. Check IV site every 30 minutes for signs of infiltration and maintenance of proper rate.

8. Measure intake and output every 8 hours including gastric losses if GI suction is being used. Replacements for gastric losses are usually given 1 cc for 1 cc

lost (5 percent dextrose in N/2 saline solution with 10 mEq potassium chloride/L is the usual replacement fluid; check hospital protocol).

INTRAOPERATIVE CONSIDERATIONS

The intraoperative period poses new stress for the surgical neonate. A baby that may already be experiencing alterations in fluid and electrolyte levels faces the potential for more large shifts of fluid and electrolyte levels during the surgical procedure itself.

The operating room's environment may be cooler than that of the nursery. This factor then affects thermoregulation and leads to increases in metabolism and increased water losses. Warming of the operating room prior to surgery, the use of warmed fluids during surgery, and warm transport of the neonate to and from the operating room to the neonatal intensive care unit (NICU) will all help alleviate thermal stress.

Another concern during surgery is the amount of water lost and the amount of fluid replaced. While fluid records are kept in operating room, no exact measurement can always be made of fluid and blood losses. The greater problem, however, is in calculating insensible water loss. Insensible water loss through the skin and pulmonary tree is affected by several factors: (1) gestational age—the more premature the greater the insensible water loss; (2) presence of clothing—a covered infant's losses are less; (3) humidity levels—the more moist the environment the less the loss; (4) fever, which increases the loss; and (5) isolettes or closed incubators, which decrease this loss (Adcock & Consolvo, 1985).

The intraoperative infant has the potential to suffer a considerable amount of insensible water loss through the cool, dry environment where the infant is usually uncovered and in an altered state of metabolism. This type of fluid loss is difficult if not impossible to calculate accurately but does affect the postoperative period. Another consideration is the metabolic response to surgery.

METABOLIC RESPONSE TO SURGERY

While it is well known that adults undergo a metabolic response to surgery, often newborns are considered different. Research has found, however, that newborns do mount a metabolic response and undergo all the changes in metabolism that adults do, but at a much more rapid pace. While it may take the adult from several weeks to several months to reach the anabolic phase, an infant may be in the phase 2-3 days following surgery. It is, therefore, imperative that a thorough and accurate assessment regarding fluid and electrolyte balance take place in the immediate postoperative peroid.

Anand et al. (1985) found that hyperglycemia occurs in newborns in the immediate postoperative period. This rise in blood glucose is a result of low circulating levels of insulin. Insulin levels usually return to normal approximately 12 hours postoperatively in full-term infants. In the premature infant these levels are less affected postoperatively. The hyperglycemia if allowed to continue can result in intraventricular bleeding and kidney damage. It may also result in osmotic diuresis. In the premature infant, Anand et al. (1985) found that high levels of lactic acid developed during surgery, possibly due to the immaturity of the liver.

In addition, vascular volume is generally lost during surgery. There is a state of hypovolemia, thus stimulating the release of AHD. The reabsorption of sodium, chloride, and water results. The renin-angiotensin cycle is triggered as well. As pressure in the renal vessels declines, renin is released. Then angiotensin is formed. The angiotensin in turn stimulates the release of aldosterone. Intravenous fluids may be given rapidly to restore the vascular volume (Filston & Izant, 1985). For more lasting effects, however, treatment should be given with volume expanders—blood, plasma, or albumin. Ringer's lactate may also be given (Filston & Izant, 1985). A combination of Ringer's lactate and albumin may be given to raise the oncotic pressure in the intravascular space.

THIRD SPACING OF FLUIDS

Another consideration is the third spacing of fluids. Newborns that have undergone surgical procedures, often on the third to fourth day postoperatively shift fluids to the third space, thus causing edema, ascites in particular. This excess fluid in the third space may be in the form of sequestered fluid or fluid contained within the cell. The extracellular fluid moves from the extracellular spaces to areas such as the bowel or serous cavities. This movement is especially great when intestinal obstructions are present and following abdominal and bowel surgeries. Plasma proteins follow this extracellular movement creating a pressure gradient that pulls more fluid into the third space (Porth, 1986). Thus the sequestered fluid increases.

Third spacing of fluids and the maintenance of fluids and electrolyte levels, coupled with the surgical procedure itself, makes close monitoring of the infant essential in the postoperative period. It is a challenge for the nurse to assess accurately and monitor the status of a postoperative newborn.

POSTOPERATIVE STABILIZATION

The goal of the postoperative period is to maintain or restore fluid volume and electrolyte balance without overhydration.

1. Monitor vital signs every 15 minutes four times, every 30 minutes four times, every hour four times, and then every 2 hours for the first 24 hours postoperatively.

2. Check serum electrolyte levels every 2-4 hours after surgery, if stable, then every 8-12 hours for the next 24 hours, and then every day for the next 3-4 days to identify any shifts in electrolyte levels and to achieve a balance.

3. Check dextrostix every 1-2 hours after surgery for 6 hours, then every 2-4 hours for the next 6-12 hours (if stable), then every 8-12 hours for the first 24-48 hours. Report results to the physician.

4. Weigh infant daily; if large fluctuations are noted, then twice daily. Remem-

ber to subtract from the calculations what equipment or dressings the infant is being weighed with, so that accurate weight comparisons can be made.

5. Maintain IV fluids at the ordered rates; large fluctuations in fluid and electrolyte levels are not well tolerated in a postoperative newborn.

    a. IV fluid orders should be reevaluated after each electrolyte determination (at least daily).

    b. IV fluids should be maintained on a pump rather than gravity to achieve greatest accuracy. It may be necessary during transport of the infant from surgery to the unit to maintain a drip IV.

6. Check IV site every 30 minutes for signs of infiltration.

7. Maintain a neutral thermal environment (see Thermoregulation in this chapter for specific guidelines).

8. Calculate intake and output every 4-8 hours to identify fluid deficits or excesses.

    a. Include the amount of gastric output if gastric suction is being used, to reflect accurately the fluid losses from this route.

    b. Replace gastric fluids in addition to the maintenance IV fluids with dextrose 5 percent in N/2 saline solution with 10 mEq potassium chloride/L: 1 cc of fluid replacing 1 cc of gastric output. Dextrose 5 percent Ringer's lactate may be used in some institutions; consult hospital protocol.

9. Monitor urine output closely, also checking specific gravity and urine dipstick to detect any alterations in fluid or glucose levels.

    a. Report urine output <1mL/kg/h or >5mL/kg/h to a physician immediately.

    b. Report high or low specific gravity values >1.015 or < 1.003.

    c. Report abnormal urine dipstick results, such glucose or protein present that might indicate altered renal function and electrolyte shifts.

10. Assess for signs of fluid overload or dehydration: see Maintenance of Fluid and Electrolytes (p. 268) in this chapter.

11. Assess the newborn thoroughly, according to the specific surgical procedure done, keeping in mind that these guidelines are general for all types of surgical procedures.

Fluid Requirements

Pat Gorgone   Susan Bondi Schilling

DESCRIPTION

The volume and distribution of body fluids make the neonate much more susceptible to fluid and electrolyte imbalances than the older child or adult. The full-term infant is between 70- and 80-percent water and ingests and excretes a relatively high water volume daily. During this process the neonate exchanges approximately half the extracellular fluid. This also results in less fluid reserve than in an adult (Metheny & Snively, 1983).

Greater fluid losses occur through the infant's skin than through the adult's because of the infant's proportionally larger body surface. Therefore any condition that alters intake or increases an output of water and electrolytes has a profound effect on the neonate.

DAILY MAINTENANCE OF FLUIDS IN THE NEONATE

Daily maintenance of fluids should be calculated as follows:

1. By body surface: 1500-1800 mL/m^2/d

2. By weight:
   a. 1-10 kg requires 100 mL/kg of fluids
   b. 11-12 kg requires 1000 mL + 50 mL/kg for each additional kilogram
Clinical and environmental factors also affect fluid needs.

FACTORS THAT AFFECT FLUID NEEDS

Increase Fluid Needs	Decrease Fluid Needs
Fever	Mist tent
Respiratory distress	High-humidity environment
Radiant warmer	Renal oliguria
Gastric fluid loss	Congestive heart failure
Blood loss	Thermal blanket
Vomiting	
Phototherapy	

Surgical neonates receiving IV fluids should have their fluids monitored for intake and output volume on a 24-hour basis. The output fluid measured includes: urine and nasogastric, ileostomy, colostomy, and chestube drainage. Urine volume > 2 mL/h and urine-specific gravity < 1.010 suggest an adequate state of hydration if renal disease is not present (Pereira & Glassman, 1986).

General Nutritional Considerations in the Surgical Neonate

Pat Gorgone   Susan Bondi Schilling

DESCRIPTION

Normally 10 percent of the neonate's birth weight is lost in the first few days of life and is then regained by about day 10. During the first 3 months the infant should gain on the average 1 ounce per day. By 5 months of age the birth weight is usually doubled and then tripled by 1 year, while at the same time the birth length has increased by 50 percent (Lowrey, 1978).

GUIDELINES

These are only guidelines helpful in monitoring infant growth, but velocity growth standards (Figs. 9-1 through 9-4) for length, weight, and head circumference are more helpful in the serial monitoring of these infants (Lebenthal, 1986). These velocity curves from infancy to 18 years of age have been developed by the National Center for Health Statistics (Hyattsville, Maryland). Several velocity curves for premature infants have also been devised (Lubchenco, 1976). Using serial monitoring and plotting these parameters on the growth curves is one way to help determine if the infant is progressing along predictable patterns or if problems in growth are appearing. Critically ill neonates or those debilitated from surgery present a challenge for those managing their caloric and metabolic needs if growth is to be promoted and maintained.

MEASUREMENT METHODS

1. Weigh infant weekly:
   a. Use the same scale each time to ensure accuracy and consistency.
   b. Weigh the infant the same time each day (prior to enteral feedings).
   c. Empty all drainage bags (e.g., ileostomy) before weighing.
   d. Subtract the weight of the equipment attached to the baby, for example, IV lines, tracheostomy tube, and dressings.

2. Measure length weekly:
   a. For greatest accuracy the infant should be measured with a length board; however, some critically ill infants may not be stable enough for placement on the board or some institutions may not have this equipment. Some measurement of length, at least with a tape measure, in the isolette or under the radiant warmer should be attempted.
   b. Measuring with the length board requires two people, one to hold the infant's head, one to stretch the legs and to hold the toes up.

3. Measure the head circumference weekly:
   a. The widest part of the occipital-frontal circumference is measured.
   b. The average of the weight, length, and circumference of the head is then used to determine caloric and fluid requirements.

Protein-Caloric Malnutrition

Pat Gorgone   Susan Bondi Schilling

DESCRIPTION

Infants that are stressed by prematurity, respiratory distress, sepsis, cardiac complications, fever, or surgery are at risk for developing protein-caloric malnutrition. It is a utilization of protein stores to meet caloric requirements to the point of catabolic response, resulting in malnourishment.

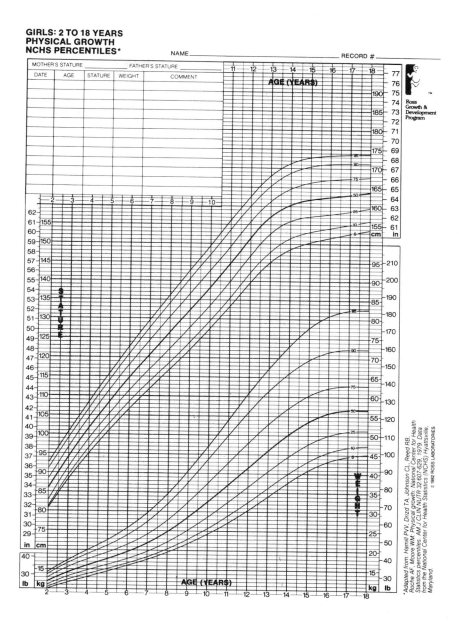

GIRLS: 2 TO 18 YEARS
PHYSICAL GROWTH
NCHS PERCENTILES*

Fig. 9-1.

275

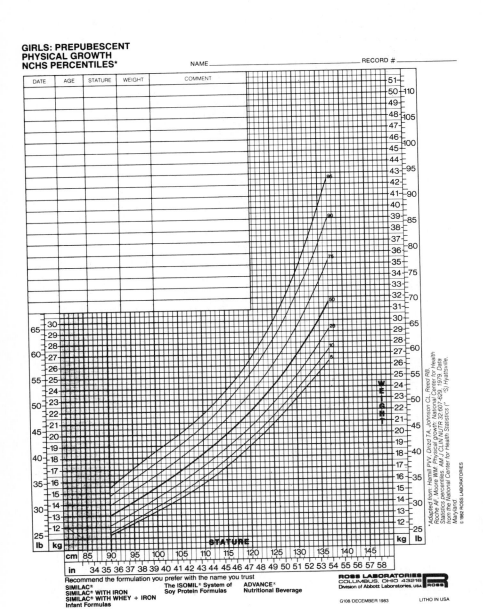

Fig. 9-2.

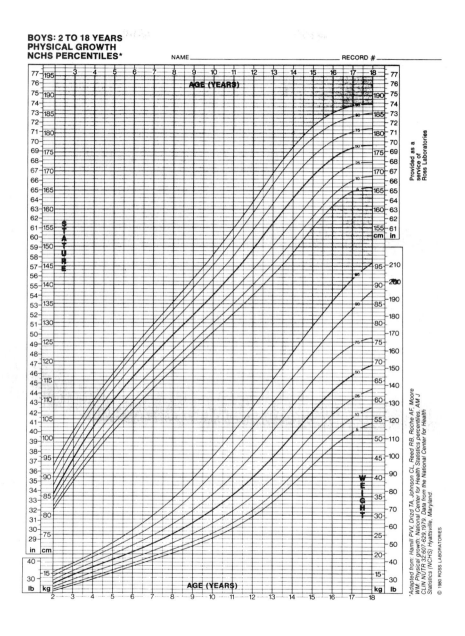

BOYS: 2 TO 18 YEARS
PHYSICAL GROWTH
NCHS PERCENTILES*

NAME_____ RECORD #_____

*Adapted from: Hamill PVV, Drizd TA, Johnson CL, Reed RB, Roche AF, Moore WM. Physical growth: National Center for Health Statistics percentiles. AM J CLIN NUTR 32:607-629,1979. Data from the National Center for Health Statistics (NCHS) Hyattsville, Maryland

© 1980 ROSS LABORATORIES

Fig. 9-3.

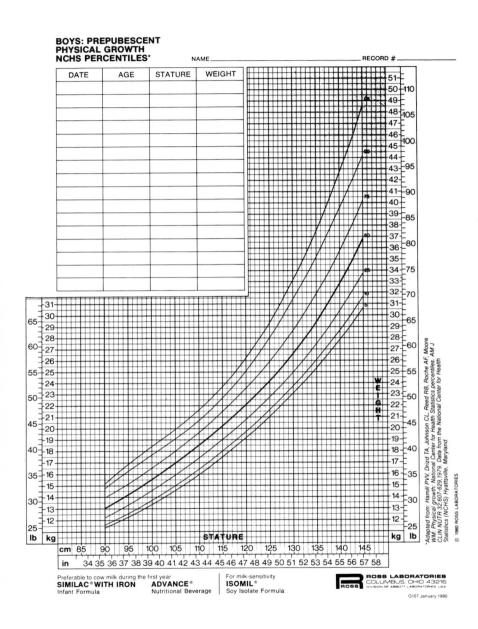

BOYS: PREPUBESCENT PHYSICAL GROWTH NCHS PERCENTILES*

Fig. 9-4.

PATHOPHYSIOLOGY

The basic metabolic rate is higher in infants because the major metabolic organs such as the brain, liver, heart, and kidneys make up a larger proportion of the body weight. This factor also creates an increased need for fluids and calories. In addition, protein requirements per kilogram are greater in infants to promote growth. A critically ill infant quickly becomes catabolic. Catabolism is the degradation of body tissues resulting in the release of energy for body utilization. Catabolism that occurs during illness results in decreased muscle mass, circulating T cells, cardiac output, fat stores, enzyme production, and increased urinary nitrogen excretion. Therefore, there is an increased need for energy, catecholamines, glucocorticoids, plasma fatty acids, keto acids, ketones, and fluid.

ENERGY AND STRESS REQUIREMENTS

Energy

1. Metabolic response to surgery:
   a. Increase in oxygen consumption
   b. Increase in urinary nitrogen excretion

2. Caloric requirements (Kerner, 1983; Cox, 1985):
   a. Premature infant: 104-130 cal/kg/d
   b. Normal neonate: 100-120 cal/kg/d
   c. Protein-caloric malnourished infant: 150-175 kcal/kg/d (needed for catch-up growth reguirements)

Infants who receive all their nutrition IV require fewer calories than those fed enterally. This is due to the problems of malabsorption, especially fat malabsorption, known to occur in the premature infant.

Stress

1. Stress factors increase caloric needs (Wesley et al., 1980):
   a. Fever: for every degree > 37 C calorie needs are increased 12 percent.
   b. Cardiac complications: caloric needs are increased up to 25 percent.
   c. Surgery: caloric needs are increased by 30 percent.
   d. Sepsis: caloric needs are increased up to 50 percent.
   e. Respiratory distress: caloric needs are increased between 50 and 75 percent.

2. The body's preferred source of energy is carbohydrate or glucose.
   a. Glucose is stored as glycogen in the liver and is only capable of providing energy for 4-6 hours after birth.
   b. Infants who are premature or small for gestational age have less glycogen stores:
      i. They may only be capable of providing energy for a short time, < 4 to 6 hours.

ii. They are not able to withstand long fasting periods (Klaus & Fanaroff, 1986).

Parenteral Nutrition: Peripheral and Total Parenteral

Pat Gorgone   Susan Bondi Schilling

DESCRIPTION

Surgical neonates with gut problems that preclude enteral feedings for long periods of time (weeks and months) receive total parenteral nutrition (TPN) via a central line.

Peripheral Nutrition

Peripheral nutrition is used to supplement neonates being enterally fed or is used postoperatively when it is anticipated that enteral feeding will be tolerated in 7-10 days.

Total Parenteral Nutrition

It has been proven that TPN successfully promotes the growth of infants, but it is also known that the tolerance levels among neonates are different. The ability to metabolize glucose is limited in neonates, especially in the premature infant. Therefore, glucose is initiated in a slow stepwise fashion to allow the infant to have an adequate response of endogenous insulin (Kerner, 1983). Blood glucose levels need to be carefully monitored, and as the infant's tolerance increases so can the glucose concentration.

To provide sufficient calories for long-term stress states, the higher dextrose concentrations ($> D_{10}W$) are needed. The high osmolarity of the solutions necessitates a central-line catheter, which is placed in a large vessel. The large volume of blood flow in these vessels dilutes the hypertonic fluids. Solutions of $D_{10}W$ and less are safely delivered in peripheral veins.

Caloric Density and Osmolarity of Dextrose Solutions

Solutions	Kcal/mL	Osmolarity
$D_{5.0}W$	0.17	252
$D_{7.5}W$	0.25	378
$D_{10.0}W$	0.34	505
$D_{12.5}W$	0.40	631
$D_{15.0}W$	0.51	758
$D_{20.0}W$	0.68	1010
$D_{25.0}W$	0.85	1263
$D_{30.0}W$	1.02	1515

CRYSTALLINE AMINO ACIDS

1. Crystalline amino acids are given to promote protein synthesis:
   a. Amino acids as a nitrogen source are given to prevent nitrogen loss or to reverse negative nitrogen balance.
   b. Neonatal amino acid requirements are 2-3 g/kg/d.

2. Concentrations of amino acids:
   a. The amino acid concentration is initiated at a low level.
   b. The BUN level is monitored to evaluate tolerance as the concentration is advanced.

FATS

1. Fats are an integral part of parenteral nutrition because of their:
   a. Essential fatty acids
   b. High caloric density
   c. Low osmolarity

2. Fats as calorie source:
   a. Fats provide 30-50 percent of the neonatal calories.
   b. A 10 percent solution yields 1.1 kcal/mL (used in infants with impaired tolerance to lipid solutions).
   c. A 20-percent solution yields 2 kcal/mL.

3. Serum triglycerides:
   a. Monitor the level 24 hours after an incremental increase.
   b. If an increase is tolerated, the fat calories can parallel the glucose advancement.

ELECTROLYTES AND MINERALS

1. Electrolytes and minerals are added to the hyperalimentation solution based on the neonate's.
   a. Serum concentrations
   b. Known fluid losses
   c. Estimated renal function

2. Vitamins and trace minerals are also added. Safe and adequate base levels are adopted from U. S. Recommended Dietary Allowances with adjustment for individual patient needs.

**Required Laboratory Tests for Neonates
Receiving Maintenance TPN**

Test	Frequency of Draw (per week)
CBC	Once
Differential	Once
Reticulocyte count	Once
Phosphorus	Twice
Magnesium	Once
Total protein	Once
Albumin	Once
Total and direct bilirubin	Once
Alkaline phosphatase	Once
SGOT	Once
SGPT	Once
Triglyceride	Once if not receiving a fat emulsion; twice if receiving fat supplements
Cholesterol	Once
Ammonia	Once
Glucose	Twice
Sodium	Twice
Potassium	Twice
Chloride	Twice
Carbon dioxide	Twice
Calcium	Twice
BUN	Twice
Creatinine	Twice
Bile acids	Once

CARBOHYDRATE COMPLICATIONS

Description

1. Glucose and fluid intolerances are the major problems that interfere with the provision of kilocalories in the low birth weight infant and the critically ill infant.

2. Provision of calories is even more difficult when the infant is in respiratory distress and receiving assisted ventilation (Kerner, 1983).

Monitoring

1. Frequent monitoring of the serum glucose level during the first 24-48 hours is mandatory.

2. Sepsis must be suspected in an infant who suddenly demonstrates glucosuria after receiving a glucose concentration previously tolerated.

3. The older infant seems to have much less difficulty with glucose intolerance. These infants have plasma insulin concentrations that increase significantly during infusion of hypertonic dextrose solutions (Kerner, 1983).

4. Close observation and monitoring is necessary to gradually advance infant to the higher concentrations and again to wean (gradually decrease) this infusion in both concentration and rate prior to stopping the solutions.

Complications

1. Hypoglycemia
   a. Profound hypoglycemia with secondary seizures and coma can result from an abrupt stopping of a hypertonic solution.
      i. This stoppage may be accidental through the breaking of the solution bottle.
      ii. It may result from clotting of the infusion line.
   b. When these problems occur a 10-percent dextrose solution should be administered immediately (Kerner, 1983).

2. Instability of glucose tolerance in surgical infants:
   a. After the major trauma of surgery, infants may be glucose intolerant due to high circulating levels of cortisol and glucagon (Kerner, 1983).
   b. It is better, therefore, to wean (gradually decrease) the infant on a 10 percent dextrose solution prior to surgery and then to wait before restarting the higher concentrations until after the immediate postoperative period.

3. Fatty infiltrates:
   a. In infants, it has been found that an excessive intake of carbohydrate seems

to result in fatty infiltrations of the liver. Studies have shown that if the carbohydrate calories are replaced by fat calories, this complication can be decreased.
   b. If respiratory function deteriorates, balance the TPN solution to include carbohydrates, proteins, and fats. The key is to balance the amount of calories coming from the glucose source, protein source, and fat source so that the bulk of the calories is not coming from just nonprotein substances. The respiratory function may then improve.
   c. Fat is a good source of nonprotein calories and causes less carbon dioxide production than its caloric equivalent in glucose (Kerner, 1983).

PROTEIN COMPLICATIONS

Description

1. Protein needs are high in the infant to promote rapid growth, but frequently the infant is not able to metabolize increased amounts of protein.

2. Thus, these infants will experience protein intolerance, hyperchloremic metabolic acidosis, azotemia, and hyperammonia.

Considerations

1. Infants with sepsis or impaired liver function are at even greater risk for protein complications.

2. Monitoring BUN and blood ammonia levels is important (Kerner, 1983).

3. Long-term complication of parenteral protein intake is cholestatic liver disease.
   a. The smaller the infant the more often it seems to occur during hyperalimentation.
   b. Enteral feedings help in the treatment of this liver dysfunction.

4. Thrombophlebitis.
   a. There is an increased risk of irritation and thrombophlebitis to peripheral veins.
   b. To decrease the risk of thrombophlebitis, amino acids in peripheral TPN should not exceed 2 percent (Kerner, 1983).

FAT COMPLICATIONS

Description

1. Enterally, infants receive about 40-50 percent of their calories as fats.

2. In the early years of TPN administration and hyperalimentation, fats were used for essential fatty acid requirements only.
   a. Recent studies, however, have shown that a positive nitrogen balance can be produced and maintained when lipids are substituted for glucose as a nonprotein energy source (Kerner, 1983).
   b. Intravenously administered fats are an excellent calorie source, tolerated well by neonates.

3. Fat calories make up 35-50 percent of the total TPN calories.
   a. The fats should be administered during a 12- to 24-hour period.
   b. The triglyceride level is important to assess if the lipids are clearing the vascular system.
   c. A decreased tolerance to IV fats is noted in the premature infant; thus, close monitoring is essential.
   d. Septic infants or any acutely ill infants may have decreased tolerance to the intralipid infusion.

DISORDERS OF BONE METABOLISM

Disorders of bone metabolism are often seen in infants receiving TPN long term. Often rickets is not seen until swelling and erythema over a long bone is noted and radiographs show a fracture. When osteoporosis is seen, care must be taken with these infants. Nursing observation will identify those infants who seem particularly irritable or fussy when touched or handled, secondary to bone pain. Special care must be taken to safeguard these infants from further fractures and provide comfort.

Formulas
Pat Gorgone   Susan Bondi Schilling

DESCRIPTION

Formulas come in a variety. Many are quite simple in composition. In the surgical neonate it is important to consider not only the size of the infant and whether the infant is in the preoperative or postoperative period, but also how well the infant is able to ingest and digest enteral formulas. In each section of this book, the particular surgical problem along with feeding considerations is addressed. The method of choice, gavage, gastrostomy, nasojejunal, or nipple feedings, is discussed in each section as well. This section includes lists of the formulas, their composition and indications for use.

STANDARD FEEDINGS

	Breast Milk	Standard Formulas		
		Similac*	Enfamil†	SMA‡
kcal/mL	0.7	0.67	0.67	0.67
Protein, g/mL	0.1	0.015	0.015	0.015
Fat, g/mL	0.045	0.036	0.038	0.036
Protein	Human whey 80%, casein 20%	Cow's milk	Cow's milk	Cow's milk, demineralized whey
Fat	Human	Soy oil, coconut oil	Soy oil, coconut oil,	Oleo, coconut oil, safflower, soy oil
Carbo-hydrate	Lactose	Lactose	Lactose	Lactose
Osmolarity	300	290	300	300
Sodium, mEq/cc	0.007	0.011	0.009	0.006
Potassium, mEq/cc	0.013	0.02	0.017	0.014
Iron, mg/cc	0.0005	0.002	0.001	0.012
Indications	Values are average since there is a wide variation in composition; supplementation with iron, fluoride, and vitamin D recommended	Normal infant feeding supplement for breast-fed infants; available with iron	Normal infant feeding supplement for breast-fed infants; available with iron	Decreased sodium and potassium levels versus other formulas; used with decreased renal and cardiovascular problems; protein type similar to breast milk

*Ross, Columbus, Ohio
†Mead Johnson, Evansville, Indiana
‡Wyeth, Philadelphia, Pennsylvania

SPECIAL FEEDINGS: SOY FORMULAS

	Isomil*	Prosobee†	Nursoy‡
kcal/mL	0.67	0.67	0.67
Protein, g/mL	0.02	0.02	0.02
Fat, g/mL	0.04	0.36	0.36
Protein	Soy isolate	Soy isolate	Soy isolate
Fat	Soy, Coconut	Soy, coconut, oleo, safflower	Soy, coconut
Carbohydrate	Corn syrup, sucrose	Corn syrup	Sucrose
Osmolarity	250	200	296
Sodium, mEq/cc	0.014	0.013	0.009
Potassium, mEq/cc	0.024	0.02	0.018
Iron, mg/cc	0.012	0.013	0.012
Indications	Hypoallergenic protein source; lactose free; recovery stage after mild/moderate diarrhea	Lactose and sucrose free	Blend of four fats

*Ross, Columbus, Ohio
†Mead Johnson, Evansville, Indiana
‡Wyeth, Philadelphia, Pennsylvania

SPECIAL FEEDINGS: ADJUSTED-CALORIE FORMULAS

	Emfamil*	Simalac-24†	SMA-24‡	Simalac 27*	SMA 27‡
kcal/mL	0.8	0.8	0.8	0.9	0.9
Protein, g/mL	0.018	0.02	0.025	0.025	0.02
Fat, g/mL	0.045	0.043	0.048	0.048	0.049
Protein	Cow's milk	Cow's milk	Cow's milk	Cow's milk	Cow's milk
Fat	Soy, coconut	Soy, coconut	Oleo, soy, coconut	Soy, coconut	Oleo, soy safflower
Carbo-hydrate	Lactose	Lactose	Lactose	Lactose	Lactose
Osmolarity	360	360	364	410	416
Sodium, mEq/cc	0.085	0.015	0.008	0.017	0.008
Potassium, mEq/cc	0.011	0.028	0.014	0.002	0.016
Iron, mg/cc	0.02	0.002	0.014	0.002	0.016
Indications	Recovery from illness that induced malnutrition, limited volume intake	Recovery from illness that induced malnutrition, limited volume intake	Increased calories	Increased calories	Casein/ whey ratio, 60:40 density and osmolarity

*Ross, Columbus, Ohio
†Mead Johnson, Evansville, Indiana
‡Wyeth, Philadelphia, Pennsylvania

SPECIAL FEEDINGS: ALTERED FORMULAS

	Pregestimil*	Nutramigen*	Portagen*	Simalac†	Isomil SF PM 60/40†	RCF†	Lofenalac*
kcal/ml	0.67	0.67	0.67	0.67	0.67	0.67	0.67
Protein, g/mL	0.019	0.02	0.024	0.016	0.02	0.02	0.02
Fat, g/mL	0.027	0.026	0.032	0.038	0.036	0.036	0.027
Carbo-hydrate	Tapioca starch	Tapioca starch, sucrose	Corn syrup sucrose	Lactose	Corn syrup	Add carbo-hydrate	Corn syrup modified tapioca starch
Osmolarity	350	480	220	260	150	Varies	360
Sodium mEq/cc	0.014	0.014	0.014	0.007	0.014	—	0.014
Potassium mEq/cc	0.019	0.017	0.021	0.015	0.02	—	0.017
Iron, mg/cc	0.013	0.013	0.013	0.002	0.012	—	0.013
Indications	Severe malab-sorption problems; recovery stage after severe diarrhea sucrose, and lactose free	Intact protein intolerance or allergies	Use when convention-al fats are not well digested or absorbed	Use with renal and cardiovas-cular prob-lems; low renal solute load; lower mineral content	Sucrose and lactose free	For intoler-ance or added to support carbohy-drates	For infants with phenyl-ketonuria

*Mead Johnson, Evansville, Indiana
†Ross, Columbus, Ohio

SPECIAL FEEDINGS: ELECTROLYTE SOLUTIONS

	Pedialyte*	Pedialyte RS*
kcal/mL	100 kcal/L	100 kcal/L
Protein, g/mL	—	—
Fat, g/mL	—	—
Protein	—	—
Fat	—	—
Carbohydrate	Dextrose	Dextrose
Osmolarity	—	—
Sodium, mEq/cc	45 mEq/L	45 mEq/L
Potassium, mEq/cc	20 mEq/L	20 mEq/L
Iron, mg/cc	—	—
Indications	Used to maintain fluid and electrolyte balance in mild/moderate diarrhea	For management of dehydration due to moderate or severe diarrhea

*Ross, Columbus, Ohio

ELECTROLYTES

See Fluid and Electrolyte Status (p. 263) in the beginning of this chapter. For specific acceptable values for serum electrolyte levels see Appendix D.

Antibiotics
Carole Kenner

DESCRIPTION

Antibiotics are often given prophylactically as well as for the treatment of a specific infectious agent. Some institutions, however, do not recommend the use of precautionary antibiotics especially in the preoperative period when neither a clear history of infection nor a potential for infection secondary to maternal history exists. Due to a rise in chlamydiae infections, overuse of antibiotics may block the effectiveness of treatment of this infection. It is the nurse's responsibility to check hospital protocol before administration of precautionary antibiotics.

Consideration must also be given as to where such drugs are detoxified. If a newborn has minimal renal output, drugs that are detoxified through the liver and kidney can produce devastating effects. Gentamicin for instance, is cleared through the kidney. If not cleared, and the drug continues to be given, then toxic levels are reached quickly, producing nephrotoxicity and ototoxicity. Levels of antibiotics, peak and trough, must be carefully monitored. In administering antibiotics, the old cliché "more is better" is not accurate. Dosages must be carefully titrated according to kilograms of body weight, renal function, and liver function. Antibiotic doses should be given 12 hours apart for at least the first week of life, due to immature kidney function and altered renal clearance.

COMMON NEONATAL ANTIBIOTICS

These are only guidelines. Consult hospital protocol and infant's physician.

Ampicillin

Indications
Infections caused by gram-positive (staphylococci, streptococcus viridans, *Streptococcus pyogenes*, and Diplococcus pneumoniae), and gram-negative (*Neisseria gonorrhoeae*, and *Neisseria meningitidis*) organisms. This antibiotic is broader in coverage than penicillin G since it treats all of the organisms that penicillin does but several other gram-negative organisms (*Escherichia coli, Hemophilus influenzae, Klebsiellae*) as well. Give ampicillin prophalactically prior to or after surgery.

Dosages IV:
Usually 100 mg/kg/d in divided doses; can be given up to 200 mg/kg/d in divided doses, IV or IM. Orally: 50-100 mg/kg/d in divided doses.

Side effects:
Vomiting, diarrhea, fine red rash (erythema), anaphylaxis, anemia, phlebitis.

Considerations
1. Should be given during a period of 30-60 minutes, IV drip, as the drug is stable for 1 hour after reconstitution.
2. Space 1 hour from any bacteriostatic antibiotic, chloramphenicol, and gentamicin, especially.
3. May be given IV push slowly over a period of 5-10 minutes.
4. Oral intake of food interferes with absorption.

Penicillin G Potassium Aqueous

Indications
Infections caused by gram-positive (staphylococci, *S. viridans, S. pyogenes*, and *D. pneumonia*) and gram-negative

organisms (*N. gonorrhea* and *N. meningitidis*). May be given before or after surgery to infants with suspected menigitis.

Dosages   IV or IM: 50,000-100,000 U/kg/d in divided doses. If menigitis is present up to 150,000 U/kg/d may be administered (Cloherty & Stark, 1985).

Side effects   Fine red rash (erythema), anaphylaxis, anemia, phlebitis.

Considerations   Space 1 hour from any bacteriostatic antibiotic, chloramphenicol, and gentamicin, especially.

Gentamicin

Indications   Severe infections, especially those due to all forms of Staphylococcus. May be given prophylactically prior to or after surgery.

Dosages   3.5-5.0 mg/kg/d in divided doses, IV, or IM. May be given up to 7.5 mg/kg/d after the first week of life, IV or IM.

Side effects   Vomiting, nephrotoxicity, ototoxicity, oliguria, proteinuria, or fine red rash (erythema).

Considerations
1. May be given by slow IV infusion after administration of a a penicillin derivative.
2. Should never be given IV push due to nephrotoxicity.
3. Should be discontinued or dose reduced in the presence of decreased urine output.
4. Monitor urine output and renal chemistries.
5. Monitor peak and trough levels closely. Peak levels should be 4-8 µg/mL 1 hour after completion of dose. Trough levels immediately prior to next dose should be 2 µg/mL or less (Cloherty & Stark, 1985).

Clindamycin or Cleocin

Indications   Used for staphlyococci, streptococci, or anaerobic infections. Dosage 8-25 mg/kg/d IV in divided doses. Usually recommended in infants 4 to 6 weeks of age or older.

Side effects   May be associated with cardiovascular complications in the newborn such as shock, cardiac compromise, and respiratory difficulty. Vomiting, diarrhea, or fine red rash (erythema).

Considerations 1. Assess infant carefully for signs of toxcity.
2. Generally do not give to renal or hepatically immature or compromised infants. Usually not given to infants < 4 weeks of age.

Amphotericin B

Indications Antifungal agent usually used for candidiasis. Use with extreme caution in infants.

Dosage 0.25mg/kg/d diluted in a dextrose solution usually of dextrose 5 percent to a concentration of 1.0 mg/10 cc, IV (Cloherty & Stark, 1985). This dosage may be gradually increased to a maximum of 1 mg/kg/d per continuous IV infusion over several hours (Cloherty & Stark, 1985).

Side effects Nephrotoxicity, azotemia, hepatotoxicity, anemia, vomiting, diarrhea, and phlebitis.

Considerations 1. Give during a period of approximately 6 hours. Some institutions use shorter periods than this, so consult hospital policy.
2. Cover medication with dark plastic or foil to prevent breakdown of drug by light. This includes IV bottle and tubing. Explain to parents why this is necessary.
3. Do not mix with other medications. It will precipitate in the presence of sodium chloride.
4. Inspect IV site frequently as medication is very irritating.
5. Monitor CBC and renal and liver chemistries closely.

REFERENCES

Fluid and Electrolyte Status:
Preoperative, Intraoperative, and Postoperative

Adcock, E. W., III, & Consolvo, C. A. (1985). Fluid and electrolyte management. In G. B. Merenstein & S. L. Gardner (Eds.), *Handbook of neonatal intensive care* (pp. 161-178). St. Louis: C. V. Mosby.

Anand, K. J. S., Brown, R. C., Causon, N. D., Christofides, S. R., Bloom, S. R., & Synsley-Green, A. (1985). Can the human neonate mount an endocrine and metabolic response to surgery? *Journal of Pediatric Surgery, 20*, 41-48.

Avery, G. B. (Ed.). (1987). *Neonatology: Pathophysiology and management of the newborn* (3rd ed.). Philadelphia: J. B. Lippincott.

Baumgart, S. (1983). Fluid and electrolyte therapy in the premature infant. In R. A. Polin & F. D. Burg (Eds.), *Workbook in practical neonatology* (pp. 25-39). Philadelphia: W. B. Saunders.

Fallon, M. (1983). Inappropriate antidiutretic hormone. *Neonatal Network, 2*(6), 46-52.

Filston, H. C., & Izant, R. (1985). *The surgical neonate: Evaluation and care.* (3rd ed.). New York: Appleton-Century-Crofts.

Johnson, T. R., & Moore, W. M., & Jeffries, J. E. (Eds.). (1978). *Children are different: Developmental physiology.*(2nd ed.). Columbus: Ross Laboratories.

José, P. A., Tina, L. U., Papadopoulou, Z. L., & Calcagno, P. L. (1981). Renal Diseases. In G. B. Avery (Ed.), *Neonatology: Pathophysiology and management of the newborn* (3rd ed.) (pp. 795-849). Philadelphia: J. B. Lippincott.

Page, E. W., Villee, C. A., & Villee, D. B. (1981). *Human reproduction: Essentials of reproductive and perinatal medicine* (3rd ed.). Philadelphia: W. B. Saunders.

Porth, C. M. (1986). *Pathophysiology: Concepts of altered health status.* Philadelphia: J. B. Lippincott Company.

Vander, A. J. (1985). *Renal physiology* (3rd ed.). New York: McGraw-Hill.

Wodniak, C., & Szwed, J. (1986). Fluids and electrolytes. In L. Abels (Ed.), *Critical care nursing: A physiologic approach* (pp. 337-420). St. Louis: C. V. Mosby.

Antibiotics

Bourcierm, K. M., & Seidler, A. J. (1987). Chlamydia and condylamata acuminata: An update for the nurse practitioner. *Journal of Obstetric, Gynecologic, and Neonatal Nursing, 16*, 17-22.

Cloherty, J. P., & Stark, A. R. (eds.). (1985). *Manual of neonatal care* (2nd ed.). (pp. 393-400). Boston: Little, Brown.

Cox, M. A. (1985). Nutrition. In J. P. Cloherty & A. R. Stark (Eds.), *Manual of neonatal care* (2nd ed.). (pp. 423-458). Boston: Little, Brown.

Kerner, J. (1983). Caloric requirements. In J. Kerner (Ed.), *Manual of pediatric parenteral nutrition* (p. 65). New York: John Wiley & Sons.

Kerner, J. (1983). Carbohydrate requirements. In J. Kerner (Ed.), *Manual of pediatric parenteral nutrition* (pp. 81-86). New York: John Wiley & Sons.

Klaus, M. H., & Fanaroff, A. A. (1986). *Care of the high risk neonate* (3rd ed.) Philadelphia: W. B. Saunders.

Lebenthal, E. (Ed.). (1986). *Total parenteral nutrition* (p. 153). New York: Raven Press.

Lowrey, G. H. (1978). *Growth and development of children.* Chicago: Year Book Medical.

Lubchenco, L. O. (1976). *The high risk infant.* Philadelphia: W. B. Saunders Company.

Metheny, N. M., & Snively, W. (1983). *Nurses' handbook of fluid balance* (p. 375). Philadelphia: J.B. Lippincott.

Pereira, G., & Glassman, M. (1986). Parenteral nutrition in neonates. In J. Rombeau & M. Caldwell (Eds.), *Parenteral nutrition, clinical nutrition* (p. 2, 706). Philadelphia: W. B. Saunders Company.

Wesley, R., Saran, P. A., & Kholdi, N., et al. (Eds.). (1980). *Parenteral enteral nutrition manual of the University of Michigan Medical Center.* Chicago: Abbott Laboratories.

BIBLIOGRAPHY

Fluid and Electrolyte Status:
Preoperative, Intraoperative, and Postoperative

Apgar, V. (1953). A proposal for a new method of evaluation of the newborn infant. *Current Researches in Anesthesia Analgesia, 32,* 260-267.

Ballard, J., Kazmaier, K., & Driver, M. (1977). A simplified assessment of gestational age. *Pediatric Research, 11,* 374.

Brück, K. (1978). Thermoregulation: Control mechanisms and neural processes. In J. Sinclair (Ed.), *Temperature regulation and energy metabolism in the newborn.* Orlando, FL: Grune & Stratton.

Chance, G. (1978). Thermal environment in transport. In J. Sinclair (Ed.), *Temperature regulation and energy metabolism in the newborn.* Orlando, FL: Grune & Stratton.

Coran, A. G., Drongowski, R. A., & Wesley, J. R. (1984). Changes in total body water and extracellular fluid volume in infants receiving total parenteral nutrition. *Journal of Pediatric Surgery, 19,* 771-775.

Dawes, G. (1968). *Fetal and neonatal physiology.* Chicago: Year Book Medical.

Dubowitz, L. M., Dubowitz, V., & Goldberg, C.(1970). Clinical assessment of gestational age in the newborn infant. *Journal of Pediatrics, 77,* 1.

Endo, A. (1981). Using computers in newborn intensive care settings. *American Journal of Nursing, 81,* 1336-1337.

Hodson, W. A., & Truog, W. E. (1983). *Critical care of the newborn.* Philadelphia: W. B. Saunders.

Johnson, T. R., Moore, W. M., & Jeffries, J. E. (eds.). (1978). *Children are different: Developmental physiology* (2nd ed.). Columbus: Ross Laboratories.

Lutz, L., & Perlstein, P. (1971). Temperature control in newborn babies. *Nursing Clinics of North America, 6,* 15-23.

Nour, B., Boudreaux, J. P., & Rowe, M. (1984). An experimental model to study thermogenesis in the neonatal surgical patient. *Journal of Pediatric Surgery, 19,* 764-769.

Page, E. W., Villee, C. A., & Villee, D. B. (1981). *Human reproduction: Essentials of reproduction and perinatal medicine* (3rd ed.). Philadelphia: W. B. Saunders.

Perez, R. H. (1981). *Protocols for perinatal nursing practice.* St. Louis: C. V. Mosby.

Perlstein, P., Edwards, N., & Sutherland, J. (1970). Apnea in premature infants and incubator-air-temperature changes. *New England Journal of Medicine, 282*, 461-466.

Perlstein, P., Hersch, C., Glueck, C., & Sutherland, J. (1974). Adaptation to cold in the first three days of life. *Pediatrics, 54*, 411-415.

Perlstein, P., Edwards, N., Atherton, H., & Sutherland, J. (1976). Computer-assisted newborn intensive care. *Pediatrics, 57*, 494-501.

Scanlon, J. W., Nelson, T., Grylack, L., & Smith, Y. F. (1979). *A system of newborn physical examination.* Baltimore: University Park Press.

Vestal, K., & McKenzie, C. A. (1983). *High risk perinatal nursing: The American association of critical care nurses.* Philadelphia: W. B. Saunders.

Antibiotics

Cashare, W. J., Sedaghatian, M. R., & Usher, R. H. (1975). Nutritional supplements with intravenously administered lipid, protein hydrolysate, and glucose in small premature infants. *Pediatrics, 56*, 88.

Hay, W. (1986). Justification for total parenteral nutrition in the premature and compromised newborn. In E. Lebenthal (Ed.), *Total parenteral nutrition* (p. 284). New York: Raven Press.

Sheard, N., & Udall, J. Immune deficiency and parenteral nutrition. In E. Lebenthal (Ed.), *Total parenteral nutrition.* (p. 355) New York: Raven Press.

Chapter 10

Ventilatory Care

Laurie Porter Gunderson   *Carole Kenner*

This chapter discusses respiratory care, which includes a thorough assessment for respiratory difficulties as well as intervention strategies to decrease respiratory or ventilatory problems. One such intervention is suctioning. A protocol for partially ventilated suctioning is described. The second and third sections of this chapter describe extracorporeal membrane oxygenation, which is an increasingly popular technique for oxygenating infants with persistent pulmonary hypertension and diaphragmatic hernia, and the use of high frequency ventilation.

Respiratory Care and Suctioning
Laurie Porter Gunderson

ASSESSMENT OF THE INFANT WITH RESPIRATORY DIFFICULTY

The purpose of assessing infant's with respiratory difficulty is to determine which infants are compensating for their respiratory difficulties and which need some type of intervention. The intervention may include suctioning the airway, increasing the fraction of inspired oxygen (FiO_2), intubation, and the initiation of mechanical ventilation.

To assess the infant, the nurse must assess three systems—the nervous system, cardiovascular system, and respiratory system—to determine how heavily the infant is stressed. The assessment of the nervous system includes noting the behavior and positioning of the infant at rest, the infant's responses to stimuli, and reflexes such as sucking and grasping.

The next system to be assessed is the cardiovascular system: the heart rate and rhythm should be determined. The peripheral pulses should be evaluated. Measurement of blood pressure and skin perfusion are also necessary in determining the efficiency of the heart action. Hepatomegaly may be noted with portal hypertension and congestive heart failure.

The respiratory system should be assessed for quality and character of respirations. Evaluate the rate, rhythm, and effort of the infant's respiratory status. Assessment of respirations includes observing for grunting, retractions (may include intercostal, supraclavicular, or subcostal), or nasal flaring. Note the position of the trachea in midline and chest expansion.

The infant's color (pink, blue, or pale) is an indicator of the effectiveness of respiratory effort. Meconium staining indicates that the infant has been stressed in utero and may be indicative of respiratory compromise if meconium is found below the cords. The assessment of breath sounds should include the evaluation of symmetry, presence of abnormal sounds, and location. The presence or absence of breath sounds may be indicative of pathology or the presence of a physical obstruction in the airway (Chart 10-A).

Assessing the breath sounds requires proper equipment and knowledge of the underlying anatomical structures. Selecting the proper stethoscope is important. When assessing an infant who weighs 1500 g or less it is best to use a stethoscope designed for premature infants. Assessment of larger infants calls for the use of an infant stethoscope. The problem with using too large a stethescope is that it is difficult to distinguish which lung field is being auscultated (Fig. 10-1). It is better to use a small stethoscope on a larger infant than a large stethoscope on a premature or small infant.

AUSCULTATION OF LUNG FIELDS

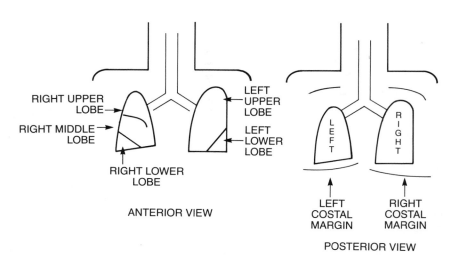

Fig. 10-1.   Ausculation of lung fields.

Chart 10-A Respiratory Care Examination

Nervous System	Cardiovascular System	Respiratory System
Posture Influenced by maturity **Tone** Flexion good near term Active—spontaneous movements Response to tactile stimulation	**Perfusion—Skin Blood Flow** **Heart Rate** **Arterial Pulsations** **Blood Pressure** **Maximal Cardiac Output**	**Color** Red—polycythemia Blue—cyanotic White—poor perfusion, shocky Green—meconium- stained Rate Slow, normal, or fast **Rhythm** Regular, periodic, gasping, or apneic **Respiratory Effort** 1. Presence of grunting 2. Retracting such as movement of soft parts • lag—movement of ribs during respiration • See-saw movement —the ribs in an inspira- tion while the abdomen moves out • Abdomen paradox 3. Nostrils flaring **Breath Sounds** Symmetry Note where breath sounds loudest Rales, rhonchi, stridor, or wheeze **Tracheal position** Midline

POSTOPERATIVE RESPIRATORY MANAGEMENT

Immediately postoperatively a thorough baseline assessment of the infant's respiratory status needs to be completed. From data gathered, the nurse can determine changes in status that may be indicative of improvement or that may signal a deteriorating condition.

Neonatal nurses need to be cognizant of the infant's position. Certain positions and placement will compromise the neonate's lung capacity. Positioning the infant on the back tends to decrease the infant's lung capacity by applying pressure on the diaphragm and limiting chest expansion. Therefore, careful choice of positions will enable the infant to have maximal lung capacity.

Infants who are premature can be further compromised by the lack of surfactant produced by the type II cells in the lungs. Surfactant decreases the surface tension in the alveoli. Essentially, surfactant prevents the alveoli from collapsing, thus aiding in the gas exchange process.

The nurse taking care of the surgical neonate needs to be cognizant not only of the normal respiratory physiology but also of the compromises that are associated with the neonate's surgical condition. Therefore, the nurse must be aware of

1. Abdominal distention

2. Diaphragmatic involvement

3. Nerve involvement

4. Anesthesia

5. Medication that the infant has received or is receiving

All of these factors may lead to respiratory compromise that may alter the infant's ability to maintain adequate ventilation.

If the neonate is incapable of maintaining minimal ventilatory assistance, supplemental FiO_2 may be necessary. The FiO_2 may be provided via oxygen hood or nasal cannula. The oxygen hood is the most common method for providing supplemental oxygen. The nurse needs to pay special attention to the concentration of oxygen within the oxygen hood. If the nurse questions the oxygen analyzer reading and believes that there may be a discrepancy between it and the actual amount of oxygen that the infant is receiving, the analyzer should be calibrated or replaced.

If the infant needs further assistance, intubation and mechanical ventilation is necessary. When caring for an infant using a ventilator, careful assessment must be carried out hourly and more frequently if the infant appears to be compromised. Maintaining a patent airway is essential. This requires suctioning of the endotracheal tube. Often the endotracheal tube is to be suctioned at set intervals. This regimented suctioning may be detrimental to the infant if not carefully monitored. The infant's respiratory status should be assessed and suctioning of the endotracheal tube should be carried out based on the infant's respiratory status and the amount and tenacity of the secretions.

SUCTIONING

Researchers advocate a method of endotracheal suctioning that does not call for the disconnection of the infant from the ventilator (Cabal et al., 1979; Zmora & Merritt, 1980; Gunderson, McPhee, & Donovan, 1986). Several adaptors are on the market that allow the infant to be partially ventilated during the endotracheal suctioning procedure (Fig. 10-2). Partial ventilation during endotracheal suctioning minimizes the risks of hypoxia and bradycardia (Cabal et al., 1979; Zmora & Merritt, 1980; Gunderson et al., 1986).

PARTIALLY VENTILATED STERILE ENDOTRACHEAL SUCTION

The purpose is to maintain a patent airway facilitating the exchange of oxygen and carbon dioxide.

Equipment

1. Sterile suction catheters: use 5/6 F with 2.5- and 3.0-mm internal diameter endotracheal tubes and 8 F with 3.5-mm internal diameter endotracheal tubes.

2. Sterile gloves.

3. Sterile cup.

4. Bottle of sterile water.

5. Source of negative pressure, with connecting tubing.

6. Backup manual resuscitation bag circuit (capable of 100 percent oxygen delivery) with warmed humidified air and pressure manometer.

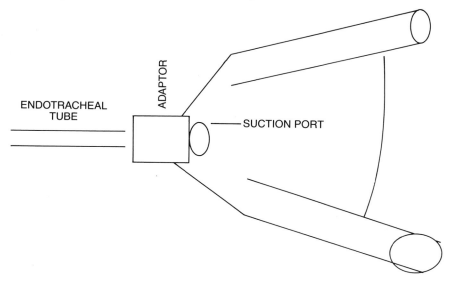

ENDOTRACHEAL TUBE FOR PARTIALLY VENTILATED SUCTION

Fig. 10-2. Endotracheal tube for partially ventilated suction.

Method

Action	Reason
1. Check the oxygen setting for the *rebreathing bag*	The oxygen setting should be congruent with the FiO_2 setting, the infant is presently on; retrolental fibroplasia is a potential side effect of high oxygen concentrations; it is best to start with the same FiO_2 and increase as needed
2. Test the *rebreathing bag* for proper inflation; keep the *Mapleson* on standby during the procedure	Checking the *rebreathing bag* will avoid potential problems such as no air flow, clamped tubing, possible hole in the bag, and improper setup
3. Turn negative pressure to suction source to the "on" position	Negative pressure to suction source should be regulated for continuous pressure, not to exceed 80-100 mm Hg for premature infants and 120 mm Hg for larger infants
4. Peel open suction catheter of appropriate size, allowing the sterile catheter to remain in package until ready for use	
5. Pour a small amount of sterile water into a sterile cup	This will be used to moisten the tip of the catheter to clear secretions from the catheter and to instill into the endotracheal tube if deemed necessary (see item 9 below)
6. Put sterile glove on dominant hand.	Other hand can manipulate necessary items
7. Pick up suction catheter with dominant gloved hand, keeping catheter tip sterile	
8. Hold connecting tubing in opposite hand and attach suction catheter	
9. Moisten the tip of the suction catheter with the sterile water	Should secretions be tenacious and the nurse believes that instilling sterile water may improve removal of secretions, then sterile water can be instilled into the endotracheal tube; the instillation will be done by sterile technique via the special adaptor; after instillation the infant is to be left on the ventilator for 15-20 seconds prior to suctioning; manual ventilation should not be performed unless bradycardia ensues
10. Open the port hole adaptor	The infant will receive rate, pressure, and FiO_2 greater than room air during the suctioning procedure
11. Insert the catheter through the port hole down the endotracheal tube until catheter clears the tip of the endotracheal tube (0.5 cm)	Negative pressure should not be applied during instillation of the suction catheter; this could cause tissue trauma, decrease FiO_2, and generate negative pressure
12. Apply thumb to suction catheter and withdraw with a rotating motion	Rotating the suction catheter increases the potential for removing the secretions from all sides of the endotracheal tube wall
13. Close the port hole	Closing the port hole reestablishes the entire rate, pressure, and FiO_2

Action	Reason
14. If secretions are copious and the patient's condition remains stable, repeat the procedure	Nursing judgment should be used in determining the actual need to repeat the procedure
15. Should apnea or bradycardia occur and persist after recommencing ventilation, hand bagging should be instituted to return the patient to baseline level	

Whenever an infant is receiving mechanical ventilatory assistance, emergency equipment needs to be available. The equipment includes a spare endotracheal tube of the appropriate diameter and laryngoscope with the proper blade size. Every time an infant is intubated a note should be made and taped to the bedside or recorded in a highly visible area as to the tube diameter and the depth of insertion; this should be noted on the tube when the tube is taped and secured. In the tracheostomy patient a spare tracheostomy tube with an obturator, if necessary, should be available at the bedside at all times. Decannulation of the trachea can occur anytime a tracheostomy is present. If the spare is used, the spare should be immediately replaced so there is always a backup tracheostomy tube available.

TRANSCUTANEOUS OXYGEN MONITORING

Transcutaneous oxygen monitoring (TCM) is a noninvasive procedure that uitilizes the phenomenon that oxygen diffuses through the skin and can be recorded in a numerical value. TCMs can be a great tool in aiding the nurse in assessing the infant's oxygen status (Norris, Campbell, & Brenkert, 1982). The transcutaneous readings are dependent upon several factors: circulation, electrode temperature, skin conditions, and electrode applications. The factors can be managed with proper calibration of the TCM, correct choice of electrode temperature, correct choice of placement site, and proper placement of electrode probe (Severinghaus, 1982). When positioning the probe, avoid areas of poor perfusion and those sites with edema present.

Pulse oximeters are also available to measure the oxygen saturation. This probe must also be placed in areas of good tissue perfusion to be accurate. Fingers, toes, ankles, and ear lobes (the latter site is difficult in the neonate) are the sites of choice for the oximeter. If these factors are controlled, then TCMs and pulse oximeters are a reliable, noninvasive method for recording transcutaneous oxygen tension and saturation.

Extracorporeal Membrane Oxgyenation

Laurie Porter Gunderson

DESCRIPTION

Extracorporeal membrane oxygenation (ECMO) is a modified heart-lung machine that allows for an individual's blood to be oxygenated outside of the body. The ECMO procedure involves the cannulation of both the right atrium via the internal jugular vein and the aortic arch via the common carotid artery. Blood is removed from the right atrium and circulated through tubing via a pumping device and then through a membrane oxygenator. There, the desaturated blood becomes oxygenated before flowing back through a heating device and into the cannula placed in the carotid artery (Bartlett, Andrews, Toomasian, Haiduc, & Gazzaniga, 1982; Bartlett et al., 1976; Bartlett et al., 1977; Bartlett et al., 1978).

METHODS OF ECMO

Several methods for ECMO bypass exist. The most common method is the venoarterial (VA) bypass method. This method calls for the cannulation of the right atrium via the right internal jugular vein and cannulation of the aortic arch via the right common carotid artery (Bartlett et al., 1982). The other method of cannulation is called venovenous (VV) bypass (Andrews, Klein, Toomasian, Roloff, & Bartlett, 1983; Andrews, Toomasian, Gram, & Bartlett, 1982). Venovenous bypass has not been as successful in the neonatal population (Bartlett et al., 1982). With VV bypass the right atrium is cannulated via the right internal jugular vein to allow for venous drainage and the oxygenated blood to be returned to a cannula placed in the femoral vein. The remainder of this section refers to VA bypass since it is the most widely used method.

The extracorporeal circuit consists of polyvinylchloride tubing, a servoregulated roller pump with a 10-mL venous reservoir bladder, a bladder box, a membrane lung, and a heat exchanger (Bartlett et al., 1982). See Fig. 10-3.

BLOOD FLOW THROUGH THE ECMO CIRCUIT

Blood is drained from the venous side of the infant's body via the right atrium. Blood flows by gravity down to the 10-mL reservoir bladder. If there is insufficient blood in the reservoir, the bladder collapses. The collapsed bladder signals the pressure-sensitive bladder box to automatically shut off the pump. Shutting off the pump prevents blood from being sucked from the infant's body. When enough blood and pressure have built up in the bladder, the bladder box signals the pump

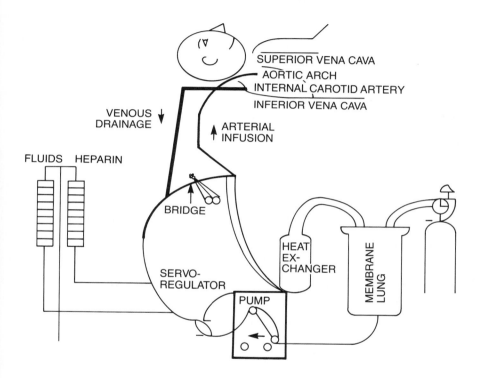

Fig. 10-3.   Extracorporeal membrane oxygenation.

to turn back on. After the blood flows through the bladder it passes into soft, pli-
able tubing to the servoregulated direct-drive roller pump. The tubing that traver-
ses through the pump is called race-way tubing.

The flexibility of the tubing allows the pump heads to compress the tubing and
surge the blood forward to the membrane oxygenator. The membrane oxygenator
has an internal meshlike structure similar in appearance to screening. The mesh-

work allows blood to flow by on one side of the meshwork and gases to pass by on the other side. The pressure of the blood compartment is greater than the gaseous side, allowing for gases to diffuse across the membrane (University of Michigan Department of Surgery, 1984).

The blood picks up oxygen and releases carbon dioxide. The blood next travels through the membrane to the heat exchanger. In the heat exchanger blood flows through the exchanger with warmed water passing by in the opposite direction. The water is warmed to approximately 37°C. The heat exchanger may be adjusted to maintain the infant's temperature. After the blood has passed through the heat exchanger, it is returned to the neonate and enters via the cannula in the right common carotid artery to the aortic arch. Once the blood has been returned to the aortic arch, the blood is pumped throughout the body via normal circulation.

SUGGESTED PATIENT SELECTION AND ENTRY CRITERIA

1. Candidates for ECMO are infants who have reversible profound respiratory disease.

2. Possible candidates are infants diagnosed with congenital diaphragmatic hernia, persistent pulmonary hypertension, and/or meconium-aspiration syndrome.

3. These infants should not have any type of congenital heart defects, ventricular hemorrhage, or overwhelming sepsis.

4. ECMO candidates are infants who have not been stabilized using conventional, maximal, intervention.

5. If the standard treatment procedures do not work, then the infant may be considered as a possible candidate for neonatal ECMO.

6. A weight of at least 2000 g is suggested in an attempt to decrease the risk of intraventricular bleeds and to eliminate the premature infant from being selected as a candidate.

The exact entry criteria may vary from institution to institution. Some institutions use the newborn pulmonary insufficiency index (NPII). The NPII is an objective measure of the severity of respiratory failure during the infant's first 24 hours of life (Bartlett et al., 1982; Krummel et al., 1982; Zapal, Snider, & Schneider, 1977). The other objective measure is the calculation of $AaDO_2$, the alveolar arterial diffusing capacity of oxygen:

$$AaDO_2 = 760 - (47 + PaCO_2 + PaO_2)$$

where 760 indicates barometric pressure at sea level and 47 indicates water pressure in the alveoli. For example, if an infant has an arterial blood gas drawn and the results are $PaO_2 = 45$; and $PaCO_2 = 50$, then

$$AaDO_2 = 760 - (47 + 50 + 45) \qquad = 760 - 142 \qquad = 618 \text{ torr}$$

Usually institutions specify that the $AaDO_2$ should be > 620 torr for the infant to receive ECMO. Specific criteria for many institutions with neonatal ECMO teams may vary somewhat. Some of the more common criteria are listed next.

Commonly Suggested Entry Criteria for ECMO

1. Birth Weight ≥ 2 kg

2. Age < 168 hours (1 week)
3. Patient using ventilator, receiving maximum optimal ventilation, $AaDO_2$ > 620 plus hypotension and a pH of < 7.15 accompanied by a base deficit

Other criteria sometimes used in addition to the above criteria are the presence of pulmonary interstitial emphysema, pneumoperitoneum or pneumopericaridum, persistent air leaks, or a mean airway pressure > 15 cm/H_2O.

Contraindications

1. Bilateral pulmonary hypoplasia

2. Intracranial/ventricular hemorrhage

3. Oliguric renal failure

4. Disseminated intravascular coagulation

5. Irreversible pulmonary damage

6. Associated uncorrectable congenital anomalies inconsistent with survival

7. Weight < 1500-2000 g (weight limit varies among institutions)

8. Cyanotic congenital heart disease

9. Uncontrolled septicemia (Nugent, 1986; University of MIchigan Department of Surgery, 1984)

Careful screening of potential ECMO candidates is necessary to determine that none of the contraindications exists. Therefore, all patients being considered for neonatal ECMO need to have the following evaluation done to rule out any contraindications:

1. Cranial ultrasonography within the past 24 hours

2. Neurological exam by consulting neurologist

3. Electrocardiogram

4. Echocardiogram

5. Chest radiograph taken in the past 24 hours (University of Michigan Department of Surgery, 1984)

All of the tests need to be completed within the past 24 hours. If any of the test results are older than 24 hours, those procedures need to be repeated.

If a patient appears to be a possible candidate for ECMO, early referral to the ECMO team in house or in the region is advised. Early detection of possible ECMO candidates may improve the outcome for that infant.

CANNULATION

Once an infant meets criteria for bypass, the actual surgical procedure of isolation and cannulation of the right common carotid artery and the right internal jugular vein can take place. The cannulation procedure is done in the nursery with the infant under local anesthesia. After the cannulation procedure is completed the infant is allowed to wake up. The infant remains in an unanesthetized state while on bypass. Therefore, the infant goes through normal changes in sleep-wake patterns. In some institutions pancuronium bromide and/or morphine may be used during this period.

As soon as the infant's right common carotid artery and internal jugular vein are cannulated the infant is ready to be placed on bypass. While the surgeons are working with the infant, a specially trained nurse perfusionist primes the ECMO circuit. The total volume of the ECMO circuit is approximately 450-500 mL (Bartlett et al., 1982). Priming of the ECMO circuit consists of filling the circuit with carbon dioxide followed by flushing the system with a crystalloid prime and lastly priming the system with freshly heparinized blood or packed RBCs (Bartlett et al., 1982).

Immediately after going on bypass the infant appears to respond quite rapidly with regard to color. The dusky cyanotic infant prior to bypass often turns bright pink within minutes. The nurse and staff must remember that the change in color is due to the membrane oxygenator providing adequate oxygen to the tissues and not as a result of sudden marked improvement in the infant's lung condition.

The infant on bypass remains intubated. The ventilator rates and settings are reduced to minimal settings. The exact method for airway management varies from institution to institution. Usually some type of tracheal lavage is performed, especially for those infants diagnosed with meconium-aspiration syndrome. Loss of an airway is not an emergency situation (Altose, Hicks, & Edwards, 1976). This is often difficult to comprehend for the NICU nurse who is trained to maintain an airway in any circumstance.

While the infant is on bypass it may be necessary to perform direct suctioning. In this instance endotracheal tubes may be electively removed to perform this direct suctioning; however, there may be an increased incidence of trauma to the trachea if multiple intubations are done. Prior to discontinuing ECMO, surgeons and physicians generally change endotracheal tubes to provide optimal airway support after bypass is discontinued.

The amount of time an infant spends on bypass is variable. The major determining factor is the infant's underlying lung pathology. To determine how well the infant's lungs are recovering, trial periods off ECMO are instituted. During these trial periods off ECMO the ventilator support is increased to maximal FiO_2 and rates with a pressure of at least 30/3 (Bartlett et al., 1982). The trial phase off ECMO allows the physician to determine lung function (Bartlett et al., 1982). The

ECMO circuit can also be regulated to allow more blood to pass through the infant's lungs as lung function appears to improve. Therefore the ECMO circuit can be reduced to minimal support or increased to maximal flow rates depending on the infant's condition.

NURSING ROLES IN ECMO

When an infant is on bypass the infant is usually managed by a nurse perfusionist who is specially trained in operating the ECMO circuit. Extensive lab time and/or clinical time is obtained prior to having the nurse perfusionist manage the ECMO circuit alone. The nurse perfusionist manages the circuit by drawing blood gases hourly from the infant as well as drawing blood gases from the circuit itself at specified intervals.

Lab values must be closely monitored and maintained. These lab values include CBC, platelet count, hemoglobin, along with electrolyte levels. Fluctuations from baseline are noted and treated accordingly by the nurse perfusionist under a physician's supervision.

Neonates on ECMO are heparinized to prevent coagulation of the blood as it transverses the ECMO circuit. The nurse perfusionist is cognizant of the infant's coagulation times, which are usually kept from 2 to 2-½ times the baby's normal pre-ECMO baseline values. To maintain the clotting times, samples of blood are analyzed hourly. If changes occur, the heparin drip, which is infusing continuously, is adjusted to maintain the clotting times. An example of the orders for the nurse perfusionist are presented next.

Orders for the Nurse Perfusionist

1. Monitor laboratory data immediately after cannulation and after bypass institution: CBC, platelet count, electrolytes, calcium, glucose, specific gravity, and chest radiographs (both anterior, posterior, and lateral).

2. When stable perfusion flow rate is reached, decrease ventilator settings to $FiO_2 + 0.3$ pressure - 15/4, rate = 10; and inspiratory/expiratory = 1.0.

3. Ideal umbilical arterial catheter gases:
   $PO_2 = 60-70$; $PCO_2 = 35-45$; pH = 7.35 - 7.45.

4. Heparin drip: given by continuous infusion. Some institutions use 75 U of heparin/cc, others up to 100 U/cc (Nugent, 1986) to maintain the clotting times between 2.0 and 2.5 times the control or baseline clotting time.

5. Routine monitoring of laboratory values:
   - Every hour: arterial blood gases and clotting times
   - Every 4 hours: CBC with platelet count and calcium levels, urine-specific gravity and pH (Nugent, 1986)
   - Every 8 hours: electrolytes, blood urea nitrogen (BUN), creatinine, glucose, and premembrane and postmembrane oxygenator blood gases

- Every day: morning chest radiographs, phosphorus and magnesium blood levels, liver function tests, plasma hemoglobin, blood cultures, fibrinogen, fibrin split products, and urinalysis.

6. One-fourth unit of packed RBCs should be available in the unit at all times and 1 U of packed RBCs in the blood bank (Nugent, 1986).

7. Administer packed RBCs to maintain the hematocrit levels between 38 and 42 percent.

8. Replace 1 cc of blood lost with 1 cc of replacement every 10 cc.

9. Maintain platelet count at > 50,000.

10. Heparin bolus with all platelet packs: 1-2 U/cc platelets to maintain clotting times 2-2.5 times control.

11. Check the ECMO system every hour and as needed.

12. Maintain venous temperature at 37.0° C.

13. Administer all medications and IV fluids into the pump circuit.

14. Assist the NICU nurse with all position changes (Nugent, 1986; University of Michigan Department of Surgery, 1984).

Along with the nurse perfusionist there is always another NICU nurse assigned to care for the infant. The nurse is generally responsible for

1. Hourly position changes.

2. Hourly checking vital signs.

3. Monitoring the blood that may be oozing from the cannulation site.

4. Strict measurements of intake and output.

5. Airway management.

6. Management of the transcutaneous oxygen monitor and the pulse oximeter.

7. The nurse must be cognizant that the infant is highly heparinized and precautions should be used with oral and endotracheal suctioning.

NICU NURSING ORDERS

1. Monitor vital signs every hour: arterial BP, heart rate, and respiratory rate.

2. Weigh infant every day.

3. No IM medications.

4. No venipunctures.

5. No heelsticks.

6. No heparin flush solutions

7. NPO: nasogastric or orogastric tube to dependent drainage
   a. Check pH every hour.
   b. Administer antacid 5 cc for pH < 6.

8. Change infant's position: reposition infant from side to side every hour.

9. Check intake and output every hour.

10. Mouth care: gently clean every 2 hours and as needed.

11. Position infant on sheepskin to protect skin.

12. Neck incision:
    a. Keep neck incision open to air to note drainage and position of cannulas.
    b. Keep dressings under neck to absorb drainage that may pool.
    c. Weigh dressings at least every hour.
    d. Replace blood: 1 cc of replacement for every 1 cc of loss. This replacement is done during a period of 4–8 hours.

13. Check urine specific gravity, pH, and test for the presence of glucose and blood every 4 hours. Note any specific gravity > 1.015 or a positive test for glucose or blood in the urine.

14. Test each stool for the presence of blood.

15. Suction endotracheal tube every 1-2 hours and as needed. Collect tracheal aspirate for culture and sensitivity every morning.

16. Umbilical arterial catheter: flush umbilical arterial catheter with an unheparinized 5 percent dextrose solution since the infant is already heparinized.

17. Transcutaneous monitor should be in a preductal position and an oximeter should be placed on a finger on the infant's left hand.

18. Neurological checks (includes pupil reactions to light, reflexes, tonus, palpate anterior fontanel, assessment of cranial sutures) should be done every hour.

19. Head circumference should be measured every shift or more frequently if bleeding is suspected.

20. One fourth of a unit of packed RBCs should be kept at the bedside at all times. An additional quantity of typed blood should be available at the blood bank at all times.

PROCEDURES

Special procedures can be carried out while an infant is on bypass. These special procedures include ultrasound, cardiac catheterization, nuclear scans, and patent ductus arteriosus ligations. Next to the ultrasound the patent ductus arteriosus ligations are one of the more common procedures at this stage. Specific guidelines have been developed for performing the ligation on a heparinized infant, therefore, decreasing the risks and complications that could be associated with anticoagulated infants (Bartlett et al., 1982; Bartlett et al., 1985).

COMPLICATIONS

Neonatal ECMO is not without risk. Both the NICU nurse and the nurse perfusionist must be aware of complications that may occur while an infant is on bypass. Problems may occur with the equipment. These problems may include disconnection, breakage of tubing, or failure of the membrane. Therefore, careful monitoring is necessary to reduce potential complications. For example, blood gases from the membrane oxygenator are closely monitored. If the blood gases indicate that the membrane oxygenator is no longer functioning adequately, the membrane should be replaced immediately.

The infant is also at risk from air emboli that can accidently enter the ECMO circuit, hemorrhage due to anticoagulation, or hemorrhage due to ruptured tubing. These are only some of the complications or problems that may arise while an infant is on bypass. Therefore, careful management and observation of both the infant and the circuit are necessary to minimize the possible risks.

DISCONTINUATION OF ECMO

Neonatal ECMO is discontinued after an infant has demonstrated recovered lung function. ECMO is not abruptly discontinued but carefully decreased to allow for increased blood flow through the lungs and adjustment of the lungs to support the infant without the assistance of ECMO. ECMO may be discontinued when the infant has sustained irreversible brain damage or irreversible organ damage (Bartlett et al., 1982).

DECANNULATION

The decannulation procedure is done in the unit with the infant under local anesthesia and paralyzed to prevent air emboli from entering during the procedure. At the time of decannulation the carotid artery and jugular vein are ligated. Therefore these infants will depend on collateral circulation to perfuse the areas once served by the carotid artery and jugular vein.

After decannulation is completed, special attention is given to maintain a clean surgical site to prevent infection. Usually these infants are weaned rapidly from the ventilatory support and extubated.

FOLLOW-UP

Infants who have been on bypass are examined at intervals to assess neurological status and lung function. Usually the infants have a neurological exam, chest radiographs, and psychometric examination (Bartlett et al., 1982).

CONCLUSION

Neonatal ECMO can be a life-saving procedure for infants who are not able to be maintained by conventional medical therapy. ECMO is not without complications or risks, but with careful medical/surgical and nursing management an infant with profound reversible lung disease can be successfully managed.

High-Frequency Ventilation
Carole Kenner

DESCRIPTION

High-frequency ventilation refers to mechanical ventilation that exceeds the normal respiratory rate by at least four times and delivers tidal volumes less than or equal to the anatomical dead-space volume. This form of ventilation differs significantly from conventional methods of mechanical ventilation. Most ventilators found in the NICU are positive-pressure ventilators that deliver oxygen in bulk flow via large tidal volume and positive pressure. During this type of ventilation the expiratory phase of respiration is generally considered passive. Mean airway pressures are usually high with the conventional ventilation methods; however, high-frequency ventilation provides adequate gas exchange with a lower mean airway pressure, and expiration may or may not be viewed as a passive process.

METHODS

There are three types of high-frequency ventilation: (1) high-frequency positive-pressure ventilation, (2) high-frequency oscillation, and (3) high-frequency jet ventilation. High-frequency positive-pressure ventilation uses a two-way flow of gases. Gas flows towards the neonate from the mechanical ventilator during the active inspiratory phase of respiration. On expiration, carbon dioxide passively flows out of the infant (Gruden, 1985). The ventilatory rates range from 50 to 150 breaths per minute.

High-frequency oscillation is a form of high-frequency ventilation where the gas molecules are oscillated or set into motion by the ultrahigh rates. Approximately 900 breaths per minute may be used (Inwood, Finley, & Fitzhardinge, 1986). The cycles are usually described in terms of hertz (1 hertz = 1 cycle/sec), and the rates may range from 180 to 2400 cycles/min (Gruden, 1985; Inwood et al., 1986). It is hypothesized that this rapid molecular movement may contribute to gas exchange at the alveolar level; however, no clear-cut determination of the exact mechanism of exchange has been found.

The exchange of oxygen and carbon dioxide can be controlled independently. In most conventional ventilation methods a change in oxygen will ultimately change the level of carbon dioxide. In high-frequency oscillation, expiration becomes an active phase. With the delivery of oxygen, even into the smallest areas, exchange is facilitated due to the molecular movement of the gases. Alveoli are kept open as long as mean airway pressure is maintained. The mean airway pressure is less than that of conventional methods. Therefore, it is postulated that even in the very premature infant with little surfactant, alveoli may remain open thus protecting the infant from lung collapse or atelectasis (Inwood et al., 1986). One important consideration, however, is that any disturbance in the system such as disconnecting the infant will result in immediate decline in the mean airway pressure. A "sustained inflation" or "sigh" pressure exceeding the mean airway pressure by 6-10 cm of water for 6-10 seconds is recommended by Inwood et al. (1986, p. 55) to avoid or resolve the potential collapse of alveoli following disconnection, especially during a suctioning procedure. The high-frequency jet type of ventilation should not be completely discontinued for suctioning. While a suction catheter is being introduced, suction should be applied (Olson, Karp, Reppucci, Solon, & Nichols, 1986; Karp, Solon, Olson, Reppucci, & Nichols, 1986).

Carbon dioxide exchange is promoted via adjustments in the amplitude pressure. This is the pressure that is determined by the stroke volume delivered by the piston-driven ventilator, pulmonary compliance of the infant, and the circuit pressure itself. It may be advantageous to adjust pressure settings based on the partial pressure of arterial carbon dioxide in the infant (Inwood et al., 1986).

High-frequency jet ventilation is the most common form of the high-frequency ventilation. It is a form of positive-pressure ventilation like conventional methods; however, its delivery system is different. It uses compressed gas or a high-pressure system of delivery through a ventilator using a solenoid or flow-regulated valve (Gruden, 1985). The gas flows in small volumes (convective streaming) during inspiration via a regular endotracheal tube at rates of 100-1200 breaths per minute. (Expiration in this system is a passive act.) The rapid jets of air create a pressure gradient forcing surrounding gases to join the gas being delivered. This pulling of gases along the gradient is called the Venturi effect or entrainment. Facilitated diffusion of gases in the alveoli is thereby improved. This system then creates a high positive-end expiratory pressure and contributes to better arterial oxygen tension (Gruden, 1985).

ADVANTAGES AND DISADVANTAGES

The advantages of high-frequency ventilation are several: (1) oxygen can be delivered at lower pressures (mean airway pressure and peak airway pressure), thus decreasing the chance of barotrauma pneumothorax or other air leaks; (2) less pressure may result in better cardiac circulation in the peripheral and central circuits; (3) improved blood flow to the renal arteries and therefore to the kidneys lessen the danger of increasing the amount of ADH released during renal circulation compromise; (4) fewer cardiac arrhythmias with less compromise of the central circulation; (5) improved gas exchange and thus better control of acid-base balance; and (6) fewer incidents of systemic complications due to hypoxemia, such as GI bleeding (Gruden, 1985).

The disadvantages are (1) limited use in human population—most trials until 1980 have been with animals; (2) limited availability of delivery systems; (3) limited numbers of trained personnel to observe for complications, either mechanical or physiological ones; (4) the cost of such ventilation; (5) the difficulty in exactly calculating the tidal volume and oxygen concentration being delivered, especially with high-frequency jet ventilation (Gruden, 1985); (6) lack of standard equipment for delivery or means for humidification in the delivery circuit; and (7) a high incidence of necrotizing tracheitis.

USES

High-frequency ventilation may be used for a variety of neonates. It is postulated to be especially effective in infants undergoing surgical procedures or infants with respiratory distress syndrome, acute respiratory failure, persistent pulmonary circulation, diaphragmatic hernia, or tracheal stenosis (Karl, Ballantine, & Snider, 1983; Southwell, 1986). While some centers have used this type of ventilation on infants of varying sizes and gestational ages, other institutions have very strict guidelines for its use. Most consider this an experimental treatment and require informed parental consent prior to placing the infant on this ventilatory method.

NURSING CONSIDERATIONS

The overriding concern for nurses is to promote gas exchange for the infant while providing safe patient care. A multidisciplinary approach is needed to provide holistic care. The team should consist of the nurse, physician, respiratory therapist, and parents. The ratio of nurse to patient should be one to one for these infants since they require close observation including hourly monitoring of vital signs, blood gases, central venous pressure, ventilatory settings (mean airway pressure, ambient oxygen, and rates). Safety features and standardization of equipment may vary, thus requiring close monitoring as well. Alarms may or may not be present on the ventilation circuit, so it is imperative that nurses and respiratory therapists work closely together to maintain the integrity of the equipment.

Assessment of the ventilation and the infant's respiratory status is essential since monitoring of arterial blood gases in the conventional manner may not be sufficient to determine subtle status changes. An arterial catheter should be in place for blood sampling. Transcutaneous monitoring of both oxygen and carbon dioxide levels is also recommended, especially for infants receiving oscillating ventilation. Respiratory rates are impossible to count especially if the oscillating form of ventilation is being used. The nurse should expect the infant's breath sounds to be high-pitched and loud. Extremely high-pitched breath sounds, however, may indicate the presence of secretions. A decrease in pitch may indicate a pulmonary air leak or atelectasis. Special attention should center on keeping the endotracheal tube in the proper position. If the tube rests along the wall of the trachea, ventilation may be impaired. In an infant receiving oscillation, the chest shaking may decrease and the pCO_2 may generally increase (Inwood et al., 1986).

If a question arises as to the respiratory status or presence of an air leak, a chest radiograph should be taken or a transillumination of the chest should be done (Karp et al., 1986). The infant receiving oscillation will need to be disconnected from the oscillator during the filming; otherwise, the film will be blurred.

Movement of gases at high rates also may have the side effect of mobilization of secretions. Promoting airway clearance via frequent suctioning may be needed. The ventilatory circuit should not be disconnected for the entire suctioning procedure but rather suction should be applied via the suction catheter while the catheter is being introduced. A triple-lumen endotracheal tube is used with the high-frequency jet ventilation and allows water to be instilled down one lumen without disruption of the system prior to actually suctioning the infant. This protocol will reduce the chance of a dramatic pressure decrease at the alveolar level and subsequent respiratory alveolar collapse (Olson et al., 1986; Karp et al., 1986). Any change in the amount or consistency of secretions should be reported to the physician immediately as this may be an early sign of necrotizing tracheitis.

Parents should be prepared for the noise level created by these ventilating systems. A continuous loud clicking noise is emitted during ventilation. Infants may seem more alert and awake than usual if they are not receiving sedation. Parents also need to understand the experimental nature of this form of ventilation.

REFERENCES

Respiratory Care and Suctioning

Cabal, L., Devaskar, S., Siassi, B., Piajstek, C., Waffern, G., Blanco, C., & Hodgman, J. (1979). New endotracheal tube adaptor reducing cardiopulmonary effects of suctioning. *Critical Care Medicine, 7*, 552-555.

Gunderson, L. P., McPhee, A. J., & Donovan, E. F. (1986). Partially ventilated endotracheal suction in newborn infants with respiratory distress syndrome. *American Journal of Diseases of Children, 140*, 462-465.

Norris, S., Campbell, L. A., & Brenkert, S. (1982). Nursing procedures and alterations in transcutaneous oxygen tension in premature infants. *Nursing Research, 31*, 330-336.

Severinghaus, J. W. (1982). Transcutaneous blood gas analysis. *Respiratory Care, 27*, 152-159.

Zmora, E., & Merritt, R. (1980). Use of side-hole endotracheal tube adaptor for tracheal aspiration. *American Journal of Diseases of Children, 134*, 250-254.

Extracorporeal Membrane Oxygenation

Altose, M. D., Hicks, R. W., & Edwards, J. W. (1976). Extracorporeal membrane oxygenation during bronchopulmonary lavage. *Archives of Surgery, 111*,1148-1153.

Andrews, A. F., Klein, M. D., Toomasian, J. M., Roloff, D. W., & Bartlett, R. H. (1983). Venovenous extracorporeal membrane oxygenation in neonates with respiratory failure. *Journal of Pediatric Surgery, 18*, 339-346.

Andrews, A. F., Toomasian, J., Gram, A., & Bartlett, R. H. (1982). Total respiratory support with venovenous (VV) ECMO. *Transactions—American Society of Artificial Internal Organs, 28*, 350-358.

Bartlett, R. H., Andrews, A.F. Toomasian, J. M., Haiduc, N. J., & Gazzaniga, A. (1982). Extracorporeal membrane oxygenation for newborn respiratory failure: Forty-five cases. *Surgery, 92*, 425-433.

Bartlett, R. H., Gazzaniga, A. B., Fong, S. W., Jefferies, M. E., Roonk, H. V., & Haiduc, N. (1978). Extracorporeal circulation for cardiopulmonary failure. *Current Problems in Surgery, 15*, 375-386.

Bartlett, R. H., Gazzaniga, A. B., Huxtable, R. F., Schippers, H. C., O'Conner, M. J., & Jefferies, M. R. (1977). Extracorporeal circulation (ECMO) in neonatal respiratory failure. *Journal of Thoracic and Cardiovascular Surgery, 74*, 826-833.

Bartlett, R. H., Gazzaniga, A. B., Jefferies, M. R., Huxtable, R. F., Haiduc, N., & Fong, S. W. (1976). Extracorporeal membrane oxygenation (ECMO) cardiopulmonary support in infancy. *Transactions—American Society for Artificial Internal Organs, 22*, 80-88.

Bartlett, R. H., Roloff, D. W., Corness, R. G., Andrews, A. F., Dillion, P. W., & Zwischenberger, J. B. (1985). Extracorporeal circulation in neonatal respiratory failure: A prospective randomized study. *Pediatrics, 76*, 479-487.

Extracorporeal Circulation Laboratory. (1984). *ECMO technical specialist manual* (7th ed.). Ann Arbor: University of Michigan Hospitals.

Krummel, U. M., Greenfield, L. J., Kirkpatrick, B. V., Mueller, D. G., Ormagabal, M., & Salzberg, A. M. (1982). Clinical use of an extracorporeal membrane oxygenator in neonatal pulmonary failure. *Journal of Pediatric Surgery, 17*, 525-531.

Nugent, J. (1986). Extracorporeal membrane oxygenation in the neonate. *Neonatal Network, 4*(5), 27-38.

Zapal, W. M., Snider, M. R., & Schneider, R. C. (1977). Extracorporeal membrane oxygenation for acute respiratory failure. *Anesthesiology, 46*, 272-285.

High-Frequency Ventilation

Gruden, M. A. (1985). High-frequency ventilation: An overview. *Critical Care Nurse, 5*, 36-40.

Inwood, S., Finley, G. A., & Fitzhardinge, P. M. (1986). High-frequency oscillation: A new mode of ventilation for the neonate. *Neonatal Network, 4*(5), 53-58.

Karl, S. R., Ballantine, T. V. N. & Snider, M. T. (1983). High-frequency ventilation at rates of 375 to 1800 cycles per minute in four neonates with congenital diaphragmatic hernia. *Journal of Pediatric Surgery, 18*, 822-827.

Karp, T. B., Solon, J. F., Olson, D. L., Reppucci, P. A., & Nichols, N. S. (1986). High frequency jet ventilation: A neonatal nursing perspective. *Neonatal Network, 4*(5), 42-50.

Olson, D. L., Karp, T. B., Reppucci, P. A., Solon, J. F., & Nichols, N. S. (1986). High frequency jet ventilation: Endotracheal suctioning procedure. *Neonatal Network, 4*(5), 66-68.

Southwell, S. (1986). Update on treatment of persistent pulmonary hypertension of the newborn. *Neonatal Network, 4*(5), 19-25.

Chapter 11

Diagnostic Tests

Jeanne Harjo

ᶾᵃ

ANGIOGRAM, CEREBRAL

DESCRIPTION

1. A radiopaque substance is injected into the brachial, carotid, subclavian, femoral, or vertebral artery for radiographic visualization of the brain's vascular system.

2. Used to identify vascular anomalies or lesions that are large enough to distort the cerebral vascular system.

3. Helpful in locating tumors, abscesses, intracranial hemorrhages, and occluded, narrowed, or thrombosed arteries.

PREPARATION

N.P.O. for 8-10 hours before procedure as general anesthesia will be used.

PROCEDURE

1. Infant is positioned supine.
   a. If a carotid injection, the neck is hyperextended with a rolled towel under the shoulders and the head is immobilized.
   b. With a brachial or femoral injection, immobilize involved extremity.

2. General anesthesia is given.

3. Injection site is shaved and cleaned with an antiseptic solution.

4. The placement of the catheter in the carotid, subclavian, or brachial arteries or aortic arch is confirmed by fluoroscopy. The contrast media is carried from these remote sites and into the vessels in the cranium.

5. A series of films is taken as the dye is injected from various angles.

6. The length of the procedure is from 30 minutes to 2 hours.

POSTPROCEDURAL CARE

1. Apply sterile dressing and pressure over injection site for 15 minutes to prevent bleeding and formation of hematoma.

2. Monitor vital signs closely as the infant is at risk for bleeding and a reaction to the contrast material itself. Each condition manifests with an alteration in baseline vital signs.
   a. Measure the temperature, pulse, respiration, and BP every 15 minutes four times, every 30 minutes four times, every 1 hour four times, every 2 hours four times, and then every 4 hours.
   b. Monitor the rate and quality of respirations to detect any respiratory distress.
   c. Observe for signs of alterations in the level of responsiveness or weak muscles on one side of the body, as this may indicate arterial blockage due to a thrombosis or hematoma.

3. Carotid or vertebral injections.
   a. Perform serial measurements of neck circumference to help detect any swelling.
   b. Any respiratory distress may indicate extravasation of contrast into the neck.

4. Femoral or brachial injections.
   a. Immobilize extremity for 4 hours.
   b. Observe site for bleeding or a hematoma.
   c. Check pulse distal to puncture site, and check color and temperature of extremity. These may help identify an arterial occlusion. An arterial occlusion, if not treated immediately, could result in the loss of an extremity or lead to a stroke.

Barium Enema

DESCRIPTION

1. Examination of the large intestine after instillation of a contrast solution, such as:

    a. Barium sulfate
    b. Meglucamine diatrizoate
2. May provide identification of
    a. Meconium ileus
    b. Meconium-plug syndrome
    c. Microcolon
    d. Hirschsprung's disease
       i. A transition zone can be located by evaluating postevacuation films.
      ii. Retention of barium is also an important sign of the disease.
3. This procedure should precede an upper gastrointestinal (GI) series as it may take several days for the barium to be cleared from the bowel, thus potentially interfering with radiographic studies.
4. May be performed through a colostomy prior to reanastomosis or if there is a suspected stricture or obstruction.

PREPARATION

1. No premedication.

2. NPO 4-6 hours before procedure.

PROCEDURE

1. Position neonate supine on x-ray table. Secure extremities and head to keep positioned for turning.

2. A rectal tube is inserted. Secure enema tip by taping neonate's buttocks together.

3. Instill the contrast solution into colon by gravity.

4. Under fluoroscopy, the flow of contrast is observed while rotating the patient to different positions.

5. When the colon is filled, the tube is removed; abdominal films are taken.

6. Postevacuation films are taken every 4-8 hours after the procedure until contrast solution is expelled completely.

7. The procedure may take from 30 to 45 minutes to perform.

POSTPROCEDURAL CARE

No special care is needed. If the barium is not easily expelled, cleansing enemas may be needed. Usually instillation of saline-solution enemas will clear the barium (Tapper, 1985).

Blood Culture

DESCRIPTION

1. Used to confirm bacterial, fungal, or viral infections.

2. Used to identify the causative organism of an infection.

PREPARATION

Obtain the following necessary equipment:

1. Tourniquet.

2. Alcohol swabs.

3. Povidone-iodine swabs.

4. One 3-cc or 6-cc syringe.

5. Needles, 1-3, depending upon the number of cultures required.

6. One butterfly or angiocatheter needle.

7. Appropriate culture bottles for bacterial (aerobic and anaerobic), fungal, or viral cultures.

8. Gauze sponges, 3 x 3 inch.

PROCEDURE

1. Clean the site for venipuncture with a rubbing alcohol swab.

2. Clean the site again with a povidone-iodine swab starting at the site and working away from it.

3. Allow the site to dry for 1 minute before performing the venipuncture.

4. Perform the venipuncture using a butterfly or angiocatheter, drawing 1-2 cc of blood for each culture desired.

5. Inject 1-2 cc of blood into each culture bottle changing the needle for each different specimen.

6. Cover the site with a sterile 3 x 3 inch gauze dressing.

7. Send specimens to the lab immediately after labeling with the proper infant identification, including the puncture site.

POSTPROCEDURAL CARE

1. Observe for hematoma at the site of the venipuncture.

2. Apply warm normal saline soaked gauze as necessary when bleeding has stopped.

Bronchogram

DESCRIPTION

1. Instillation of radiopaque material into the trachea and bronchi to allow x-ray visualization of the entire tracheobronchial tree.

2. Evaluation of congenital defects or airway problems that may have resulted in damaged pulmonary structures.

3. May detect recurrent pneumonia, bronchiectasis, bronchial obstructions, pulmonary tumors, or cysts.

PREPARATION

1. NPO 4 hours prior to procedure.

2. Atropine may be given to decrease secretions.

3. A narcotic analgesic may be given for sedation and to potentiate anesthesia.

PROCEDURE

1. An endotracheal airway is inserted and general anesthesia is given.

2. An opaque catheter is inserted through the endotracheal tube.

3. A small amount of contrast solution, usually 0.5 cc of barium that has been diluted, is instilled under fluoroscopy, so that the material is placed into selected areas and in the quantities desired (Heller & Kirchner, 1979).

4. The infant is tilted into various positions to allow the contrast to run throughout the entire tracheobronchial tree.

5. A series of spot films are taken.

6. This entire procedure takes about 1 hour.

POSTPROCEDURAL CARE

1. Prevent aspiration:
   a. NPO 4-6 hours after the procedure.
   b. Position the infant from side to side every 2 hours.
   c. Perform postural drainage, chest physiotherapy, and suction every 2 hours.

2. Observe for atelectasis or bacterial or chemical pneumonia. Monitor vital signs every 1 hour four times. Check for:
   a. Increased temperature
   b. Rales or rhonchi
   c. Chest retractions

3. Observe for laryngeal spasms or edema, indicated by:
   a. Retractions
   b. Hoarseness
   c. Stridor

Bronchoscopy

DESCRIPTION

1. The tracheobronchial tree can be directly visualized with the introduction of a special lighted fiberoptic scope.

2. Congenital anomalies, obstructions, or tumors can be evaluated.

3. Samples for cultures or biopsy specimens of lung tissue can be obtained.

4. Bleeding sites can be located.

5. Mucus plugs can be removed.

PREPARATION

1. NPO 4-6 hours prior to procedure.

2. Adminster atropine:
   a. Decreases bronchial secretions
   b. Relaxes bronchial smooth muscle
   c. Lessens risks of postbronchoscopy laryngospasm

3. Administer narcotic analgesia:
   a. Sedates and relaxes the infant
   b. Alleviates coughing and gagging

4. Perform clotting studies if biopsy is to be done.

PROCEDURE

1. Anesthesia is given.

2. Position infant supine with neck hyperextended and with head slightly elevated.

3. Bronchoscope is inserted into the trachea and newborn's head is moved from side to side to ease passage into the two main bronchi.

4. The trachea and the bronchi are inspected and the carina is checked for position and mobility.

5. The infant's color, pulse, and respirations are carefully monitored as hypoxia may occur.

6. The procedure will usually take 30 minutes.

POSTPROCEDURAL CARE

1. NPO until awake and bowel sounds return in 6-8 hours.

2. Monitor vital signs, especially respiratory effort, every 15 minutes four times, every 30 minutes four times, every 1 hour four times, every 2 hours four times, and then every 4 hours.

3. Observe for laryngeal spasms or laryngeal edema:
   a. Stridor
   b. Chest retractions
   c. Either cool or warm mist may be used to lessen postbronchoscopy edema. The choice of warm or cool mist is up to the physician's discretion as opinions differ on the best treatment.

4. Observe for pneumothorax:
   a. Chest retractions
   b. Cyanosis
   c. Decreased breath sounds

5. Observe for bronchospasms:
   a. Chest retractions
   b. Wheezing

6. Observe for bleeding:
   a. There may be slightly blood-tinged secretions.
   b. Frank bleeding is not normal.

Cardiac Catheterization

DESCRIPTION

1. Introduction of a radiopaque catheter into the right or left side of the heart.

2. Catheter is inserted into an arm or leg vessel by percutaneous puncture or cutdown and is passed under flouroscopy into the heart.

3. Allows collection of blood samples to check oxygen saturation.

4. Allows intracardiac pressures to be recorded.

5. Facilitates injection of radiopaque dye into the selected chambers and vessels of the heart to help diagnose and clarify congenital heart defects.

PREPARATION

1. NPO 4-6 hours prior to procedure.

2. Infant may require sedation.

PROCEDURE

1. Position infant in supine position and restrain as needed.

2. Place electrocardiographic electrodes for continuous monitoring during procedure.

3. Administer lidocaine or other local anesthesia to chosen site.

4. Percutaneous puncture or cutdown is performed at site and catheter inserted.

5. Catheter is guided by flouroscopy to the chambers of the heart and to the vessels of the heart.

6. When the catheter is in place, contrast media is injected to visualize the cardiac vessels and the cardiac structures.

7. When all the necessary information is obtained, the catheter is removed.
   a. The cutdown vein is ligated and the skin is sutured.
   b. An arterial cutdown requires repair of the artery and skin with sutures.
   c. If the vessel was entered by a percutaneous puncture, pressure over the entry site is required to form a clot at the site.

8. The length of this procedure is from 30 minutes to 3 hours.

POSTPROCEDURAL CARE

1. Monitor vital signs every 15 minutes four times, every 30 minutes four times, every hour four times, every 2 hours four times, and then every 4 hours. Check BP and heart rate for signs of hypotension related to blood loss and dysrhythmic heart patterns due to the disturbance of the pacemaker of the heart.

2. Restrain the catheterized limb and keep straight for 6-8 hours.

3. Apply antibiotic ointment at the entry site and cover with a sterile 3 x 3 inch gauze pressure dressing to prevent bleeding and infection.
   a. Check site for hematoma or bleeding.
   b. Change dressings every 2-4 hours as needed.

4. Check color, skin temperature, pulses, and capillary refill distal to puncture site.

5. Assess infant for signs of complications secondary to the procedure. Common complications include bleeding and infection at the site of catheter entry, as mentioned above. But other complications include fluid shifts, hypotension, vascular compromise, and metabolic disturbance—especially acidosis and dysrhythmia due to placement of catheter and disturbance of the sinoatrial node.
   a. The contrast dye may be hyperosmotic in nature thus pulling fluid into the vascular space. An osmotic gradient is created and diuresis may take place.
   b. Administration of peripheral fluids may be necessary to compensate for this fluid loss and shift the fluid from vascular space.
   c. Renal function must be monitored in the form of accurate intake and output along with specific gravity since it is the kidney that detoxifies the dye.

6. Monitor arterial gases at least hourly in the immediate postprocedural period. Monitor gases more frequently if hypoxemia or acidosis is present or was present prior to the catheterization.

Cerebral Computed Tomographic Scanning

DESCRIPTION

1. The scanner passes over the infant to obtain a series of radiation-intensity measurements. Information is fed into a computer that reconstructs it into a three-dimensional image.

2. Water-soluble contrast media may be injected IV to improve the visualization of suspected anomalies.

3. Areas of lower density are found in edema of the brain as found in infarcts or contusions.

4. High-density areas:
   a. Cerebral hemorrhage
   b. Calcifications
   c. Solid or vascular tumors
   d. Vascular malformations
   e. Abscesses

PREPARATION

1. NPO 4-6 hours prior to procedure.

2. Newborn may require sedation 20-30 minutes prior to procedure to minimize movements that may prevent accurate scanning.

PROCEDURE

1. Place the infant in a supine position.

2. Immobilize the infant with a strap fitted snugly around the infant's head.

3. Restrain the extremities as necessary.

4. Scanner is rotated slowly 180° around infant's head in different planes, and readings are taken at every degree.

5. Contrast media is injected and scanner repeats as above. Observe for reaction to contrast, such as rash or respiratory distress.

6. Absorption density of the tissues is recorded.

7. When the scan is completed, the computer produces an image from the densities presented.

8. Photographs are taken of the image on the screen for a permanent record that can later be interpreted.

POSTPROCEDURAL CARE

1. Resume feedings upon the infant's return to the unit.

2. No other special care is required.

Cystoscopy

DESCRIPTION

1. Allows direct visualization of the bladder, urethra, and urethral orifices.

2. Used to evaluate congenital abnormalities or acquired lesions in the bladder and the lower urinary tract.

PREPARATION

1. NPO 4-6 hours prior to procedure
2. Preoperative sedation to enhance general anesthesia

PROCEDURE

1. Insertion of IV line and administration of anesthesia.
2. Position infant on the cystoscopy table.
3. Prepare the urethral orifice with an antiseptic solution and apply sterile drapes.
4. The lubricated cystoscope is inserted into the bladder through the urethra.
5. Visualization of the bladder, urethra, and urethral orifices is performed.
6. Cystoscope is then removed.
7. The procedure will last from 15-45 minutes depending upon the problems and difficulties encountered in insertion of the cystoscope.

POSTPROCEDURAL CARE

1. Monitor vital signs every 15 minutes four times, every 30 minutes four times, every 1 hour four times, every 2 hours four times, and then every 4 hours.
2. Monitor urine output every 1-2 hours.
   a. Report any output < 1 cc/ kg/ h.
   b. Note any hematuria.
3. Resume feedings when newborn is awake and bowel sounds return.

Echocardiogram

DESCRIPTION

1. Using high-frequency sound wave vibrations sent into the heart through the chest wall, recordings are made of the motion of the mitral, aortic, tricuspid, and pulmonic valves. The intraventricular septum and the left and right ventricles are evaluated.
2. It is a diagnostic tool for congenital heart disease, congestive heart failure,

atrial or ventricular septal defects, cardiac valve problems, vegetation due to infection, intracardiac tumors or hematoma, and patent ductus ateriosus.

3. Assesses the results of cardiac surgery.

4. May determine the timing of cardiac catheterization.

PREPARATION

1. No premedications required.

2. No dietary restrictions.

PROCEDURE

1. Place newborn in supine position.

2. Supply a pacifier to help minimize movement.

3. A water-soluble gel is applied to the skin of the chest wall and to the face of the transducer.

4. The transducer is placed firmly on the chest and moved back and forth in various directions and at different angles.

POSTPROCEDURAL CARE

1. Resume previous care.

2. Completely remove gel from skin.

Electroencephalogram

DESCRIPTION

1. Electrical activity of the brain is recorded.

2. May aid in diagnosis of intracranial lesions such as abscesses or tumors.

3. Valuable in localizing focal point of seizures.

4. Determines damaged or nonfunctioning areas of the brain.

5. Follows progress after an infection such as meningitis or encephalitis.

6. Used to confirm brain death.

PREPARATION

1. Newborn should not be made NPO. Hypoglycemia may alter a normal electrical pattern.

2. If ordered, withhold anticonvulsant medications 24-48 hours prior to procedure.

3. Infant may require sedation to prevent crying and excessive activity during the procedure.

4. Maintain the newborn's normal body temperature, as hypothermia can alter results.

PROCEDURE

1. Place infant in a supine position.

2. Use a room that is dimly lit and with external distractions at a minimum.

3. Ten to 20 electrodes are secured to the head with collodion or paste evenly distributed over the entire scalp.

4. Give a feeding or a pacifier to keep the infant still.

5. Readings are taken while infant is awake and continue as child falls asleep.

6. Recordings taken when child is hyperventilating at rates >60/min for 3 minutes may be helpful. The resulting alkalolsis may accentuate any abnormal brain activity.

7. If there is a history of seizures, monitor closely for this activity. Be prepared to administer phenobarbital or phenytoin (Dilantin) as needed.

POSTPROCEDURAL CARE

1. Resume medications as ordered.

2. Observe for seizure activity.

3. Remove electrode paste.

Excretory Urogram and Intravenous Pyleogram

DESCRIPTION

1. Radiographic examination of the kidneys, ureters, and bladder after IV injection of contrast media.

2. It is usually the initial investigation of any suspected urological problem.

3. The contrast substance is excreted by the kidneys, making the urinary tract visible in radiographic films.

4. The size, shape, and position of organs are revealed in addition to the rate of excretion of the media.

PREPARATION

1. NPO 6-8 hours prior to procedure.

2. Feces or gas in the GI tract or a recent barium study result in films of poor quality and cause inaccurate interpretation. Cleansing enemas with a saline solution may be necessary to evacuate the barium (Tapper, 1985).

PROCEDURE

1. Place the infant in the supine position and restrain as needed.

2. A small amount of media is injected IV.

3. Films are taken after the newborn voids. This gives information about renal mobility and the ability of the kidneys and bladder to empty.

POSTPROCEDURAL CARE

1. No special care.

2. Resume feedings.

INTERPRETATION

1. Bilateral enlarged renal shadows are seen in nephrotic syndrome and polycystic disease.

2. Small kidneys suggest congenital dysplasia.

3. A single enlarged kidney may be the result of a partial ureteral obstruction, inflammatory disease, bleeding, tumor, or unilateral cystic disease.

4. One small kidney shows dysplasia or atrophy.

Laryngoscopy

DESCRIPTION

1. Direct visualization of the larynx using a laryngoscope, a hollow, rigid tube lighted at the distal end.

2. Evaluation of stridor and determination of the presence of inflammation.

3. Allows the biopsy of tissue or removal of mucus plugs.

4. Insertion of an endotracheal tube.

PREPARATION

1. Position the newborn supine with head slightly extended with jaw thrust forward, avoiding excessive extension.

2. General anesthesia is administered.

3. Laryngoscope is passed into the right side of the mouth and down to the larynx under direct vision.

4. The larynx is examined and a biopsy is performed or mucus plugs are removed.

5. An endotracheal tube is passed between the vocal cords under direct vision.

POSTPROCEDURAL CARE

See Bronchoscopy (p. 325) in this chapter.

Lumbar Puncture

DESCRIPTION

1. A hollow needle (spinal needle with stylet, size 22 gauge, 1 ½ inch) is inserted into the lumbar space of the spinal cord. Cerebrospinal fluid (CSF) is withdrawn for diagnostic and therapeutic purposes.

2. This is one of the simplest and most informative neurological diagnostic tests.
   a. Used to evaluate and relieve intracranial pressure.
   b. Cerebrospinal fluid can be obtained for culture, cell count, and sugar and protein counts.
   c. Used to identify intracranial hemorrhage.

PREPARATION

1. No premedication

2. No dietary restriction, although one feeding may be withheld prior to the procedure

PROCEDURE

1. Position the newborn in the sitting position or lateral recumbent.

2. Restraint is imperative for the success of this procedure.

3. Position the newborn with knees flexed on abdomen and head flexed with chin to chest. This separates the vertebrae and increases the position between them.

4. The skin is cleansed with povidone-iodine and rubbing alcohol. Sterile drapes are positioned. The physician wears sterile gloves and maintains sterile technique.

5. The spinal needle is inserted between the third and fourth lumbar vertebrae. Once the needle is positioned, the stylet is removed and fluid is allowed to drip into three sterile test tubes placing 1 cc in each tube. Pressure may be measured with a manometer before and after removal of CSF.

6. After the necessary specimens and pressures are obtained, the needle is quickly withdrawn and pressure is applied for several minutes with sterile gauze. A bandage is placed over the puncture site.

7. Monitor respiratory status closely and administer oxygen as necessary.

POSTPROCEDURAL CARE

1. Reposition the newborn in normal alignment.

2. Resume feedings.

3. Observe and report any leakage from puncture site.

4. The procedure will take between 10 and 30 minutes depending upon the difficulty of placing the needle and the speed at which CSF drips from the spinal canal.

Pneumoencephalogram

DESCRIPTION

1. Withdrawal of CSF and injection of air by lumbar puncture.

2. Since air is lighter than CSF it rises into the ventricular system.

3. Diagnostic of degenerative cerebral atrophy and detects masses along the brain stem or at the base of the brain, areas not seen well on CT scan.

4. This test is not used as frequently now that CT scans are available.

5. The disadvantages are (1) it is an invasive technique; (2) it requires a lumbar puncture with all its risks of infection or damage to the neurological function; (3) if increased intracranial pressure is present, injection of air into these areas may be difficult if not impossible since the space for the air is already filled with CSF; and (4) any time air is injected there is a risk of an air embolus.

6. Contraindications: the physician may suggest that the test not be done if increased intracranial pressure or meningitis is present or if a central nervous system infection is suspected.

PREPARATION

1. Preoperative sedation may be necessary.

2. NPO for 6-8 hours.

PROCEDURE

1. General anesthesia may be used.

2. The infant is positioned and prepared as for a lumbar puncture.

3. Free flow of CSF is established and air is injected in 5- 10-cc increments. Injection of air is continued until 20-30 cc has been injected to allow adequate filling of the ventricular system.

4. The needle is removed as with a lumbar puncture.

5. Radiographs are taken with the infant's position rotated from head up to head down to allow the air to flow from one ventricle to another.

6. This procedure takes 2-4 hours.

POSTPROCEDURAL CARE

1. Keep the newborn flat for 24 hours. Turn the newborn from side to side every 2 hours to help disperse the air.

2. Monitor vital signs and check neurological signs every 30 minutes for 2 hours, then every 1-2 hours for a 24-hour period, and then every 4 hours.

3. Minimal handling is important to decrease external stimuli as increased irritability to stimuli may follow this test.

Radioisotope Brain Scan

DESCRIPTION

1. Intravenous injection of radioactive solution and application of a radiation counter to scan the brain, showing an increased uptake of the radioactive material at the site of pathology.

2. Test material tends to accumulate in areas of tumors and around abscesses.
   a. Detects certain local brain lesions.
   b. Detects abscesses from central nervous system infections such as candidiasis.

3. Positive uptake with encephalitis, subdural hematomas, and cerebral infarcts due to vascular occlusion.

4. Allows evaluation of seizures and other neurological symptoms that could indicate central nervous system disease.

5. Results may be compared with those of a CT scan.

PREPARATION

1. No premedication required.

2. No dietary restrictions.

3. Many institutions require an informed consent any time radioisotopes are to be injected. Consult hospital policy.

PROCEDURE

1. Intravenous injection of the material.
2. Position the newborn supine and restrain to keep still.

3. Multiple imaging views are taken at 10, 30, and 60 minutes. Views of frontal, posterior and both lateral positions are recorded.

4. Delayed imaging is done 2 hours after injection.

5. Early scans show information concerning cerebral blood flow.

6. Late scans define alterations in blood-brain permeability. Normal brain tissue does not allow passage of radioactive material from the plasma.

7. The length of the procedure is from 1 to 2 hours.

POSTPROCEDURAL CARE

No special care is needed.

Radioisotope Renal Scan

DESCRIPTION

1. After IV injection of the radioisotope, sites over both kidneys are monitored with radioactive counters.

2. Records the difference between the two kidneys with respect to blood flow, tubular function, and excretion.

3. Delineates the structure and function of the kidneys without disturbing normal physiological processes.

PREPARATION

1. No premedication needed.

2. No dietary restrictions.

3. Informed consent may be required for the injection of radioisotopes. Consult hospital policy.

PROCEDURES

1. Intravenous injection of the radioactive material.

2. Position infant and restrain as necessary.

3. Serial films are taken every 3-5 minutes for a period of 30 minutes.

4. Delayed films are taken several hours after injection to visualize poorly functioning kidneys.

POSTPROCEDURAL CARE

1. Wear gloves when changing diapers within 24 hours after the procedure.
2. Use special containers for linens and trash for the first 24 hours after the procedure.

Rectal Suction Biopsy

DESCRIPTION

1. Identifies the absences of or a reduction in ganglion cells in the bowel.
2. Diagnostic test for Hirschsprung's disease.

PREPARATION

1. No premedication required. While more research is being done regarding neonatal pain and the use of pain medications, no pain medication is used for neonates at many institutions even if the procedure is done at the bedside. This procedure may be carried out in the operating room, however, where an anesthetic most likely will be used.
2. No special dietary restrictions are necessary unless the infant is to have anesthesia. If anesthesia is to be used, the infant should be NPO for at least 4 hours prior to the test.

PROCEDURE

1. Infant is positioned supine and legs held up toward abdomen.
2. Using suction apparatus, small pieces of rectal tissue are excised.
   a. These pieces are taken for the mucosa and submucosa specimens.
   b. Specimens are taken from varying depths.
3. The specimens are taken to pathology where they are examined microscopically to determine the absence or presence of ganglion cells.

POSTPROCEDURAL CARE

1. Observe and report any rectal bleeding.
   a. This may occur for 2-3 stools after the procedure.
   b. Report any massive bleeding that may require rectal packing to stop bleeding.

2. Watch for signs of intestinal perforation or sepsis:
   a. Fever
   b. Increased heart rate
   c. Decreased BP
   d. Abdominal distention, firmness, or redness
   e. Guaiac-positive stools persisting
   f. Rectal bleeding

Retrograde Pyelogram

DESCRIPTION

1. Injection of radiopaque material through the ureteral catheter during a cystoscopy.
2. Examination of the entire renal collecting system.

PREPARATION

1. If general anesthesia is used, preoperative sedative may be given.
2. NPO 6-8 hours if general anesthesia is used.

PROCEDURE

1. General anesthesia is given.
2. Cystoscopy is performed and one or both ureters are catheterized with opaque catheters, depending upon the condition or abnormalities suspected. This allows for correct positioning of catheter tip in the renal pelvis.
3. The kidney is emptied and 4-5 cc of contrast material is injected through the catheters.
4. When adequate filling has occurred, anterioposterior, lateral, and oblique films are taken.

5. After examination of the renal pelvis is complete, 1-2 cc of contrast solution is injected to outline the ureters as the catheters are slowly withdrawn.

6. Delayed films taken at 10-15 minutes after the catheter is completely removed to check for retention.

7. If ureteral obstruction is found, ureteral catheters may be kept in place and with a Foley catheter are connected to gravity drainage systems until urinary flow returns to normal.

8. The procedure takes about 1 hour.

POSTPROCEDURAL CARE

1. Monitor vital signs every 15 minutes four times, every 30 minutes four times, every 1 hour four times, every 2 hours until stable, and then every 4 hours.

2. Monitor urinary output closely:
   a. Measure output and report any urine < 1 cc/kg/h.
   b. Check urine for blood. If bleeding occurs after the third void, this is abnormal and should be reported.
   c. Notify the physician if the infant has not voided in 4-8 hours or if the bladder becomes distended.

3. Secure catheters and position to allow drainage by gravity.

4. Observe and report any signs of sepsis:
   a. Fever
   b. Increased heart rate
   c. Decreased BP
   d. Cloudy urine

Suprapubic Tap

DESCRIPTION

1. Bladder aspiration for obtaining urinary cultures.

2. Some physicians feel this procedure is a safe, easy procedure without the complications associated with catheterization.

PREPARATION

1. No special preparation.

2. Do not perform if the infant has just voided.

3. Do not attempt if the infant has dilated bowel loops.

PROCEDURE

1. Infant is placed supine with restraints as needed.

2. The lower abdomen is cleaned with an antiseptic solution as for any venipuncture.

3. Locate the symphysis pubis.

4. Puncture the abdomen:
   a. Use a 3-, 6-, or 12-cc syringe with a size 22 gauge, 1-inch needle.
   b. Puncture in the midline approximately 1-2 cm above the symphysis.
   c. Angle the needle about 30° toward the fundus and advance into the bladder.

5. Withdraw the urine needed:
   a. Minimal pressure is needed to withdraw the urine.
   b. Needle is withdrawn.
   c. Apply pressure until any bleeding stops.

POSTPROCEDURAL CARE

1. No dressing is usually needed.

2. Observe for blood in urine—abnormal if seen after the third void.

Sweat Chloride—Iontophoresis

DESCRIPTION

1. Measurement of chloride and sodium in sweat

2. Diagnostic for cystic fibrosis

3. The safest and most reliable test for testing the neonate for cystic fibrosis

PREPARATION

1. No special premedication.

2. No dietary restrictions.

3. The most reliable results are usually obtained after 6 weeks of age when the infant produces more sweat.

PROCEDURE

1. Clean the area on the infant to be used—the thigh, forearm, or back—with sterile water.
2. An electrical current drives pilocarpine into the skin.
   a. Done for 5-10 minutes to stimulate local sweating
   b. May need external heat sources to increase sweat production
3. The specimen is absorbed into gauze or filter paper that has been previously weighed so that the amount of sweat can be accurately determined.
4. The gauze is returned to the lab and chloride and sodium values are measured. Care must be taken to avoid contamination or evaporation of the specimen.
5. Test results of sweat chloride > 60 mEq/L are consistent with cystic fibrosis.

POSTPROCEDURAL CARE

No special care is required.

Ultrasound

DESCRIPTION

1. Sound waves are emitted by a transducer and travel through the tissues. Their echoes are reflected back to the transducer, which also functions as a receiver. These echoes are displayed on an oscilloscope, on photographic paper or film.
2. Abdominal ultrasonogram.
   a. Detects space containing lesions of the abdomen.
   b. Evaluates the liver, gallbladder, and biliary system.
3. Head ultrasonogram.
   a. Shows ventricular size.
   b. Detects intracranial hemorrhage.
   c. Locates masses.
4. Renal ultrasonogram.

a. Shows the size, shape, and position of the kidneys.
b. Locates urinary obstruction.
c. Detects abnormal accumulation of fluid such as residual urine in the bladder.
d. Differentiates between solid masses and cystic lesions.
e. Shows hydronephrosis or dysplasia.

PREPARATION

1. No premedication.

2. No dietary restrictions except if the gallbladder is being evaluated; then NPO 4-6 hours prior to procedure.

PROCEDURE

1. Position the patient:
   a. Supine for abdominal and head ultrasonograms.
   b. Prone, if possible, for kidney ultrasonograms.

2. Warm water-soluble gel is applied to area to be evaluated. The transducer is placed over the prepared area and is passed vertically and horizontally until the needed information is obtained.

POSTPROCEDURAL CARE

1. Remove gel from area tested.

2. Resume diet if NPO.

Upper Gastrointestinal Series with Small Bowel Follow Through

---

DESCRIPTION

1. Barium sulfate or other water-soluble contrast solution is swallowed for study of the upper GI tract.

2. Evaluation of the esophagus:
   a. Patency and diameter are examined.
   b. May indicate anatomical or functional obstruction.

   c. Gastroesophageal reflux can be found.

   d. Esophageal atresia, stenosis, or fistula can be identified.

   e. Shows abnormal swallowing mechanisms.

3. Examination of the stomach:
   a. Patency, motility, and thickness of the gastric wall can be evaluated.
   b. Anatomic abnormalities such as perforation or pyloric stenosis are seen.

4. The small intestine is studied:
   a. Visualizes the duodenum, jejunum, and ileum.
   b. Stenosis, atresia, or perforation can be seen.

PROCEDURE

1. Contrast media is ingested by swallowing or through a nasogastric tube. If a tracheoesophageal fistula is suspected, give no more than 0.5 cc of contrast solution to avoid tracheal aspiration.

2. Follow-up films are needed at half-hour intervals to determine the rate of gastric emptying and the degree of small bowel motility.

3. The procedure takes between 30 minutes to 4 hours depending upon the small bowel follow through.

POSTPROCEDURAL CARE

1. Infant may resume diet after small bowel follow through is finished.

2. No further special care is needed.

Voiding Cystourethorogram

DESCRIPTION

1. Instillation of a radiopaque contrast material through a catheter to visualize the lower urinary tract

2. Evaluations:
   a. Neurogenic bladder with urinary retention
   b. Vesicoureteral reflux
   c. Posterior ureteral valve obstruction

PREPARATION

1. No premedication
2. No dietary restrictions

PROCEDURE

1. After the neonate voids and bladder is empty, a urinary catheter is inserted into the bladder and the bladder is emptied completely.
2. Radiopaque material is slowly instilled through the catheter and the catheter is removed.
3. Films are taken during and after voiding usually with fluoroscopy:
   a. In supine position to provide anterioposterior (AP) view
   b. Left-to-right semilateral positions
   c. After bladder is completely emptied to show any retention of the contrast or if any has refluxed into the kidney

POSTPROCEDURAL CARE

1. Watch for signs of infection from catheterization:
   a. Fever
   b. Increased heart rate
   c. Cloudy urine
2. Observe for blood in urine—abnormal after the third void.
3. Report if the infant has not voided after 8 hours.

REFERENCES

Behrman, R., & Vaughan,V. (1983). *Nelson's textbook of pediatrics.* Philadelphia: W. B. Saunders.

Droske, S., & Francis, S. (1981). *Pediatric diagnostic procedures.* New York: John Wiley & Sons.

Filston, H. (1982). *Surgical problems in children: Recognition and referral.* St. Louis: C. V. Mosby.

Heller, R. M., & Kirchner, S. G. (1979). *Advanced exercises in diagnostic radiology.* Philadelphia: W. B. Saunders.

Klaus, M., & Fanaroff, A. (1986). *Care of the high risk neonate* (3rd ed.). Philadelphia: W. B. Saunders.

Professional Education Committee (1974). *Guide to Diagnosis and Management of Cystic Fibrosis.* Atlanta: Cystic Fibrosis Foundation.

Tapper, D. (1985). Surgical emergencies in the newborn. In J. P. Cloherty & A.R Stark (Eds.). *Manual of neonatal care* (pp. 395-408). Boston: Little, Brown & Co.

The Nurse's Reference Library—Diagnostics. (1981). Nursing '81 Books. Springhouse, PA: Intermed Communication.

Chapter 12

Procedures

Jeanne Harjo   *Ann Brueggemeyer*
Patricia Gorgone

This chapter describes procedures that might be required for the care of the newborn while in the hospital or once discharged to home. Some of these procedures may need to be taught to the parents in preparation for discharge. This is not meant to be an all-inclusive set of procedures but represents the most common ones.

Gastrostomy Care
Jeanne Harjo

There are several types of gastrostomy tubes available for the neonate. The most common are the mushroom (with basket device to hold tube in place) or the Foley catheter. Other tubes include the percutaneous transpyloric tube and The Button® tube. These tubes are currently used less frequently in the very small infant. The Button® gastrostomy is used mostly for long-term gastrostomy patients. Its appearance resembles a button with a cylinder that slips directly into the stoma. Initially this device is inserted with an obturator. The button is the only visible part of the device on the infant. This button is then removed whenever a feeding tube is attached. The main advantage is that the the infant does not need extra tubing dangling from the stoma unless a feeding is taking place. There is an internal valve that prevents reflux of formula. This tube may be used for gastric decompression as well as feeding. The disadvantage to this system is that a specialized decompression or feeding tube must be purchased. At present this Button® comes in sizes for the pediatric population that may be too large for the very small infant. The cost of the total system is around $150.

Neonatal Surgery: A Nursing Perspective
ISBN 0-8089-1893-1

The transpyloric tube may be used in an infant who is experiencing symptoms of upper bowel obstruction secondary to tube slippage. A second consideration of this tube is the inclusion of a plastic support ring that may help to prevent pressure on the abdominal site and allows air to circulate around the gastrostomy site. (MIC® Gastrostomy Tube is of this variety.) But more importantly this ring locks the tube in place. A balloon is inflated at the tube's end to further ensure the tube's placement and prevents reflux of formula around the tube. This tube may be used for decompression as well as feedings. The cost of this system is around $40.

Other infants experiencing problems with abdominal skin breakdown may benefit from the use of a new type of gastrostomy tube that adheres to the skin via an adhesive shield much like skin barriers used for colostomy bags. One disadvantage of this type is that the adhesive shield is relatively large in relation to the abdominal surface area of a small infant.

When preparing parents for the infant's discharge, consideration should also be given to cost. Most manufacturers of gastrostomy tubes have toll-free numbers available so that questions regarding product information and cost can be easily obtained.

Tube Care

1. Equipment (some new tubes on the market are designed so as not to require a dressing):
   a. Tape: ½-inch adhesive tape (2-3 strips each approximately 3 inches long), 1-inch paper tape (5-6 strips each approximately 3 inches long)
   b. Hydrogen peroxide
   c. Cotton-tipped applicators
   d. Soft washcloth or gauze
   e. Sterile, disposable infant bottle nipple
   f. Scissors
   g. Small, clean container for hydrogen peroxide
   h. Split 2 X 2 inch gauze dressing
   i. A skin barrier to avoid skin irritation, if needed

2. Preparation:
   a. Wash hands.
   b. Cut tape strips.
   c. Pour a small amount of hydrogen peroxide into sterile container.
   d. Cut sterile, disposable nipple (standard infant formula nipple) for use as support, using only the rubber portion:
      i. Cut off tip of nipple providing hole large enough to thread gastrostomy tube through it.
      ii. Cut small holes on opposite sides of the nipple to allow for air circulation.

3. Procedure:
   a. Remove tapes, dressings, and rubber nipple from infant:
      i. Stabilize gastrostomy tube while carefully removing tapes and dressing.
     ii. Remove old adhesive tape by pulling off from top to bottom to prevent accidental removal of tube.
   b. Clean baby's skin and tube with hydrogen peroxide, using applicators until drainage and mucus is removed.
   c. Dry the skin with a clean cloth and apply skin barrier if needed.
   d. Apply strips of adhesive tape along the tube and over the abdomen. Do not spiral the tape around the tube. Bend adhesive tape back on itself at the top for approximately 1 cm to allow a tab for easy removal.
   e. Apply dry gauze split dressing around tube if necessary.
   f. Slide rubber nipple in place over tube and secure over abdomen or dressing with paper tape. This may prevent the tube from bending on itself or becoming dislodged. Some new tubes may not require this support if the tube itself has a built-in support ring.
   g. Tape junction of rubber nipple and tube to help keep baby from pulling out the tube. (See Fig. 12-1.)

4. The baby may lay prone to sleep unless otherwise indicated.

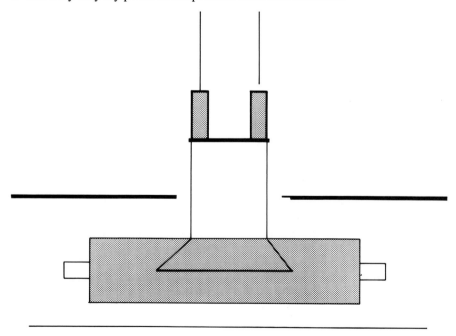

GASTROSTOMY TUBE AND DRESSING

Fig. 12-1.　Gastrostomy tube and dressing.

Note: Sometimes granulation tissue grows up around the base of the gastrostomy tube. This may have an increased discharge or may bleed when touched. Placing dry gauze around this tissue will help dry it. A green mucousy discharge is normal. If you find it increasing in amount or becoming foul-smelling clean the gastrostomy tube two or three times a day instead of once a day until the discharge improves. These changes should be reported to the physician.

When the tube is unintentionally removed, it must be replaced. This situation is not life-threatening; however, the longer the tube is out, the more difficult it is to replace without trauma. If this occurs in the hospital, follow hospital protocol (e.g., call the physician or reinsert the tube yourself). Parents may be taught to reinsert the tube at home if according to the physician's preference. If the infant must return to hospital or clinic for tube reinsertion, then a clean dressing should cover the opening. It is not unusual for formula to leak from the opening. The old tube should be brought from home to replace it with the same size tube.

Tube Feeding

1. Equipment:
   a. 35-cc catheter tipped syringe or large syringe with adaptor
   b. Formula

2. Preparation:
   a. Wash hands.
   b. Make sure the baby is clean and dry.

3. Procedure:
   a. Connect gastrostomy tube to syringe while clamp is still in place.
   b. Open clamp and pull back on plunger of syringe to aspirate contents of the stomach.
   c. Reinsert aspirate. If there is more than one fourth of the amount of the last feeding, reinsert formula and recheck in 1 hour. If a large amount persists, skip one feeding. If this happens frequently, call the physician. Large aspirate that persists may be an indication of impending illness.
   d. Reclamp tube and remove syringe from tube.
   e. Remove plunger and put empty syringe barrel on gastrostomy tube and unclamp tube.
   f. Pour formula into the syringe. Formula should flow into tube. If not, use a plunger to give a gentle push to start the formula flowing, but do not continue to push. Remove the plunger.
      i. Formula should flow slowly by gravity over 20 minutes.
      ii. Control flow rate by the height of the syringe; elevate to flow faster and lower to flow slower. If needed to slow the flow more, pinch tube with fingers. Feeding the baby too fast may cause diarrhea or vomiting.
   g. Observe the infant closely during feeding.
   h. Rinse the tube with 5 cc of water after feeding.

i. Reclamp gastrostomy tube if no gagging or vomiting has occurred.
j. Offer a pacifier during the feeding to encourage sucking, correlating oral stimulation and satiation of hunger.
k. Burp infant after feeding.
l. Wash equipment with hot soapy water and rinse well—syringes may be reused.

Note: Solids may also be included in feeding the infant. Any solids used must be fully mixed with formula before they are placed into the gastrostomy tube. If solids are used, it may slow the flow of the feeding and require the use of the plunger to push the solution through the tube. Never push hard or fast, and stop feeding if the infant's abdomen becomes distended or the infant becomes fussy.

Central-Venous Line Care

Patricia Gorgone

DESCRIPTION AND TYPE OF FLUIDS

A central venous catheter is defined as an indwelling catheter with the tip in a major vessel. This includes catheters inserted via the umbilical vein. The most common central line is a percutaneously tunneled silastic catheter whose tip is in the superior vena cava. This catheter is used for long-term parenteral therapy. The fluid may be dextrose ≥ 10 percent with amino acids, multivitamins, and trace elements—hyperalimentation fluids as well as 10-20 percent intralipids. The duration for a central venous line is between 1 month and 1 year. Umbilical lines are used for short-term therapy of approximately 5 days.

COMPLICATIONS

1. Septicemia (an infection of the blood):
   a. Symptoms: generally fever or temperature instability is the first sign.
   b. Diagnosis: Positive blood culture results and a fever spike without other source of infection.
   c. Treatment:
      i. Antibiotic therapy or line removal or both.
      ii. Treatment depends on the type of microorganism and patient's response to therapy.
   d. Prevention:
      i. Nurses that are responsible for central-line care should participate in a central-line workshop that includes a skill's performance evaluation.

    ii. Strict adherence to a central-line protocol and handwashing before and after all central line procedures.

2. Catheter site infection (localized infection of the catheter exit site):
   a. Symptoms: inflammation around exit site.
   b. Diagnosis: positive site culture results.
   c. Treatment:
      i. Daily dressing changes may help to reduce the chance of infection.
      ii. Antibiotic therapy is given if necessary. If the patient is not septic, catheter removal is not necessary, but the situation should be closely monitored.
   d. Prevention:
      i. Always maintain an occlusive dressing over the site.
      ii. Strict adherence to central-line dressing procedure (see Procedure section on pp. 353-354).

3. Catheter perforation (catheter perforates vessel and parenteral fluid is delivered into tissue):
   a. Symptoms:
      i. Swelling in upper chest and neck
      ii. Respiratory distress
      iii. Blood cannot be withdrawn from catheter
   b. Diagnosis: radiograph confirmation of line position.
   c. Prevention: early identification minimizes complications.
   d. Management: catheter is removed.

4. Leaking central line at exit site (catheter has a hole usually around cuff area):
   a. Symptoms:
      i. Central line dressing is wet.
      ii. Swelling along the tract.
   b. Diagnosis:
      i. Contrast studies with confirmed hole.
      ii. Dextrose sticks are glucose-positive for leaking fluid.
   c. Prevention:
      i. Irrigation of catheter prior to insertion to test for holes
      ii. Appropriate technique when tunneling catheter
   d. Management: catheter is removed.

5. External damage to catheter (catheter has a visible hole or crack at hub):
   a. Symptoms: fluid is leaking on skin or clothing.
   b. Prevention:
      i. Clamps used on catheter should be padded.
      ii. Do not use clamps on catheter hub or on central line tubing itself.
      iii. Attachment of IV apparatus to catheter hub should be secure but not so tight to strip Luer Lok or crack hub.
   c. Management: most externally damaged central lines can be repaired with an appropriate central-line repair kit.

INTRAVENOUS TUBING CHANGE

Change tube daily utilizing sterile technique with mask, sterile gloves, and sterile towel or field. The goal is to minimize line-opening to once a day to prevent infection.

1. Equipment:
   a. Pump tubing according to hospital protocol
   b. Povidone-iodine
   c. 10% percent rubbing alcohol
   d. Mask
   e. Sterile gloves
   f. Sterile towel or barrier
   g. Sterile gauze pads (3 x 3 inch), four packages

2. Procedure:
   a. Wash hands and put on mask.
   b. Prepare sterile field:
      i. Open and place each package of sterile gauze pads on sterile field.
      ii. Saturate one set of gauze pads with povidone-iodine and one with rubbing alcohol.
   c. Put on sterile gloves.
   d. Scrub junction of catheter and IV tubing.
      i. Hold line with dry gauze pad in nondominant hand.
      ii. Scrub junction with povidone-iodine-soaked gauze pad in dominant hand for 1 minute.
      iii. Allow junction to air dry for 1 minute.
      iv. Scrub junction with alcohol-soaked gauze pad in dominant hand for one minute.
   e. Pinch clamp line with dry gauze pad in dominant hand.
   f. Remove used fluid lines and discard.
   g. Pick up new tubing with nondominant hand and drip new fluids into hub of catheter to fill catheter with fluid.
   h. Attach tubing to catheter and unclamp line.
   i. Set infusion pump according to ordered rates and amounts.
   j. Tape all junctions if IV tubing is without Luer Lok.

DRESSING CHANGE

1. Indication for dressing changes:
   a. Dressing on Silastic catheters is changed once a week on nonimmunosuppressed patients.
   b. Any central-line dressing that becomes loose or soiled is changed, not reinforced.
   c. Perform culture of insertion site for symptoms of localized infection.
   d. An infected site requires daily dressing changes until clear.

2. Equipment: a custom dressing tray is preferred to ensure sterility of equipment and to reduce nursing time in gathering supplies.
   a. Hydrogen peroxide: used in place of acetone alcohol, which is very irritating to the neonate's skin.
   b. Povidone-iodine is used to cleanse the skin.
   c. Povidone-iodine ointment is used on the exit site.
   d. Transparent dressing is preferred to allow visualization of site.
   e. Slit tape in center to slide under catheter to secure transparent tape to skin.

3. Procedure
   a. Cleanse infant's skin with hydrogen peroxide.
   b. Use povidone-iodine to cleanse the skin again.
   c. Povidone-iodine ointment is then used on the exit site.
   d. A transparent dressing such as Tagaderm® is used over the line insertion site.
   e. A tape with a slit in the center is placed at the edge of the transparent dressing and slid under the catheter to secure transparent tape to skin.
   f. Place a piece of tape cut in the shape of a chevron around catheter to secure it.
   g. Secure chevron-shaped tape with another strip of tape (Fig. 12-2.).

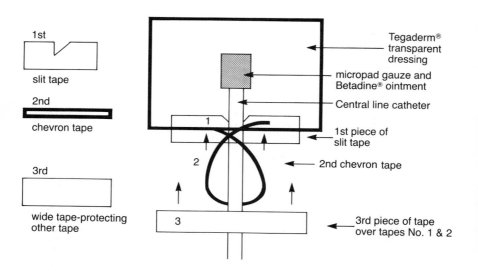

Fig. 12-2.   Central line dressing.

CAPPING AND HEPARINIZATION

1. Capping:
   a. Purpose: an injection cap is changed weekly when a central line is not used for infusing fluids.
   b. Equipment:
      i. Mask
      ii. Sterile gloves
      iii. Sterile field
      iv. Povidone-iodine
      v. 10-percent rubbing alcohol
      vi. Heparinized saline solution: the heparin concentration in the neonatal unit is 2 U/cc. The volume is 2 mL.
      vii. 2- or 3-cc syringe and separate needle
      viii. Sterile gauze pads, four packages of 3 x 3 inch
      ix. Injection cap
   c. Procedure:
      i. Prepare sterile field. See Intravenous Tubing Change (p. 353.) in this section. Add syringe and injection cap to sterile field. Place needle at edge of sterile field.
      ii. Glove one hand to hold sterile syringe and use ungloved hand to place the needle on the syringe and to hold vial of heparinized saline solution.
      iii. Fill syringe with 2 cc of heparinized saline solution and place on sterile field with needle in place.
      iv. Glove other hand.
      v. Fill injection cap with heparinized saline solution carefully removing all air bubbles.
      vi. Prepare the junction of catheter and injection cap. Hold catheter line with dry gauze pad in nondominant hand. Scrub junction with povidone-iodine-soaked gauze pad in dominant hand for 1 minute. Allow to air dry for 1 minute. Scrub junction with rubbing-alcohol-soaked gauze pad in dominant hand for 1 minute.
      vii. Clamp or pinch catheter.
      viii. Using a sterile 4 x 4 inch gauze pad remove old injection cap.
      ix. Drip several drops of heparinized saline solution into catheter to avoid air entering the catheter.
      x. Attach new injection port to the catheter and unclamp or unpinch.
      xi. Inject heparinized saline solution into the catheter.
      xii. As the last $\frac{1}{4}$ mL of flushing solution is infused, slowly withdraw the needle from the injection cap.
      xiii. Tape junction of catheter and injection cap.
      xiv. Secure catheter to patient in an upright position.

2. Heparinization:
   a. Purpose of heparinizing line is to maintain patency of central line when it is not used to infuse fluids; it is done once every 24 hours.

  b. Equipment:
     i. Heparinized saline solution: the heparin concentration in the neonatal unit is 2 U/cc. The volume is 2 mL.
     ii. Sterile gauze pads or prepared swab sticks.
     iii. Povidone-iodine swabs
     iv. 10 percent rubbing alcohol
     v. 2- or 3-cc syringe with needle to inject heparinized saline solution.
  c. Procedure:
     i. Prepare central line cap with swab sticks, soaking for 1 minute with povidone-iodine, allowing 1 minute to air dry, and soaking for 1 minute with alcohol.
     ii. Inject heparinized saline solution into injection cap.
     iii. As the last ¼ mL of flushing solution is infused, slowly withdraw the needle from the injection cap.
     iv. Secure catheter to patient and tape catheter in an upright position.

EMERGENCY: CLOTTED CENTRAL LINE

1. Causes:
  a. A very low flow rate combined with kinked tubing.
  b. Pumps not functioning.
  c. Pump pressures set too low if a variable pressure pump is used.

2. Treatment: aspiration of clot to safely aspirate clot and restore patency of line.

3. Equipment:
  a. Sterile field.
  b. Sterile gloves.
  c. Tuberculin syringes: 2- and 3-cc syringes with 2 separate needles.
  d. Heparinized saline solution: the heparin concentration in the neonatal unit is 2 U/cc. The volume is 2 mL.
  e. Sterile gauze pad, four packages.

4. Procedure:
  a. Use sterile technique and set up a sterile field as described in Intravenous Tubing Change (p. 353) in this section. Add tuberculin syringes, 2 and 3 cc, to the sterile field. Place extra needles at edge of field.
  b. Glove one hand to hold syringe and one ungloved hand to attach needle and to hold heparinized saline solution vial.
  c. Fill syringe with 2 cc of heparinized saline solution, remove needle, and place syringe on sterile field.
  d. Glove other hand.
  e. Prepare junction of catheter and IV tubing with povidone-iodine for 1 minute, air dry for 1 minute, and swab with alcohol for 1 minute.
  f. Clamp or pinch catheter.

g. Using a sterile 4 x 4 inch gauze pad disconnect IV tubing and place needle over tubing to maintain sterility.

h. Attach tuberculin syringe to the catheter.

i. Unclamp or unpinch tubing.

j. Slowly aspirate clot.

k. Clamp or pinch tubing.

l. Remove clot-filled syringe.

m. Drip several drops of heparinized saline solution into the catheter to avoid air entering the catheter.

n. Attach syringe containing heparinized saline solution to the catheter.

o. Unclamp catheter.

p. Flush catheter with heparinized saline solution.

q. Clamp or pinch catheter.

r. Drip several drops of fluid into catheter hub to avoid air entering into catheter and attach IV tubing and unclamp.

5. If unable to aspirate a clot:

a. Clamp or pinch catheter.

b. Remove tuberculin syringe.

c. Attach heparinized saline solution syringe and fill catheter hub.

d. Unclamp or unpinch catheter. Never push fluid into the catheter against resistance without consulting with the physician.

e. Slowly inject with minimum pressure the heparinized saline solution into the catheter until met with resistance, then aspirate back. These two steps may be repeated several times. If still unable to aspirate clot, clamp the line leaving the syringe in the end of catheter. Wrap a secure sterile 4 x 4 inch gauze pad around the catheter hub and notify the physician.

MANIFOLD SYSTEM

When a neonate has a Silastic central line, usually other compatible parenteral solutions are delivered simultaneously with the nutritional solution. To reduce the risk of infection when multiple solutions are used, a 24-hour closed delivery system is used called a manifold system. This means that fluid and medication needs are identified for 24 hours. Fluids and medications are then ordered as a special multiple solution with a special order form to decrease confusion of orders. A pharmacist reviews compatibility and stability of the components and then makes up a 24-hour volume of solution. A manifold is incorporated into the IV delivery system. A manifold is a device made of molded plastic that encases three to five stopcock parts. A specific solution can be given by simply opening the stopcock at that part. A flushing solution is also incorporated into the system. Each solution is color coded by colored tape being wrapped around the drip chamber, the IV cassette, and the manifold part for easy identification. This visual aid is a safety precaution to decrease the risk of opening the wrong port and delivering an incorrect solution. See Fig. 12-3.

MANIFOLD SYSTEM

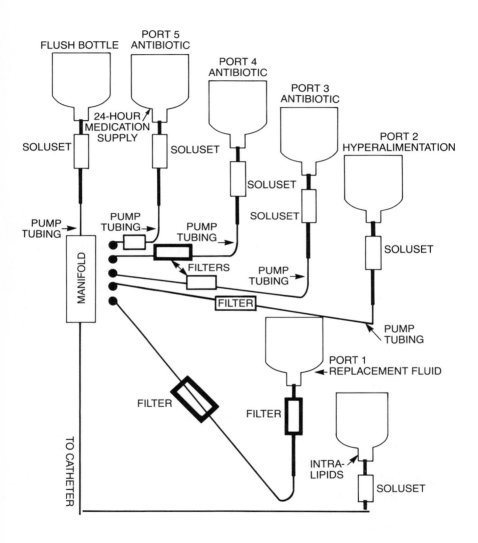

Fig. 12-3. Manifold system.

Dilation: Rectal and Esophageal
Jeanne Harjo

RECTAL DILATION

1. Indications:
   a. Allows rectal stimulation when the rectum is complete but the anus is covered by a membrane.
   b. Used to dilate rectal fistula.
   c. Dilation of rectal stenosis can be accomplished.

2. Equipment:
   a. Sizes 8-10, 12-14, and 16-18 red rubber catheters.
   b. Lubricating gel.
   c. Examination gloves.

3. Procedure:
   a. Catheters are lubricated and inserted into the area to be dilated by the physician.
   b. Gradually increase the size of catheter until the desired effect has been achieved.

4. Postprocedural care:
   a. Observe and report any excessive bleeding.
   b. Observe for passage of stool.

ESOPHAGEAL DILATION

1. Indications:
   a. Used when stenosis at the site of anastomosis of esophageal atresia repair is encountered.
   b. May be needed weeks to months after repair.
   c. May need occasional dilation for 1 or 2 years.

2. Equipment:
   a. Graduated sizes of tapered metal or rubber dilators.
   b. Espophageal string (black surgical suture material).
   c. Lubricating gel.

3. Preparation:
   a. NPO for 4-6 hours prior to procedure.
   b. Preoperative sedation as indicated.

4. Procedure:
   a. General anesthesia may be given.

b. Dilators are guided through the nose or mouth down the esophagus and out the gastrostomy tube. The size of the dilator catheter is increased after each dilation attempt.

c. Gastrostomy tube may be kept in place and an esophageal string is passed through the nose or mouth, down the esophagus, and out the gastrostomy tube to guide the dilators.

    i. Dilators can then be passed through the gastrostomy and up the esophagus to be removed.

    ii. Secure the string at the infant's face and at the gastrostomy tube to keep in place for future dilations.

5. Postprocedural care:

a. Monitor vital signs every 15 minutes four times, every 30 minutes four times, every 1 hour four times, every 2 hours until stable, and then every 4 hours.

b. Resume infant's preoperative diet when awake. The esophagus string, if in place, will not disrupt oral feedings.

Tracheostomy Suctioning at Home

Ann Brueggemeyer

---

1. Special considerations:

a. Infants with tracheostomy tubes will have thick secretions unless provision is made to humidify inspired air. Room vaporizers or humidifiers may be used in whichever room the infant is in.

b. If oxygen is used, special precautions must be taken to avoid combustion. Smoking should not be allowed in the room. Open flames as from a stove or fireplace should not be permitted in the room.

c. Because the tracheostomy bypasses the vocal cords, the infant will not be able to vocalize. Observe the infant frequently to make sure there are no problems such as cyanosis, poor respiratory effort, or a loosened tracheostomy.

d. If restlessness, signs of congestion, or gasping for air are present, the infant may need to be suctioned.

e. If suction, oxygen, or monitoring equipment is being used, notify the power company and local emergency services to ensure prompt response in case of problems.

f. Keep an extra supply of all equipment on hand at all times.

g. Pay special attention to food, fluid, and small objects in the presence of the infant. The tracheostomy is a direct opening into the lungs. Aspiration must be prevented.

2. Equipment:

a. Portable suction machine and connector hoses.

    b. Suction catheters, sizes 8 and 10 F. The catheter size should not exceed half the inner diameter of the tracheostomy tube.

    c. Sterile normal saline solution or water in a sterile container for irrigation. (The solution can be purchased or made at home using 1 teaspoon of salt for every half pint of water.)

    d. Dropper or syringe for irrigation.

    e. Manual resuscitator bag with adaptor.

    f. Sterile container (may use a small jar that has been cleaned and sterilized).

    g. Tracheostomy dressings (presplit gauze).

    h. Twill tape.

    i. Hydrogen peroxide.

    j. Extra tracheostomy tube, neonatal sizes 00, 0 and 1.

    k. Applicator swabs.

    l. Vaporizer or humidifier.

    m. Pipe cleaners if using metal tracheostomy tubes.

3. Preparation:

    a. Wash hands well. The use of sterile gloves at home is not recommended.

    b. Open packages and containers so that applicators, suction catheter, hydrogen peroxide, water solution, and tracheostomy dressings are available.

    c. Turn on suction machine.

    d. Have manual resuscitator bag available.

4. Procedure: The infant should be suctioned whenever secretions need to be cleared. The infant should be suctioned at least 3-4 times a day. Usually, infants require suctioning every few hours during the day and often at least once during the night.

    a. Remove inner cannula if one is being used, and place in sterile container to soak (may use saline solution and hydrogen peroxide).

    b. Connect sterile suction catheter to machine and test suction.

    c. If secretions are thick, place a few drops of water or saline solution into the tracheostomy.

    d. Moisten tip of catheter using sterile water or saline solution.

    e. Pass catheter into tracheostomy until slight resistance is met. Do not apply suction during insertion.

    f. Withdraw catheter about 1 cm before applying suction.

    g. Apply suction as catheter is slowly withdrawn. This procedure should not be any longer than 15 seconds.

    h. Allow the infant time to take several breaths before repeating the suctioning. If the infant is unable to breathe easily, assist the breathing with the manual resuscitation bag several times before proceeding.

    i. If inner cannula is used, clean before reinserting:

        i. Hold cannula by outer rim only.

        ii. Insert pipe cleaner into upper opening and pull through lower opening.

        iii. Rinse inner and outer edges. Shake off excess moisture. Do not attempt to dry.

        iv. Reinsert inner cannula into tracheostomy tube.

   j. Dispose of all equipment used unless it can be effectively sterilized.

5. Tracheostomy care:
   a. Stoma care, performed twice a day or more often if needed:
      i. Use applicators to clean stoma area with hydrogen peroxide. Do not soak the area so that solution does not enter tracheostomy tube.
      ii. Place sterile gauze pads around stoma, being careful not to dislodge the tracheostomy tube.
   b. Change tracheostomy ties as needed (always change ties when a second person is available to assist).
      i. Cut two pieces of twill tape to about 12 inches.
      ii. Ends should be cut at an angle to prevent ravelling.
      iii. Secure new tapes on tracheostomy tube without removing old tapes. Various types of knots may be used. Refer to hospital or physician's protocol.
      iv. Tie new tape around the infant's neck, securing at the side of the neck using double square knot. Make sure knot is secure. Tapes should be tight enough to hold tube in place with one finger able to slip under tape. A second variation of tying a tracheostomy tape is the slit-tape method. This involves cutting two lengths of twill tape long enough to be secured around the tube and tied to the side of the infant's neck. The ends are cut at a right angle to avoid fraying edges. A small slit is made approximately 1 inch from one end of each tie. This end is threaded through the opening on the plastic or metal securing wing of the tracheostomy. The free end of the tape is then threaded through the slit and pulled securely against the securing wing of the tracheostomy. This method may be more difficult to perform and can result in dislodgement of the tracheostomy tube. A third type of tracheostomy tying involves the use of a single tape. Each end of the tape is used to thread through one of the securing wings of the tracheostomy tube from the back of the neck. The ends are then tied together at the back or side of the infant's neck. The tape should only extend from the securing wings to the back or side position for tying. The tape should not encircle the infant's entire neck in a front to back fashion. Since this method results in two separate strands of tape that are not secured at the securing wings, this is rarely the method of choice. A further disadvantage is the increased chance of tube dislodgement.
      v. Cut and remove the old tape.

Intermittent Catheterization at Home
Jeanne Harjo

---

1. Equipment:
   a. Cotton balls, at least three.

b. Povidine-iodine solution.

c. Infant feeding tube, size 5 or 8 F (sterile).

d. Leg restraints.

e. Clean diaper.

f. Pacifier or bottle to quiet the infant.

g. Container for urine: paper or plastic cup.

h. Soap and water with washcloth.

2. Procedure:

a. Wash hands with soap and water.

b. Remove diaper and restrain the infant's legs.

c. Prepare equipment:

    i. Pour povidone-iodine over cotton balls.

    ii. Open catheter.

d. Cleanse baby with soap and water.

e. Wash hands with povidone-iodine solution.

f. Rinse hands and shake excess water from hands.

g. Cleanse baby with povidone-iodine solution, cleaning entire area well, using at least three cotton balls. For a female newborn, spread the labia to expose urethra; for a male newborn, retract the foreskin to expose urethra.

h. Povidone-iodine solution must remain in continuous contact with baby for at least 15 seconds.

i. With dominant hand, touching nothing else, pick up the catheter to within 1½ to 2 inches from the tip, or whatever distance allows control of the catheter.

j. Spread newborn's labia or retract foreskin with the opposite hand.

k. Gently insert catheter directly into the urethra until urine is obtained. If the catheter touches anything else, start the procedure over again after obtaining a new catheter; rescrub and insert the catheter.

l. Withdraw the catheter slowly to permit the bladder to empty completely. It may be helpful to apply gentle pressure over the pubic area.

m. Cleanse povidone-iodine off newborn's skin to prevent irritation after the catheter is removed.

n. Immediately after using catheter, rinse it with hot water—not soap.

3. Sterilization of catheter:

a. Coil the plastic catheter into a circle and wrap in an aluminum-foil square.

b. Place in clean pan with lid, preferably a new pan that has not been used for cooking (for catheters only).

c. Cover catheter with water and bring to a boil.

d. Boil for ½ hour.

e. Drain off water from catheter "pack."

f. Keep catheter wrapped in foil until used.

g. Place in refrigerator to help retard bacterial growth.

h. Resterilize catheter after each use; unused catheter should be resterilized at least every 24 hours.

i. Do not use a catheter that was sterilized more than 24 hours before.

Colostomy Care
Jeanne Harjo

1. Colostomy dressing to be used postoperatively in the hospital or at home if skin becomes excoriated.
   a. Equipment:
      i. Gauze dressings, squares, or rolls.
      ii. Soap and water; towel and washcloth.
      iii. Protective cream.
      iv. Surgical tie mask with wire removed to secure dressings in place; a securing device may be used.
   b. Preparation:
      i. Wash hands.
      ii. Unfold gauze squares; if using gauze roll, unroll as needed.
      iii. Remove any metal strips from surgical mask.
   c. Procedure:
      i. Carefully remove old dressings, may need to moisten with water if they have adhered to the stoma.
      ii. Clean area around stoma without excessive friction. Area may be dark and crusty and may bleed easily if site is not healed.
      iii. Apply protective cream liberally around stoma.
      iv. Observe condition of stoma and report to physician any excessive bleeding or skin breakdown.
      v. Place gauze dressings around and over stoma.
      vi. Secure dressings with mask or ties.

2. Colostomy bag (pouch): apply pouch as soon as infant is forming stools.
   a. Equipment:
      i. Byram® premie pouch or one that has a collar that can be cut to fit around an incision or fistula.
      ii. Stomahesive® squares.
      iii. Stomahesive Paste® if needed.
      iv. Sharp scissors.
      v. Pattern for stoma size.
      vi. Skin preparation pads.
      vii. Soap and water; towel and washcloth.
      viii. Clamp to secure bottom of bag, may use clamp from previous bag.
   b. Procedure: change bag when loose or leaking.
      i. Wash hands.
      ii. Carefully remove old bag by gently pulling from skin.
      iii. Clean around stoma with soap and water. Rinse well and dry.
      iv. Apply skin preparation around stoma and allow to dry.
      v. Measure stoma and draw pattern for the outline of the stoma on

Stomahesive® and pouch. Save pattern for subsequent bag changes. Holes should be slightly larger ($\frac{1}{16}$ inch) than stoma.

vi. Cut holes in Stomahesive® and pouch. External edge of Stomahesive may be trimmed to size of bag faceplate.

vii. Remove paper from adhesive on pouch. Apply to shiny side of Stomahesive®.

viii. Remove paper backing from Stomahesive® and apply pouch over stoma. Stomahesive Paste® may be used on skin before applying pouch. Moisten finger and apply paste in thin layer around stoma. Allow to dry for 1 minute before applying pouch.

ix. Fold bottom of pouch several times and apply clamp.

c. Emptying bag:

i. Empty bag when full or at least once a day.

ii. Open clamp and unfold bottom of the bag to let out contents.

iii. When emptying, clean the bottom of the bag inside and out.

iv. Report to physician any change in color, consistency, or amount of stool.

BIBLIOGRAPHY

Ahmann, E. (1986). *Home care for the high risk infant: A holistic guide to using technology.* Rockville, MD: Aspen.

American Endoscopy Inc. (1985). *Long term confidence in gastrostomy feeding: The Button.* Mentor, OH: Product Information.

Kennedy, A., Johnson, W., & Sturdevant, E. (1982). An educational program for families of children with tracheostomies. *Maternal-Child Nursing Journal, 7,* 42-49.

Lichtenstein, M. A. (1986). Pediatric home tracheostomy care: A parent's care. *Pediatric Nursing, 12,* 41-48, 69.

Medical Innovations Corporation. (1985). *The MIC gastrostomy tube.* San Jose, CA: Product Information.

Wills, J. (1983). Concerns and needs of mothers providing home care for children with tracheostomies. *Maternal-Child Nursing Journal, 12,* 89-107.

Chapter 13

Resources for Home Care

Jeanne Harjo *Ann Brueggemeyer*
Carole Kenner

ᶜᵃ

Support Groups

Association for the Care of
  Children's Health
3615 Wisconsin Avenue, NW
Washington, DC 20016
(202) 244-1801

Cystic Fibrosis Foundation
6000 Executive Boulevard
Suite 309
Rockville, MD 20852
(301) 881-9130

La Leche League International, Inc.
9616 Minneapolis Avenue
Franklin Park, IL 60131
(312) 455-7730

Local Infant Stimulation Programs
(available through individual state's
crippled children's programs or the National Easter Seal Society—see above)

National Cystic Fibrosis Research
  Foundation
3379 Peachtree Road, NE
Atlanta, GA 30326
(404) 325-6973

National Down's Syndrome Society
146 East 57th Street
New York, NY 10022
(212) 460-9330 or (800) 221-4602

The National Easter Seal Society for
  Crippled Children and Adults
2023 West Ogden Avenue
Chicago IL 60612
(312) 243-8400

The National Foundation of the
  March of Dimes
P.O. Box 2000
White Plains, NY 10602
(914) 428-7100

Neonatal Surgery: A Nursing Perspective
ISBN 0-8089-1893-1

National Genetics Foundation, Inc.
555 West 57th Street
New York, NY 10019
(212) 586-5800

National Kidney Foundation
116 East 27th Street
New York, NY 10010
(212) 889-2210 or (212) 683-1088

Parentele
1301 East 38th Street
Indianapolis, IN 46205
(317) 926-4142

Parents Helping Parents
47 Maro Drive
San Jose, CA 95127
(408) 272-4774

Parents of Premature and High-Risk
Infants, International, Inc.
33 West 42nd Street
New York, NY 10036
(606) 277-0008

Spina Bifida Association of America
343 South Dearborn Street, Room 317
Chicago, IL 60604
(312) 663-1562

United Cerebral Palsy Association, Inc.
66 East 34th Street
New York, NY 10016
(212) 481-6300

Financial Assistance

National associations for financial assistance are not listed here. Local organizations should be contacted directly. Other services may be available in your area.

1. Bureau of Crippled Children Services

2. Women-Infant-Children

3. Social Security: Aid to Dependent Children and Aid to Dependent Families and Children

4. Religious organizations and charities

5. Salvation Army

6. City or county social services departments

Supplies and Equipment

1. Surgical pharmacies should be consulted for ostomy supplies, feeding supplies, and special formulas.

2. Local community organizations may lend extra supplies.

3. Local religious and charity organizations may subsidize the cost of supplies and equipment.

BIBLIOGRAPHY

Ahman, E. (1986). *Home care for the high risk infant: A holistic guide to using technology.* Rockville, MD: Aspen.

Chapter 14

Perinatal Ethical Issues

Ann Brueggemeyer

Ethics has been a concern in the health profession since the advent of organized health care. Physicians and nurses alike have pondered the meaning of life and their role to play in the preservation of life. There are no clearly defined standards that nurses can call on to identify the appropriate actions to be taken.

Ethical issues in health care are concerned with identifying and understanding the basis of our moral judgments (Schröck, 1981). The health team member attempts to document reasons for conduct in relation to actions in certain situations (Curtin, 1977).

Our value system plays a large role in our interpretation of ethical dilemmas and centers on our cognitive development (Ketefian, 1983). Ethical decision making is based on personal values. These values cannot be forced on others.

ETHICAL DILEMMAS

Ethical dilemmas arise when there is a choice in what ought to be done. These choices may have various outcomes with differing levels of harm or benefit (Aroskar, 1980). Types of ethical issues have changed over the years, yet the solutions still do not come easy.

The complex issues facing the perinatal nurse cannot be dealt with on a purely technical basis. Many factors must be considered in dealing with the types of ethical decisions that are made in regard to infants. Legal factors often play a role in what decisions are made. Financial considerations are often a major determining factor when ethical decisions are made in relation to infants. The health care team can influence parental and legal decisions. Parents' rights are often considered but may not be the ultimate factor in decision making.

There are many factors that influence why ethical decision making is so difficult. Curtin (1977) describes four factors that influence the decision making.

Neonatal Surgery: A Nursing Perspective
ISBN 0-8089-1893-1

First, there is a very narrow concept of morality. This places strict interpretations on what is right and wrong. Second, many times the decision is rationalized. Decisions are made and then reasons are determined for why the particular decision was made. Third, there is often a strong emotional appeal involved in choosing the action to take. Personal value systems influence our behavior. Last, we work very hard to determine guidelines that will encompass all situations to the point that they then become meaningless.

DECISION MAKING

Problem-solving techniques help to enhance our ability to interpret ethical decisions. All aspects of the problem should be completely analyzed before decision making takes place. Several positions on ethical decision making can help guide us.

The first position looks at the consequences of the actions. Decision making is determined by the greatest amount of good or the least amount of harm (Aroskar, 1980). This method of decision making also looks at how the decision will affect not only the patient, but the family, the community, and society in general. The decision, then, may not deal with what is best for the patient but what is best for the family.

The second position deals with the personal benefits of the choices available. The solution that is chosen is the one that is best for the decision maker. The decision may or may not be what is actually best for the patient (Aroskar, 1980).

A third position deals with the formal structure of the moral decision. The outcome of the decision is what is important. The means for achieving it is irrelevant. Decisions are based on seeking outcomes as determined by what is universally considered "right."

A fourth position encompasses the concept of justice. It suggests that determinations of outcomes be based on what would be fair to others in a similar position. These decisions must be applicable to a wide variety of people and situations. Perelman (in Lumpp, 1982) identifies justice in regard to distribution of resources. The distribution follows six principles: (1) to each the same, (2) to each according to his or her merits, (3) to each according to his or her work, (4) to each according to his or her need, (5) to each according to his or her rank, and (6) to each according to his or her legal right.

Identifying decision makers is an equally difficult task. This is true especially in the treatment of infants. Although parents have often had the right to determine the outcomes of their children, recent cases have removed the parents as legal guardians if it was determined that they were not acting in the best interest of the child. In these cases, it is the legal system that then decides what is best for the child. Several questions arise when parents become the decision maker in regard to the care of their children (Muyskens, 1982). Are they the the most qualified to identify what is best for the child? Do they have the interests of the child at heart, or their own self-interests? Do they have legal control over the child? Do outside factors play too big a role in influencing their decision? Financial burden and family considerations often play a major role in what decisions are made.

Parents do not make decisions in isolation. The health care team is a powerful influence in these decisions. How the team members present the alternatives can affect the way the parents interpret the outcomes. The personal value systems of the individuals who are working with the family will influence how the choices are offered. Parents may be heavily influenced by the health team if the parents view the health care team as the ultimate experts. Previous experiences and religious beliefs may alter both the interpretation of the choices offered and the final choice the family makes. Life-or-death decision making may be too much to expect from a family already in crisis.

The health care team can also affect patient outcome (Homer, 1984). How quickly or fully the nurse carries out prescribed treatment may affect long-term survival. At times, alternatives to treatment are not discussed with the family, which places the ultimate decision making in the hands of the health care team. Lack of complete disclosure can complicate the moral issue (Fromer, 1981).

ETHICAL ISSUES IN FETAL THERAPY

Many congenital and hereditary problems can be diagnosed in the fetal period. Treatment of some of these problems is becoming more common. In some cases, treatment for some genetic defects would mean therapeutic abortion. That issue is not addressed here.

Ethical considerations in fetal intervention include: fetal outcome, maternal risk, and the difference between innovative treatment and research (Fletcher, 1985). Fetal surgery for such problems as obstructive uropathies, hydrocephalus, and hemolytic disease have become common. Risk to the mother is less than the risk of not treating the fetus. Despite the relative ease of diagnosis and treatment for these disorders, it is not clear what the legal rights of the fetus are over the rights of the body integrity of the mother (Robertson, 1985).

THE PRETERM AND LOW BIRTH WEIGHT INFANT

Technology has made it possible to care for smaller infants than was possible even a few years ago. The survival rate of preterm infants has improved. With this technology and advancement has come an added burden. Health care costs continue to rise, especially in treatment involving high technology. The added financial burden is shared by all. Ethical decisions in relation to the treatment of all preterm infants may soon reflect this spiraling cost.

As health care costs rise, discussions arise as to the quality of life. Certain factors play a role in identifying risk factors for long-term morbidity. Artificial ventilation often increases the risk for morbidity in the newborn at a high-risk perinatal center (Roncoli & Brooten, 1985). Although regionalization of health care services helps to hold down costs, will further cutbacks prevent us from treating every infant who needs care?

THE SURGICAL NEONATE

The surgical neonate presents a whole new set of ethical dilemmas. The decision to treat or not to treat becomes more complicated. Many congenital anomalies are readily correctable. Once corrected, however, they may then require a lifetime of chronic medical care. Should the cost of medical care determine whether or not the infant is treated?

Some proponents of the "not treat" group use the concept of quality of life. They feel that the life of the child and the family would be so burdensome that treatment is not in the baby's best interest. In the case of physically handicapped newborns, who determines what is quality of life? Is the quality of life for a child who cannot walk any less than for a child who does not use normal capabilities to the fullest? The decision to allow the handicapped infant to die was once a personal one. Legal considerations have begun to surface. The rights of the child are weighed against the rights of the parents. The withholding of treatment is justified when those treatments would not change the course of the infant's life. Treatment is not justified when the only outcome is continued suffering for all involved (Curtin, 1983). But any action taken to hasten death cannot be justified.

The infants abused by withholding treatment are often unwanted for nonmedical reasons (Manney & Blattner, 1985). The reasons often expressed are financial or emotional burdens to the family. Quality of life may be interpreted to mean how well the child will fit into the norms of family life.

The importance of hospital ethics committees cannot be ignored. Their purpose is to provide guidance in the process of making these important decisions. Often, the committee is made up of a variety of disciplines within the confines of the institution. Physicians, nurses, and chaplains provide input to the committee to give a well-rounded view of each situation. Theory-based decision making also helps the caretakers make decisions that provide the best care for each infant.

PAIN MEDICATION

The use of pain medication in the neonate is a source of controversy. It becomes an ethical dilemma as nurses and physicians may disagree over the need for such medications in the neonate. Parents may become involved as they may interpret the infant's behavior as an indication of pain. They may seek relief of pain in their infant as a means of being involved in the care of their infant.

In the past, health care workers have denied the existence of pain in the neonate. These decisions may have been based on the inability of the infants to verbalize their pain. Nurses now recognize nonverbal expressions of pain through alterations in vital signs, facial expressions, and other bodily appearances of discomfort. Some health team members have also suggested the lack of long-term memory of the pain as a reason for not administering medications to relieve pain. Perception of pain in the neonate has also been used as a reason for withholding pain medication as many health care workers do not believe that pain perception is the same in the infant as it is in the adult.

Concerns about depressing the compromised respiratory status of the infant may be invalid as many mild to moderate pain medications will not compromise the infant. Infants who are receiving assisted ventilation should not need to have this concern addressed. In an infant who is experiencing pain, respiratory compromise may occur as the infant attempts to compensate by altering the effectiveness of ventilation due to splinting.

The nurse must identify concerns and risks before making decisions about the administration of pain medications. No clear-cut answers can be given. Each infant must be evaluated within the context of the surgical procedure and any other influencing factors. The parents should be active partners in decision making. Current trends may indicate an increase in concern over the use of pain medications in the neonate. Liberal use of pain medications in the postoperative period is already being practiced in some institutions. Like all other controversial neonatal issues, the potential exists for legal action to be instituted over the lack of attention paid to neonatal pain.

CONCLUSION

The perinatal nurse will be exposed to many ethical dilemmas during the course of his or her practice. The nurse must analyze his or her own value system and live by it. When decisions are made that do not seem to be in the child's best interest, the nurse must act on his or her convictions. The nurse as care giver has a right to participate in ethical decisions that affect the patients.

The parents traditionally have had the right to be the final decision makers. Their decisions should be respected. But the nurse has the responsibility to see that every attempt has been made to fully educate the parents as to the significance of their decisions (Roberts, 1979). The legal system reserves the right to intervene when the parents' decisions are not in line with accepted medical and moral practice.

REFERENCES

Aroskar, M. (1980). Anatomy of an ethical dilemma: The theory. *American Journal of Nursing*, April *80*, 658-663.

Curtin, L. (1977). Update on Ethics. *1*, 1-28.

Curtin, L. (1983). The babies Doe: Common sense and common decency. *Nursing Management, 14*(12), 7-8.

Fletcher, J. (1985). Ethical considerations in and beyond experimental fetal therapy. *Seminars in Perinatology, 9*, 130-135.

Fromer, M. (1981). *Ethical issues in health care*. St. Louis: C.V. Mosby.

Homer, M. (1984). Selective treatment. *American Journal of Nursing, 84*, 309-312.

Ketefian, S. (1983). Judging ethical issues in nursing: Research strategy and selected correlates. In N. Chaska (Ed.), *The nursing profession: A time to speak* (pp. 237-249). New York: McGraw-Hill.

Lumpp, F., Sr. (1982). Is health care a right? In. L. Curtin & M. Flaherty (Eds.), *Nursing ethics* (pp. 25-36). Bowie, MD: Robert J. Brady.

Manney, J., & Blattner, J. (1985). Infanticide: Murder or mercy? *Journal of Christian Nursing, 2*, 10-14.

Muyskens, J. (1982). *Moral problems in nursing* (pp. 73-74). Totowa, NJ: Rowman & Littlefield.

Roberts, C. (1979). Ethical issues in the treatment of neonates with severe anomalies. *Nursing Forum, 18*, 352-365.

Robertson, J. (1985). Legal issues in fetal therapy. *Seminars in Perinatology, 9*, 136-142.

Roncoli, M., & Brooten, D. (1985). Low-birthweight infants: Balancing the scales of care. *Nursing and Health Care, 6*, 198-201.

Schröck, R. (1981). Philosophical issues. In L. Hockey, *Current issues in nursing*. New York: Churchill Livingstone.

Appendix A

Transport

Ann Brueggemeyer   *Jeanne Harjo*

Carole Kenner

1. Keep the infant in a warmed transport isolette to maintain an axillary temperature between 36.5° and 37°C.

2. Support the respiratory status as required: give warm, humidified oxygen to keep pink and allow for easy respirations. Some teams have transcutaneous monitors that may be transported. Use this equipment to follow the level of oxygenation as warranted by the infant's condition.

3. Provide fluids and electrolytes as needed. See Fluid Requirements and General Nutritional Considerations (pp. 263-280) in Chapter 9.

4. Monitor vital signs at least every 15 minutes.
   a. Infant should be constantly observed during transport.
   b. Keep resuscitation equipment available at all times during transport.

5. Visit the parents before the transport to explain the problem and the upcoming transfer as simply as possible. These explanations will require repetition as the parents are under a great deal of stress.

6. Allow the parents to see and touch the baby prior to transfer, if the condition will permit.

7. Encourage the parents to call and visit the baby once transported.

Neonatal Surgery: A Nursing Perspective
ISBN 0-8089-1893-1

Appendix B

Regular Admission Setup

Ann Brueggemeyer   *Jeanne Harjo*
                    Carole Kenner

ADMISSION SETUP

1. Oxygen equipment:
   a. Inflatable oxygen bag (anesthesia bag) or rebreathing bags (capable of delivering 100-percent oxygen)
   b. Manometer with T-piece
   c. Masks: sizes premie, infant, and child
   d. Flow meter
   e. Humidification chamber
   f. Oxygen analyzer
   g. Mixbox (blender for delivering specific oxygen concentrations up to 100 percent)
   h. Oxygen connector tubing
   i. Oxygen hood to keep infant pink and breathing easily
   j. Positive-pressure ventilator
   k. Transcutaneous oxygen monitor or pulse oximeter if available

2. Suction equipment:
   a. Vacuum source with regulator head (pressure dial)
   b. Drainage bottle
   c. Connector tubing
   d. Sterile suction catheters: sizes 5/6, 8, and 10 F
   e. Sterile gloves if not prepackaged with suction catheter
   f. Sterile water or normal saline solution (0.9 percent) for irrigation according to hospital protocol (See Ventilatory Care, Chapter 10, p. 297-304).

3. Warmer beds (to maintain axillary temperature of 36.5°-37°C):
   a. Isolettes: for infants weighing <1800 g
   b. Radiant warmer (with light source): for infants weighing >1800 g

Neonatal Surgery: A Nursing Perspective
ISBN 0-8089-1893-1

4. Cardiopulmonary monitoring device with BP measuring capabilities:
   a. Lead wires
   b. Electrode pads with moist conduction gel

5. Intravenous access equipment:
   a. Sizes 23 and 25 butterfly needles.
   b. Sizes 22 and 24 angiocath.
   c. Tape.
   d. Armboard.
   e. Rubbing alcohol pads and 3 x 3 inch gauze pads.
   f. Fluids: see Fluid Requirements and General Nutritional Considerations, Chapter 9.
   g. Infusion pump capable of infusing low volumes.
   h. Intravenous tubing to include pump tubing and delivery setup.

6. Blood drawing equipment:
   a. Microtainers or collection tubes
   b. Sizes 23 and 25 butterfly needles
   c. Lancets
   d. Skin preparation swabs (rubbing alcohol preparations or other anti-microbial solution)
   e. 3 x 3 inch gauze pads
   f. Heparinized needle and syringe for arterial blood gas analysis

7. Diagnostic/lab tests
   a. Blood gas analysis, preferably arterial sample for baseline measurements
   b. Complete blood cell count with differential
   c. Blood type and crossmatch
   d. Chest radiograph
   e. Urinalysis
   f. Baseline serum electrolyte measurements and other lab tests as indicated

REGULAR UNIT SETUP

1. Stethoscope.

2. Thermometer.

3. Blood pressure cuff, using electronic machine, standard sphygmomanometer, or flush method. Flush method may be inaccurate. Electronic measurement should be used whenever possible.

4. Tape measure.

5. Infant scale.

6. Urine collection bag.

7. Linens:
   a. Diapers
   b. Bed coverings
   c. T-shirts: if neonate is not under radiant warmer
   d. Blankets

8. Chart equipment:
   a. Nursing notes
   b. Progress notes
   c. Physician's order sheets
   d. Informed consent forms
   e. Lab slips
   f. Radiograph requisitions
   g. Medical history and physical forms
   h. Kardex or nursing process tool

9. Oxygen and suction setup as needed at bedside.

10. Soft restraints and safety pins as needed.

Appendix C

Normal Parameters for Infant Assessment

Ann Brueggemeyer   *Jeanne Harjo*
Carole Kenner

Blood Pressure

	28-32 weeks	33-37 weeks	38 weeks-Full Term
Systolic (Torr)	48-52	55-62	62-68

Heart Rate

Newborn average: 120-160 beats per minute.

Respiratory Rate

Newborn average: 40-60 breaths per minute.

Temperature

Newborn average: maintain skin temperature at 35.5° C-36.5° C: Rectal temperature should range from 36.5° to 37.5° C.

Premature: may maintain < 36.5° C rectally but should not be < 35.0° C on the average. If skin temperature and core temperature of any infant varies more than 1.0° C, sepsis should be considered.

Neonatal Surgery: A Nursing Perspective
ISBN 0-8089-1893-1

Head Circumference

28-30 weeks	31-34 weeks	35-37 weeks	Full Term
24-31 cm	26-34 cm	29-35 cm	31-36 cm

These values are based on the range from the 10th to 90th percentiles for each category.

Length

28-30 weeks	31-34 weeks	35-37 weeks	Full Term
32-44 cm	37-49 cm	41-51 cm	44 -53 cm

These values are based on the range from the 10th to 90th percentiles for each category.

Weight

28-30 weeks	31-34 weeks	35-37 weeks	Full Term
800-1800 g	1200-2800 g	1600-3400 g	2200-3800 g

These values are based on the range from the 10th to 90th percentiles for each category.

Appendix D

Normal Blood Chemistries, Blood Gases, and Hematologic Values

Ann Brueggemeyer   *Jeanne Harjo*
                          Carole Kenner

BLOOD CHEMISTRIES

1. Alkaline phosphatase: 3.0-24.0 IU

2. Bilirubin, total:
   a. < 1
   b. Peaks at 4-15 after several days
   c. > 5 at birth indicates hemolytic disease

3. Blood urea nitrogen:
   a. Premature: 3.0-20.0 mg/dL
   b. Term: 6.0-30.0 mg/dL

4. Calcium, total in term infant: 7-10 mg/dL

5. Carbon dioxide, term: 20-25 mEq/L

6. Chloride, term: 95-110 mEq/L

7. Creatinine:
   a. Premature: 0.8-1.5 mg/dL
   b. Term: 0.2-0.9 mg/dL

8. Glucose, term: 40-97 mg/dL

9. Magnesium, term: 1.5-2.5 mEq/L

Neonatal Surgery: A Nursing Perspective
ISBN 0-8089-1893-1

10. Potassium:
    a. Premature: 4.5-6.5 mEq/L
    b. Term: 4.5-6.8 mEq/L

11. SGOT, term: 16-74 IU

12. SGPT, term: 0-24 IU

13. Sodium:
    a. Premature: 130-145 mEq/L
    b. Term: 135-145 mEq/L

ARTERIAL BLOOD GASES

pH 7.35-7.45
pCO_2 35-45
pO_2 70-90 mm Hg
Base excess 2.5-4.0
Sodium bicarbonate 20-25 mEq/L

If the newborn is breathing room air, the pO_2 for a term infant should be > 75 mm Hg and for a premature infant, > 55 mm Hg.

HEMATOLOGIC VALUES

Hemoglobin

	28 weeks	35 weeks	Full Term
3 days	17 g/dL	18 g/dL	19 g/dL
1 week	14 g/dL	15 g/dL	17 g/dL

Hematocrit

	28 weeks	35 weeks	Full Term
3 days	52	58	58
1 week	47	50	50

Reticulocyte (percentage)

	28 weeks	35 weeks	Full Term
3 days	7	5	4
1 week	3	3	3

BIBLIOGRAPHY

Cloherty, J. P., & Stark, A. R. (1985). *Manual of neonatal care* (2nd. ed.). Boston: Little, Brown.

Schaffer, A. J., & Avery, M. E. (1971). *Diseases of the newborn*. Philadelphia: W. B. Saunders.

Streeter, N. S. (1986). *High-risk neonatal care*. Rockville, MD: Aspen.

Index